Dr. Henry R. Porter

Dr. Henry R. Porter

*The Surgeon Who
Survived Little Bighorn*

L.G. WALKER, JR., M.D.

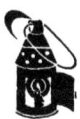

McFarland & Company, Inc., Publishers
Jefferson, North Carolina, and London

LIBRARY OF CONGRESS CATALOGUING-IN-PUBLICATION DATA

Walker, L.G., 1931–
　　Dr. Henry R. Porter : the surgeon who survived Little Bighorn / L.G. Walker, Jr.
　　　　p.　　cm.
　　Includes bibliographical references and index.

　　ISBN-13: 978-0-7864-3171-7
　　softcover : 50# alkaline paper ∞

　　1. Porter, Henry R., 1848–1903.　2. Physicians—United States—Biography.　3. Surgeons—United States—Biography.　4. Little Bighorn, Battle of the, Mont. 1876.　I. Title.
　　[DNLM: 1. Porter, Henry R., 1848–1903.　2. Physicians—Montana—Biography.　3. Physicians—North Dakota—Biography.　4. History, 19th Century—Montana—Biography.　5. History, 19th Century—North Dakota—Biography.　6. Military Medicine—history—Montana.　7. Military Medicine—history—North Dakota.　8. Military Personnel—history—Montana.　9. Military Personnel—history—North Dakota.　10. Surgery—history—Montana—Biography.　11. Surgery—history—North Dakota—Biography. WZ 100 P8456W　2008]
R154.P74W35　2008
610.92—dc22　　　　　　　　　　　　　　　　2007041480
[B]

British Library cataloguing data are available

©2008 L.G. Walker, Jr. All rights reserved

No part of this book may be reproduced or transmitted in any form or by any means, electronic or mechanical, including photocopying or recording, or by any information storage and retrieval system, without permission in writing from the publisher.

On the cover: Dr. Henry R. Porter (Photograph by B.F. Barry)

Manufactured in the United States of America

McFarland & Company, Inc., Publishers
　Box 611, Jefferson, North Carolina 28640
　　www.mcfarlandpub.com

For Dianne Melton Walker

Acknowledgments

I am greatly indebted to Cathy Davis, Elizabeth Goss, and Bill Goss of White Stone, Virginia. Elizabeth Goss is Henry Rinaldo Porter's great-niece. Also, my thanks go to Barbara Frost Wyman, North Sandwich, New Hampshire, great-niece of Charlotte Viets Porter and granddaughter of George H. Fairchild; and Lucy Wyman, her daughter of Lancaster, New Hampshire; and her sons, Burleigh and Bradford Wyman of Jefferson and West Dummer, New Hampshire. All have been generous in providing access to family letters, photographs, and memorabilia.

Mark J. Halvorson, curator of collections research, State Historical Society of North Dakota, has been extremely helpful in showing me Porter's large collections of medical equipment and personal possessions housed in the Historical Society Museum. His knowledge of North Dakota history and his suggestions after reading an earlier version of the manuscript have been invaluable.

Others who deserve my sincerest thanks for their untiring assistance and interest in the project are: Shane A. Molander, reference specialist, State Historical Society of North Dakota; Brian Shovers, reference historian, Montana Historical Society; Sandy Slater, head of Elwin B. Robinson Department of Special Collections, Chester Fritz Library, University of North Dakota; Malgorzata Myc, reference assistant, Bentley Historical Library, University of Michigan; Steven Solomon, public affairs officer, National Museum of Health and Medicine, Washington, DC; Paul Sledzik, curator of anatomical collections, National Museum of Health and Medicine, Washington, DC; Lynn Conway, university archivist, Georgetown University; and John A. Doerner, chief historian, Little Bighorn Battlefield National Monument, Crow Agency, Montana.

Librarians and staff assistants have been most helpful at Oneida County Historical Society, Utica, New York; Oberlin College Library, Oberlin, Ohio; New York State Historical Association Library, Cooperstown, New York; North Dakota Institute for Regional Studies, North Dakota State University, Fargo, North Dakota; and the National Archives I and II, Washington, DC, and College Park, Maryland.

My thanks go to readers of early versions of the manuscript for their helpful suggestions. They are: Dr. Richard Anderson, Harry Barr, Dr. Robert Lackey, Dr. Jerry Petty, Dr. Charles Reaves, Dr. Phillip Walker, Dr. Bob Brawley, Bo Walker, Jane Parrish, and Lisa Walker. William W. Walker, Jr., rendered valuable assistance to me with his legal evaluation of Dr. H.R. Porter's will. My thanks also go to Susan Cheek for seeking photographs of Porter and battle and to Patricia Braswell for obtaining photographs and assisting with research. I thank Cissy Swartz for her special advice and untiring assistance in reviewing the manuscript.

Finally, I am most grateful to Dianne Melton Walker, my wife, for all her assistance in the four years of research and in preparation of the manuscript for publication.

Table of Contents

Acknowledgments   vii
Preface   1

Chapter 1	Early Life and Education	3
Chapter 2	Medical School Adventures	8
Chapter 3	Western Adventures	19
Chapter 4	Bismarck, on the Frontier	30
Chapter 5	The Road to Little Bighorn	42
Chapter 6	The Battle as Seen by Porter	54
Chapter 7	After the Battle	61
Chapter 8	Recalling the Battle	66
Chapter 9	Return to Bismarck	76
Chapter 10	Hail to the Chief	83
Chapter 11	Early Business Ventures	91
Chapter 12	The Reno Inquiry	96
Chapter 13	Banking on Bismarck	105
Chapter 14	A Capital Matter	110
Chapter 15	Farewell to Lottie	119
Chapter 16	Banking Business	128
Chapter 17	Travels Abroad	133
Chapter 18	Italian Journey	141
Chapter 19	Up the Nile	147
Chapter 20	Travels to the Holy Land and Around the Mediterranean	153

Chapter 21	Washington and Bismarck	162
Chapter 22	Final Years	170
Chapter 23	Forgotten Hero	180

Epilogue   184

Appendix A — Holdings of Dr. H.R. Porter Items,
    North Dakota Historical Society, Bismarck   185

Appendix B — Porter Lineage   189

Chapter Notes   191

Bibliography   209

Index   215

Preface

Henry Rinaldo Porter was one of those nineteenth century young Americans who went west, neither to dodge the law nor to get a new start, but to seek the risks and rewards of the frontier. He deliberately embarked on a career that was dangerous and exciting.

As the son of a country doctor from New York State, he had the opportunity to practice in a community in the East as had his father, grandfather, and great-grandfather before him. Instead of settling down as a family physician he entered into contracts with the U.S. Army as an acting assistant surgeon after he completed his medical education.

As such he rode with the cavalry and treated soldiers in the Territories of Arizona, Dakota, and Montana during the Indian Wars. He was at Little Bighorn with Custer and lived to tell about it; two other surgeons did not. It was here, as a visitor to the battlefield, that I learned of Porter. This led me, as a surgeon, to follow his amazing story.

He arrived at Bismarck, Dakota Territory, in 1873 at its beginning; he lived and practiced medicine there off and on for the next thirty years. As the second doctor to arrive, he was part of Bismarck's history during its early years of economic and political turmoil. Bismarck began at the end of the

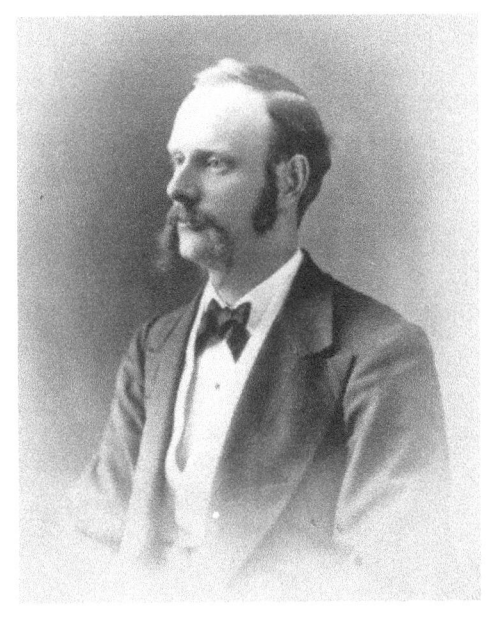

Dr. H.R. Porter at Fort Abraham Lincoln c. 1876. Photograph by O.S. Goff (State Historical Society of North Dakota 0264–08).

Northern Pacific Railroad line, which awaited completion of a bridge to cross the Missouri River. Steamboats carried passengers and freight up and down the river making stops there. Stagecoaches ran regularly between Bismarck and Deadwood City in the Black Hills where gold had been found. Settlers came in droves to farm the countryside surrounding Bismarck.

Porter's story is important for several reasons. He was an eye-witness participant of the Battle of Little Bighorn. Second, he is important in the medical history of the frontier. Third, he was an entrepreneur and an active participant in Bismarck's and the Dakota Territory's economic development. Fourth, he traveled widely and wrote interesting accounts of late nineteenth century travel for the land-locked residents of the Dakotas.

Porter lived at a time of expansion of the country westward. He amassed a fortune while others struggled. At times he was ruthless, but he was always a healer and a humanitarian. He could be tough and he could be gentle, but he was honest, courageous, and beloved by his community.

The reader may be aware that higher military ranks obtained during the Civil War were often used as a matter of protocol in discourse during the Indian Wars in place of the actual rank of the office at the time. For example, Custer achieved the rank of major general in the Civil War and was officially only a lieutenant colonel at Little Bighorn; Gibbon was a major general in the Civil War and colonel at Little Bighorn. Benteen and Reno were colonels before reverting to captain and major, respectively, in the regular army. Thus throughout this biography you may see different ranks for certain officers.

Chapter 1

Early Life and Education

> Men who live in democratic countries do not naturally have a military spirit: they sometimes take it up when they are brought despite themselves onto the fields of battle; but to rise en masse by oneself and to expose oneself voluntarily to the miseries of war, and above all those that civil war brings, is an option to which man in democracies does not resolve himself. It is only the most adventurous citizens who consent to throw themselves into a hazard like this; the mass of the population remains unmoved.
>
> Alexis de Tocqueville[1]

Henry R. Porter was born in Lee Center, Oneida County, New York, February 13, 1848. James K. Polk was then president. The Treaty of Guadalupe Hidalgo had just been signed earlier the same month by the United States and Mexico making the Rio Grande the boundary between the two countries and recognizing Texas, New Mexico, and California as a part of the United States in return for a fifteen million dollar payment. On January 24, nineteen days before he was born, gold was discovered at Sutter's Mill in California. Henry Rinaldo Porter seemed destined to be a part of the westward expansion of the country.

There is some confusion in recent publications about his birthplace and date of birth. All biographical sketches published during his lifetime clearly indicate Lee Center as his birthplace. Various later articles, in print and online, have him born on February 3, in New York Mills, New York, a town that his parents moved to in 1862 when Henry was fourteen years old.[2] His father was Dr. Henry Norton Porter, a physician and native of Oneida County. His mother was a Scottish immigrant, Helen Fulton Polson, a native of Ayrshire on the shores of the Firth of Clyde west of Kilmarnock. Helen came to New York State in 1825 as a seven-year-old orphan from Saltcoats, the town being named for the houses along the beach where its citizens had once extracted salt from seawater in their "salt cots." Other industries there included fishing, ship building, and textile weaving. Her father was John Polson, a weaver. Her mother, Helen Workman, died in 1821, after childbirth, when Helen Polson was only three.

Henry Rinaldo had two sisters, Sarah Elizabeth and Frances Emogene, ages five and two when he was born in 1848. Dr. Norton Porter, Henry Rinaldo's grandfather, was one of the first doctors, possibly even the first, to settle in Oneida County, New York. He was born in Abington, Massachusetts, in 1771, studied at Vermont Medical College, and immigrated to the village of Westmoreland, Oneida County, in 1791, five years after the first settler arrived. He was present at the first meeting of the Oneida County Medical Society held in 1806.[3] He practiced there and around the countryside for some forty years before dying at the home of his son, Dr. Henry Norton Porter, in 1852 at the age of eighty-one.[4]

The Porters had come to America from Weymouth, England. Richard Porter, age thirty, born in Dorset, England, came over with the Reverend Joseph Hull and twenty-one families in what was called the Hull Company and settled in Wessagusset near Plymouth Colony in 1635. With the influx of 106 people who came with Hull, the town was renamed and incorporated as Weymouth the same year.[5] There he grew reeds used for thatching houses.[6] His son, Sergeant John Porter, built the first sawmill in 1693 at what is now South Abington, Massachusetts, at a place called Little Comfort. He was said to have held at one time or other all the town offices in Weymouth. Samuel Porter, son of Sergeant John, was a town officer in Weymouth as well as being a schoolmaster and a shoemaker. His son Jacob, who was born in 1704, was a prominent citizen of Abington, Massachusetts, where he built the first mill on Beaver Creek. His wife was Esther Ford and his son was Noah Porter of Cummington, Massachusetts. Noah, born August 16, 1744, was Henry Rinaldo Porter's great-grandfather, the first physician in a line that extended for four generations. Noah's son, already mentioned, was Dr. Norton Porter, Henry's grandfather.

Dr. Henry Norton Porter, Henry's father, was born in Westmoreland, New York, in 1816 and served as apprentice to Dr. Whiting Smith of Whitesboro, New York, from 1835 to 1836, before graduating from Geneva College of Medicine in 1841. He practiced in Lee Center until 1862 when he moved his practice to New York Mills, a town known for the production of fine muslin, some twenty miles to the south just below the Erie Canal in the Mohawk River Valley near Utica. Dr. Henry Norton Porter was an active participant in the Anti-Slavery Society; the Temperance Society; the Oneida County Medical Association, of which he was president in 1870; the New York State Medical Association; and local church activities. He was quite interested in the health benefits of Sylvester Graham's bread and of a vegetarian diet.

Whoever selected the middle name of Rinaldo for young Henry could not have been more prescient. It was not a family name; it was the name of one of the illustrious and legendary knights or paladins of Charlemagne who subdued the horse Bayard, a powerful and magical beast that participated in his adventures and later saved his life.[7] Henry Rinaldo would always love adventure and fine horses. One such animal saved his life at Little Bighorn as it mounted the bluffs overlooking the river. Porter, unarmed, clung tightly "with superhuman strength" to its neck as the powerful black horse struggled to achieve the heights "running a gauntlet where the chances of death were a thousand to one."[8]

Henry grew up in Lee Center, a village north of Rome, New York, ten miles from the Erie Canal, situated on the banks of Canada Creek, which was the source of power for a gristmill and a sawmill during the town's early days. A church called the North Meeting House, the Harmony Library, a post office (established in 1827), two or three dozen houses, and two general stores lined the main street at the time. A turning mill, sawmill, and a small tannery were on side streets. Express stage lines ran twice daily between Lee Center and Rome. Early settlers from Lee, Massachusetts, gave the village its name. With the opening of the Erie Canal in 1825, the area experienced rapid economic expansion and population growth.

When Henry was ten years old there were two blacksmiths, two harness makers, a lawyer, a justice, a miller, a cooper, a painter, a small manufacturer of stoves, and two doctors, his father being one and Dr. J. Cornish the other. Dr. Porter's office was in a building next to his home. Directly across the street was School Number 3.[9]

Young Henry Rinaldo Porter received his early education in Lee Center, and when he was sixteen years old, his parents enrolled him in Whitestown Seminary in the village of Whitestown, three miles west of Utica. The school's 1869 catalogue described it as being "on the line of the New York Central Railroad. Street railroad cars pass[ed] every twenty minutes to and from the city."[10] The Reverend George Washington Gale, D.D., and the Reverend John Frost founded the seminary, originally called the Oneida Institute of Science and Industry, in 1827. It opened for students in 1828 with a philosophy of combining manual labor on a farm with "mental instruction."[11] Students were not particularly pleased with the farming aspects of their school and were ridiculed by some of their friends as "onion grubbers." It was a time of religious revivalism known as the Second Great Awakening. The institute became not only a college preparatory school but also a theological seminary. The students were swept up in the New England abolitionist movement and from the early days of the school published an anti-slavery newspaper, *Friend of Man*. Dr. Gale, the co-founder, left in 1837 to start Knox College in what became the town of Galesburg, Illinois.

Oneida Institute "did not prosper as had been expected" probably due to the combination of mental instruction with manual labor, as well as to the theological department's conflicts with Auburn Theological Seminary. The Presbyterian Education Society withdrew its support and Clinton Seminary, a Free Will Baptist institution, acquired the property leading to a charter of the Whitestown Seminary in 1845.

The school maintained rigid discipline and high academic standards and expected no less than exemplary conduct of its students. Study hours were from rising until 7 A.M., from 9 to noon, from 1 to 4 P.M., and from 7 P.M. until bedtime. Regulations included "no indecent, profane, or boisterous language, scuffling, or dancing allowed at any time in the Seminary buildings. All [were] prohibited from playing cards, or similar games of chance, at anytime. Also, all [were] prohibited from using tobacco in any form or intoxicating drinks as a beverage or frequenting places where such drinks are sold. All [were] required to attend public worship at least twice during the day and evening of each Sabbath, to avoid visiting other student's rooms, and to spend the day in a manner appropriate to its sacredness.... The gentlemen [were] prohibited from visiting the ladies' rooms, or the ladies, the gentlemen's rooms at any time."[12]

There is no evidence that Porter excelled in this school. His name appears nowhere on the academic prize list in the catalogues during his enrollment. In fact, he was listed as a second year student for four straight years in the English and Scientific Course, 1865, 1866, 1867, 1868, until he achieved third and final year class standing in 1869. Nevertheless, we can conclude that Porter had an excellent education by the time he completed his studies at this institution. His diligence as a student is open to question.

Published curriculum for the English and Scientific Course for gentlemen included:

First Year — Reading, Intellectual and Written Arithmetic, Grammar, Natural Philosophy, Algebra, U.S. History, Physical Geography.
Second Year–Bookkeeping, General History, Astronomy, Physiology, Geometry, Plane and Spherical Trigonometry, Mensuration, Chemistry.
Third Year — Surveying, Civil Engineering, Botany, Intellectual Philosophy, Political Economy, Science of Government, Rhetoric, Geology, (French and German optional).[13]

Tuition was eight, nine, or ten dollars per term of fourteen weeks depending on the level of the student. Board was two dollars and seventy-five cents per week; room rent was three dollars per term. There were three terms each academic year.

A much more rigorous three-year classics curriculum devoted almost entirely to Latin and Greek studies was available for college preparation, mainly for ministers. Entry to medical schools did not require classics study.

During Porter's final year, there were 522 students enrolled; 313 men and 209 women. There was a faculty of ten and one librarian. The library had 2,000 books. As public secondary education became more widely available, enrollment at this private school declined until its doors closed in 1885.[14]

Chapter 2

Medical School Adventures

Ann Arbor's streets were unpaved and muddy when Henry R. Porter arrived in 1869 to enter the Medical Department of the University of Michigan. Hitching posts lined Main Street.[1] The department was relatively new, having opened in 1850 with ninety-one students. In 1869 there were 350 in the Department of Medicine and Surgery and a total of 1,089 in the university.[2] The medical building, completed that year, was a sandstone "Greek Temple" housing three stories of laboratories, lecture rooms, and "a large amphitheater on the third floor lighted by a small dome."[3] The latter was most likely used for anatomical demonstrations and lectures and not for surgical operations as were other famous domed amphitheaters such as the Ether Dome at Massachusetts General Hospital in Boston. It was not until 1876 that the first University Hospital at Michigan was completed, six years after Porter had left.[4] This hospital did have an amphitheater in the Surgical Ward where surgical procedures were performed.[5]

A faculty member when the school opened, Dr. Moses Gunn, Geneva Medical College, class of 1846, was professor of anatomy. He was followed by Dr. Corydon L. Ford, Geneva Medical College, class of 1842, as professor of anatomy to replace Gunn when he became professor of surgery.[6] This connection with Geneva Medical College, New York, probably explains why Henry was enrolled there by his father, a member of the class of 1841, Geneva Medical College. Gunn left Ann Arbor for Rush Medical School in Chicago in 1867, before Henry Porter arrived, but Ford remained.

The medical department rapidly expanded. Porter, who had come from a strict, religious background, was exposed to a rowdy student body at Michigan, the likes of which he had probably never seen. There were brawls, chapel disturbances, and bonfire celebrations that consumed sections of the town's wooden sidewalks.[7] In April of the year that Porter was in Ann Arbor, a newspaper reported the following: "The freshmen students at the university in Ann Arbor made their annual raid upon the wooden sidewalks the other night, while the sophomores tore off the wheel of the university bell and battered South College Pretty boys."[8] The faculty brought in women students with the hope that [they] "might improve the manners of the men students." In 1870 there were thirty women students enrolled in the university.⁹

Alcohol consumption was rampant and created major problems. Student rules stated, "No student shall be allowed to frequent gaming houses, play at cards, or practice any species of gambling, or attend gaming or drinking saloons, or be guilty of profaneness, or any act of violence, or keep the company of persons of ill repute or be guilty of any other vice." Drinking intoxicating drinks was named a vice. These regulations were honored primarily in the breach.¹⁰ There were at the time six breweries in Ann Arbor. A student two years before Porter enrolled reported "a revival of temperance societies in town which are going to shut up all the whiskey cellars and so-called restaurants in town. There are fifty-five such places here." As for this prediction, two years after Porter left, there were still forty-nine saloons listed in the Ann Arbor city directory. Nothing points toward Porter drinking alcohol at this time and letters to his father the following year suggest that he avoided it based upon his religious scruples.

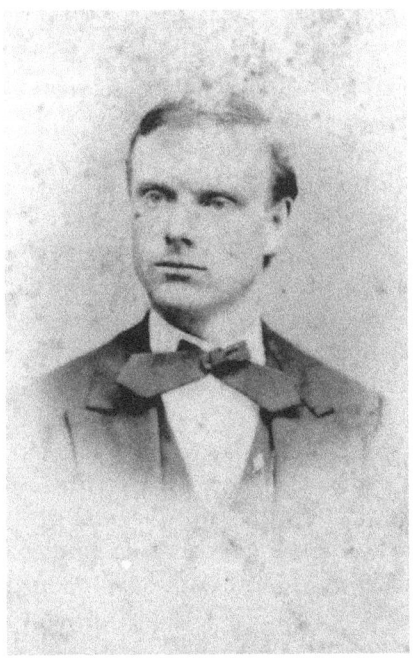

Henry R. Porter at the University of Michigan as a medical student, 1869–70. Photograph by D.P. Groves, Ann Arbor, Michigan (State Historical Society of North Dakota 0264–12).

We have no accounts of Porter's social or academic activities at Ann Arbor, but there is a photograph, a carte de visite of him at age 21 or 22 made by "D.P. Groves, Photographer, Opposite Cook's Hotel, Ann Arbor, Mich."¹¹

In the image he appears serious and intense. His face is thin and clean-shaven, his complexion fair, and his hair light colored. He wears a white shirt, a coat, a vest, and a rather large bow tie.

Though there is no evidence that he had academic problems, he failed to return to Ann Arbor to medical school the next year (1870–71). The reason for his departure is easily discovered. He simply was not interested in medicine and did not want to become a doctor. Perhaps he had been the recipient of undue family pressure to follow in the footsteps of his great-grandfather, grandfather, and father, all physicians. His niece, Helen Workman

Davis, who collected and transcribed the letters that he wrote home from Scotland in the fall of 1870 while he visited his mother's relatives, states that his "sudden trip" to Scotland occurred when he "reluctantly turned his back on his home [rather than] to face a year of study for the profession, which at that time he heartily disliked."[12] She appears to have been his favorite niece and was the one with whom he corresponded from time to time.

Henry left New York on the Anchor Line S/S *Australia* at noon, Saturday, September 17, 1870, bound for Glasgow, Scotland, an action totally unknown to his parents who believed that he was going to New York City for another year of medical studies. Anchor Line Steamers sailed every Saturday and on alternate Wednesdays from Pier 20 on North River. The *Australia* was a steamship of 1,999 gross tonnage that had been launched January 20 of the same year in Glasgow and was completing its fifth round-trip voyage on the Glasgow–New York route.[13] It had one stack, three masts, a single screw, and reached a speed of twelve knots. Rates of passage for Anchor Line ships between New York and Glasgow were $130 for best cabin accommodations, $65 and $75 first class, $33 intermediate, and $28 steerage.[14] After fourteen days he arrived in Glasgow on Saturday, October 1.[15] At the time, the Anchor Line operated a feeder route between Scandinavian ports and Scotland for its transatlantic steamer service between Glasgow and New York that became the path of many immigrants to the United States.

As always, Henry had the knack for turning a bad situation into a great opportunity. He made connections in Scotland with his mother's cousins in the Saltcoats area who further connected him with other cousins who were shipping magnates and they, in turn, introduced him to other shipping magnates who were some of the richest people in Europe. The Allans who entertained him owned the Allan Line, a precursor of the Cunard Line, which sailed from Glasgow and Liverpool and carried more young immigrants to Canada than any other line.[16] Porter visited in the home of Alexander Allan, the youngest of the five sons of Alexander Allan Sr., founder of the company. The Robert Smiths, relatives and ship owners, arranged for him to tour the Scottish highlands and took him to Belfast where they visited the Corrys of the Corry and Company shipping line at the home of the future chairman, Sir William Corry, baronet.

Henry's revolt against parental authority was a turning point in his life. He became his own man. His love of travel and his habit of sending letters back continued throughout his life. Many of his later letters were published in newspapers telling readers about his travels and adventures. The following letters have not previously been published.

His first letter from Scotland tells the story:

2. Medical School Adventures

> Kilwinning, Scotland
> October 3, 1870

Dear Folks,

I wrote you a letter while I was at sea and intended to mail it at Londonderry [Anchor Line ships stopped there between New York and Glasgow], but I have it in my pocket yet and I will now write a few more lines and send it all at once.

I don't know why I ever came away as I did, but I am here and do not know how I will ever get back and I hardly dare to come if I could. I want to hear from you. I never felt my dependence on you as I do now and never realized what a good home I had and what a chance I have lost.

I am going to Saltcoats tomorrow, the place where Mother was born. I would like to hear from Father and if you write, direct [it] to Glasgow Post Office, Scotland, to be called for, put that all on or I will not get it.

If I had gone to college as I ought and not played the liar as I have, I now would have been all right. But here I am in a fix. All I can do is to ask your forgiveness, and that I do. There are lots of things I could write about but I am not in a writing mood. You will not get this letter in less than two weeks [the length of Porter's cruise between New York and Glasgow] and if you write to me it will not get to Glasgow in less than a month and where I will be then, God only knows, but I will get the letter someway.

I am now at Kilwinning, which is only three miles from Saltcoats; I am stopping at Captain Brown's. His wife is Helen Workman, the last of a family of twenty. She says to tell you that she remembers the last Sabbath you were in Scotland; she also tells me many other things to tell you but I can not write them now. If I come home would Father ever trust me again? I suppose I can make out to live some way, but I find 'tis not so fine to be in a strange, foreign land after all. I had thought that I would not send the letter that I wrote at sea for the reason that I am ashamed of some of it, but I will send some of it.

Hoping to hear from you, I am your truant Son,

> H.R. Porter[17]

Porter's next letter was to his mother.

> [Auchengouer] Cove, [Scotland]
> October 17, 1870

Dear Mother,

I wrote a letter home while I was at Mrs. Captain John Brown's. I think you must have the letter by this time but, of course, there has not been time for me to receive an answer.

I was at Mrs. Brown's and had a splendid time. Mrs. Smith thinks she is very much like you in looks but I don't see the resemblance, but I can tell you she is a whole-souled woman, and one who tries to do all she can to make it pleasant and not make a show about it.

We went all over the country while I was there. We went to Saltcoats; saw the house you used to live in, and went to the grave yard; saw the place where your mother is buried and a number of relatives. I have a copy of all the inscriptions upon the stones. We also walked along the beach and gathered shells, so that I have a small collection.

We called upon a Mrs. Richie who is well acquainted with Mrs. Henderson. It seemed that Mrs. Henderson made her a visit a few years ago. She wished me to remember her to Mrs. Henderson. We also called upon Mr. Ronald who is the same old minister that used to preach to you, and several old women. They all remembered you, and took a great interest in me. They flocked around me to see Helen Polson's only son like small boys around a trained monkey.

We went to Kilwinning, and from there to Fenwick where Mr. Orr lives, and remained there all night. He remembered you and gave me a pair of slippers to wear for your sake.

We made a trip to Burns' monument [near Alloway in Ayrshire] and saw the place where the great poet was born and the bed he lay in. It is a very old house made of stone with a thatched roof, and there has been an addition made to it for the purpose of keeping a sort of drinking saloon and where they keep photos and other things to sell. Mrs. Brown bought a small case to put pins and, etc. in for Frank [H. R. Porter's sister, Frances Emogene], the covers are made of wood cut from trees on the banks of the river Doon which is nearby. We saw Kirk Alloway and the window in the gable and where Tam O'Shanter saw the devil playing for the witches. We were also at Ayr where the Brigs [bridges] are that Burns speaks about. All these places are in Ayrshire where the noted Ayrshire cows come from. I could buy as good a cow as any the company has for 20 pounds or about 60 dollars.

"Cove" is Mrs. Smith's summer residence and it is one of the finest places that I ever saw; they always come here to stay during the summer. They return to Glasgow next Friday, their residence there is one of the finest in the city. (Glasgow has a population of half a million). The place at Cove is on the coast and is 180 feet above the sea. Just opposite are mountains which rise to the height of two or three thousand feet. At the left are three ranges of hills which are seen in the distance and present a view which is magnificent and grand.

It is about thirty miles to Glasgow and to get there they ride in the carriage a distance of two miles, then take a steamer to Greenock, then the cars to the city. Mr. Allan and Mr. [Robert] Smith make the trip every day, so they ride sixty miles every day.

Mrs. Smith has company all the time — at present Mr. and Mrs. Greenhorn from London are here. He is agent for the Allan Steamers in London. Mrs. [Robert] Smith introduces me as her cousin from America who has just finished his education and is traveling. So you see, I am constantly in contact with the big guns of England and Scotland and I am seeing and learning things that I never knew of. You ought to see the dinners we have, such style I never dreamed of.

Mrs. Smith sent me to Loch Lomond which is in the highlands and it was a splendid sight. I talk of going to Edinburgh next week, and as soon as they get tired of me here or as soon as I see any signs of it, I want to go to France as an assistant surgeon if I can get a chance. You may smile at this, but the main thing that will hinder me is the want of money. If I could go there and stay a few months I would learn a great deal in Surgery. I have got some seeds of shrubs for you and some sweet peas which are very pretty.

Old Mr. Service, Mrs. Smith's father, is alive and is eighty-nine years old. He is blind and has been for sixteen years but he is very smart for his age and very set in his ways, and gets so mad at Mrs. Smith at times that he trembles all over. He and Mrs. Smith send their love. 'Tis well they don't know the manner that I left America.

Love to all, your son,
Harry[18]

Porter forwarded to his mother information about her family that he had recorded from tombstones. In Saltcoats he found the following sad story of the death of an infant and its young mother, his grandmother:

Erected by John Polson [his mother's father], weaver, in Saltcoats in memory of his beloved wife Helen Workman who departed this life the 26th of July 1821 age 32 years. Also his daughter Janet Stewart Polson who departed this life the 4th of August 1821 age 2 months and 25 days.

This explains why Henry R. Porter's mother came to America when she was a child of seven. Her mother died when she was only three years old after the birth of another child leaving her an orphan.

On another stone was:

Erected by Robert Workman [his mother's grandfather] in memory of his beloved spouse Eliza Boyd [his mother's grandmother] who died January 13, 1814 age 64 and their children
Eliza who died October 5, 1796, age 23 years
Mary, June 11, 1811, age 27
Jean Ellen and Ann who died in infancy
Here is interred the above Robert Workman who died February 23, 1836 in his 87th year. Also his children William, Fulton, Thomas, and William who died in infancy and Elizabeth Stewart relict [widow] of said Robert Workman who died December 16, 1850, age 58.

Descendants of the Henry Norton Porter family in America have been grateful for Henry's unexpected genealogical research of his mother's family in Scotland.

Henry's next letter was sent to his sister and her husband and expands on his situation and his thinking at the time.

October 24, 1870 15 Woodside Terrace
Glasgow, Scotland

To   Sarah Porter Davis and
     her husband, David Melling Davis
     1613 19th Street, Washington, D.C.

Dear Brother and Sister
I suppose I did a wild thing when I left New York City for Glasgow instead of

remaining there and attending Lectures. However, that may be, here I am and "what can't be cured must be endured." I have seen something of human nature and had a chance to study it since leaving New York, and I think I will have a very good chance to study it more fully before I get home.

I arrived in Glasgow on Saturday the 1st of October, stopped at a hotel until Monday.[19] Since that time I have been visiting at Captain John Brown's, Mrs. Robert Smith's and Mrs. Allan's. While at Mrs. Brown's, she and I went to Saltcoats, also the place where Mother was born, the room where her mother used to weave, etc. We also went to the cemetery where her relatives are buried. I have a copy of all the inscriptions on the stones. In Mrs. Brown's house, also in Mrs. Allan's, are large oil paintings. Mrs. Brown's father, Mother's grandfather, and your great grandfather are all the same [person]. [Therefore, Mrs. Brown was H.R. Porter's great aunt.] We also visited Robert Burns' home, monument, in Ayrshire.

I was at Mrs. Brown's house ten days and nearly every day we were at some place of interest, and I had a splendid time. Since then I have been at Mrs. Smith's at Auchengouer Cove on the coast. They live in a magnificent house and in splendid style. I will not attempt to describe it, and both her and her daughter's house in Glasgow, where we are now, are the nicest houses in the city and are fitted up in the most beautiful style.

Mrs. Smith sent Robert Allan and I off Friday morning on one of the most beautiful trips in Scotland. We got back Saturday night and I never enjoyed myself more. We left Glasgow in the morning on the cars, drove about fifty miles, then took a steamer up Loch Lomond, then a high stage to Loch Katrine, then by stage through the Trossachs, cars to Callander, and home by way of Daenleane [Dunblane] and Stirling. The scenery in and around Loch Lomond is grand and beautiful beyond description. And in Loch Katrine is Ellen's Isle and the silver strand that Scott speaks of in the *Lady of the Lake*. I have some books and pictures that describe and show the scenery better than I can tell you, so I will not tell you any more but will show them to you.

Robert Smith has thirty-eight ships and is now building four new steamers for the Suez Canal trade. Each ship costs 100,000 pounds, over half a million dollars, so you may know that he is worth something. Both he and Allan have money pouring in so fast they don't know what to do with it hardly. The women make considerable of it disappear and they have all they can use for the asking of it. Mrs. Smith has company all the time from London and other places and she introduces me as her cousin from America who has just finished his education and is traveling. Yes, I am traveling and I have four shillings of British money in the world. Nevertheless, I am traveling and have been for the last three weeks on that, and in first class style. My next move is to Edinburgh, then to Belfast and London. If I knew your friends in Wales, I would give them a call. Friends are a fine thing to have when you are in a strange country. I wish I had some in London where I could stay a week or so.

I see by the paper that one of the Anchor Line steamers went down — the same line I came on. Our Captain was in a very dangerous position near the same place one night, but he put out to sea and the next morning we were 200 miles out from land and came into Londonderry in the daytime.[20]

How are Charles, Hannah, and Jane? I hope you and Sarah are well. If you write which I hope you will, direct it to London, to be called for at the Post Office.

> With love to all,
> I am Yours truly,
> H.R. Porter[21]

The following letter is to his sister from Glasgow:

> Scotland
> October 31, 1870

Dear Sister,

... Last week I spent a day in Edinburgh which is the finest city in Scotland, also the capital, as you well know. Here are a great many places of interest. Walter Scott's Monument, the Old Castle, the Royal Museum, Holyrood Palace, etc. The latter named place is where the Queen stays when she is in Edinburgh. I went through the Palace, and saw the room and bed that Mary of Scots used to occupy, also her private stair and dining room, and Lord Darnley's room, and a great many other things and places too numerous to mention. At Stirling, I saw Stirling Castle which is over a thousand years old. There are a great many Scotch soldiers here and it would be a hard matter to take the Castle now, even with the improved guns.

The weather here is miserable, rain, fog and smoke all the time. It is very pleasant just now, but it will rain before night, if it does not 'twill be an exception. There is no cold weather here, not enough for skating even. The grass is as green now as ever.

Last Friday I was invited to dinner at Mr. George Smith's home. They had quite a large party and I did not want to go, but of course I had to, and in fact I had a good time. I have got so now that I know what finger glasses and fish knives are, and can use them all right. The way they live here is like this: breakfast at eight; lunch at one; dinner at five, and tea at eight in the evening. Dinner is the great meal of the day, and the every day fare is something like this—fish, beef roast, and cold fowl. I have forgotten to mention that the first thing is always soup. Then they have two kinds of puddings and after that American apples, French grapes and pears, figs, nuts, and raisins, several kinds of cake, and lemonade.

Yesterday there was a Norwegian spent the day here. He is one that Mr. and Mrs. Allan became acquainted with while they were traveling. I had to stop to ride with Mrs. Smith and have just returned and will proceed to finish. She has a pair of blacks and a nice carriage and a driver in livery. Mrs. Allan lives at 2 Park Gardens, about five minutes walk from 15 Woodside Terrace. My ride has just upset me, for I can think of nothing to write about, so I will put the letter by until my ideas come more readily.

[Continuing] Belfast, Ireland

> November 3, 1870

We came here yesterday morning at four o'clock. Got up at half past six and found Mr. Corry's [later Sir William Corry] carriage waiting for us. I had thought I had seen a nice house and one that was furnished in as good style as it could be, but Mr. Corry's beats everything I have seen. 'Tis a new one and they have not lived in it but a few months. All the woodwork is polished pitch pine and a rare kind of wood from India, which is very beautiful.

Yesterday we all took tea at Robert Workman's, and tomorrow evening there is to be a great party there of young people. Mother has got more relatives here than you could shake a stick at and they are all very rich and very close with their money which is a very good thing.

Since I have been here I have seen so much of style, etiquette, and formality that I am sick of it and long to breathe free once more.

Tomorrow, or next day, I am going to see the Giant's Causeway.

Give my regards to my friends,

Your Brother,

Henry[22]

[postscript]
The weather here seems to be much better than in Scotland, 'tis clearer. The farmers are getting in the potatoes and the Emerald Isle is as green as some of its people.

The next letter is a response to a letter from his father:

To Dr. Henry Norton Porter
Jewin Crescent
London, England

November 16, 1870

Dear Father,

I received your letter as soon as I returned from Ireland, and think you gave me some very good advice which I will try to keep in mind. I did not wish to withdraw from the Lodge because I intended to break my obligations, but for other reasons. I have been to fashionable dinner parties where they all took wine but myself. The ladies all drank and after the dinner was over, they retired and the men drank wine until their eyes sparkled, their blood ran faster and they would rub their hands and tell their experiences with great enthusiasm.

I left Glasgow yesterday at 2:10 P.M. and arrived in London at six this morning and have just returned from sightseeing, and am so cold I can hardly write. I started from Blackfriars Bridge and went to see the South Kensington Museum. I went by the Underground Railroad; have also seen Saint Paul's.

It was my intention to go to France or Prussia — if I could not go any other way, to go as a soldier. But since I received your letter I have abandoned that entirely. As soon as I have seen London I am going back to Glasgow.

You seem to have had a good crop of potatoes and apples; more potatoes than I thought you would get from that small patch.

'Tis very dirty here and the fog is very heavy, and the atmosphere is so full of dirt that it is almost impossible to keep your face clean. There was a frost last night and it was not very comfortable riding from Glasgow to London in a [rail] car without any stove. None of the cars here have stoves in them, and they are not equal to the American cars in any respect.

2. Medical School Adventures

You tell me to come home when I have had enough of this kind of roving. I will do so if I can get home, if not, I will do the next best thing whatever it is. I don't think I will be any the worse for this trip. I always wanted to cross the ocean and I never would have been satisfied until I had. I am well aware that I did wrong in leaving as I did, but that is done and can't be undone now.

I hope no one will get swamped in the matrimonial swells you speak of. They are very dangerous, more so than any I experienced in crossing, though they were bad enough.

Mrs. Robert Workman of Belfast says she remembers going to the ship at Greenock to see Mother start for America. While I was in Belfast I went to Queens College, which is a very fine one, and listened to a lecture by the professor of Chemistry, also one on Anatomy and Physiology. I went in the dissecting room and in some respects it is superior to ours.

I think I told you to direct your letters to London, in one of my letters. I shall not be here more than a week or two, and if you have not written I'll not get them. If you write again, direct the same as the other. I may get it and I may not, as I am on the wing so that it is hard to say where I will be by the time you will answer this. I will write to you often so that you will know where I am, and I hope I may live to see America again, and all of you well and right side up with care.

Love to Mother and Frank,
I am your affectionate Son,

Henry[23]

The previous letter foreshadows Porter's career as an adventurer and traveler. It also indicates a reconciliation of sorts with his father over his abandonment of medical school and his trip abroad. Henry happily reported to his father his teetotal behavior and his intentions to avoid the marital trap that his father called the "matrimonial swells."

The following letter is the final letter of the series so far as we know before his return to the United States.

To Dr. and Mrs. Henry Norton Porter

#6 Pyrland Road
London, England
November 25, 1870

Dear Father and Mother,

'Tis raining so that I do not care to attend church this evening. I don't know as I can spend the evening any better than to write you and let you know how I am getting on, as the Scotch say.

I have attended service twice every Sabbath but one since I landed in Glasgow. I have been to Spurgeon's Tabernacle today to hear the great [Charles Haddon] Spurgeon [1834–1892, great Victorian preacher] spurge, heard him and was very much pleased. He took his text from 1st Corinthians 6:17. His sermons are printed and I will send you a few of the one I heard today and you can give them to your friends. His tabernacle holds only six thousand and was full, as it always is. Spurgeon is a stout man, does not shave, black hair and whiskers, short neck, and a round John Bull face. He talks very distinctly and 'tis a pleasure to listen to him. I took tea this afternoon with a Dr. Crummings and he gave me a ticket to visit the Surgeon's Museum. I intend to visit it tomorrow.

Since I wrote you, I have been to the Crystal Palace [built for the Great Exhibition of 1851], the Zoological Gardens, Hyde and Regents Parks, Westminster Abbey, House of Parliament, etc. The Palace is a wonderful place. Almost everything is here in the known world. The Zoological Gardens are a fine place to spend a day for anyone who likes to see animals. I was there when the lions were fed which was worth seeing. There are animals, reptiles, fowls, and fish here from every country. Even trout from America.

At Westminster Abbey I saw all that was to be seen, which is the graves of the kings, queens and poets. Queen Mary and Queen Elizabeth, Henry II and various other kings are buried here. In the Poet's Corner I saw Charles Dickens's stone. On Mr. Dickens's stone is simply his name, and when he was born and died. This is all that marks the resting place of the author of *Pickwick* and *Copperfield*.

Tuesday, I am going to see London Tower, and in the evening, to the Spurgeon Tabernacle to hear an entertainment he gave a notice of today. 'Tis the "Bell Ringers" and said to be very fine. The money is for some good purpose.

Pyrland Road is about three miles from the heart of the city. As I was coming here Friday night in a bus, a dense fog came on, so dense that we could not see lamp posts and finally it got so dark they would not run any further.[24] The passengers had to get out and find their way the best way they could. I could not find Pyrland Road nor any one else and after a time found a place, a dirty place, to stay the night. In the morning I found my way well enough. These fogs are a fine thing for pickpockets. They can walk up and rob you without any fear of being caught.

There seems to be some reason to think there may be a war between England and Russia, if so 'twill be a good time for America, or rather, the United States, to step in and take her Alabama claims.[25] The British soldiers strut around here with their red coats and canes as if they were lions. I think the Yanks could take the tuck out of some of them and show the Queen how an eagle can whip a lion.

Henry R. Porter[26]

This ended an important phase in his life. He had completed his rebellion, had satisfied his desire for travel and adventure, for the present, and was now ready to pursue his career.

Chapter 3

Western Adventures

Forgiven for his indiscretions, Henry Rinaldo returned to New York Mills to his parents' home after his lark in Great Britain and acted temporarily as an apprentice to his father. He studied and gained practical experience until his return to medical school in the fall of 1871.

Fortunately, his sister, Sarah, and her husband, David Melling Davis, lived in Washington, DC, 1613 19th Street NW, where David was employed in the Bureau of Engraving and Printing. It was an ideal situation for Porter to have family members who lived near one of the better medical schools. Henry entered October 3rd as a senior in the Medical Department of Georgetown College on the corner of Tenth and E Streets in Washington, DC. At that time, the medical college was in its twenty-third session with a faculty of ten, twenty senior students, forty-one juniors, and one pharmacy doctoral candidate for a total of sixty-two students.[1]

Lectures were held at 5:30 P.M. daily making it convenient for students to attend, especially those "employed in various Government Departments." There was ample opportunity for clinical instruction as well as "abundant accommodations and materials afforded ... for the prosecution of this branch of medical science [dissections] in a large, convenient, and well-ventilated apartment furnished with gas and water." The Army Medical Museum was adjacent to the college buildings and contained specimens in anatomy, natural history, and pathology.

Tuition for the full course was one hundred thirty-five dollars plus fees. There were four requirements for the degree of doctor of medicine: good moral character, three years of study with two being full courses of medical education in a recognized school of medicine, one course of practical anatomy and one course of clinical instruction, and a written thesis in the candidate's own hand followed by the successful completion of an examination.[2]

Porter wrote his thesis on "Medical Diagnosis." In the list of graduates he listed his hometown as Utica, New York, near New York Mills where his parents lived.

Graduation was held on the afternoon of March 6, 1872, at the National

Theatre where there were addresses by Johnson Eliott, professor of surgery; Herbert Boardman, valedictorian; and R.D. DeL. French for the alumni.[3] It was a time of elevated sentiments, reference to the classics, a bow to medical history, and an emphasis on devotion to duty and responsibility to God, mankind, and to the profession. The president of Georgetown, the Rev. John Early, S.J., before conferring the degrees "delivered a brief but impressive address in the course of which, with more than usual emphasis, he admonished the class that it would be a duty incumbent upon them as Christian practitioners of medicine to remind patients when in danger of death — especially in cases where they [the patients] were negligent or indifferent — that *they had souls to be saved.*"[4]

Dr. Henry R. Porter then took an internship for three months after graduation at Columbia Hospital for Women and Lying-in Asylum at 25th and L Streets NW, just off Pennsylvania Avenue in Washington. Originally it had opened in 1866 on Thomas Circle NW, to give medical care for widows of Civil War soldiers, and moved to the above address in 1870. The eighty-six-bed hospital closed in 2002.[5]

At the time Porter finished his internship, a military solution to the Indian problem in the Arizona Territory was being fashioned in Washington. Despite President Grant's efforts to make peace with the Apache Indians, atrocities by both Indians and settlers continued. General George Crook was preparing an all-out campaign against the Tonto Apaches.

Porter agreed to travel to the Arizona Territory as a contract surgeon with the U.S. Army by signing at the surgeon general's office in Washington, DC, on June 26, 1872, at a salary of one hundred twenty-five dollars a month.[6] The contract was for one year, if not less, with an allowance for fuel and quarters of an assistant surgeon of the rank of first lieutenant with mileage back to the place where the contract was made.

Places in the regular army were limited by the decline in personnel due to severe budgetary cuts by Congress following the Civil War. For the few billets available, stringent written exams of medical knowledge were required as well as certification by the Army Medical Board. With no opportunity for advancement, the medical men on duty were in a stagnant corps that made contract surgeons between 1869 and 1874 of "particular importance" and much needed according to Wengert.[7] This was the beginning of another adventure for Porter.

Porter crossed the country by train from Washington to the West Coast and reached San Francisco on July 5. He wrote to his father from the Brooklyn Hotel on Bush Street the next morning:

> I had no idea what a vast country this of ours was and no one can have until they have traveled across it. To ride day after day and night after night almost without stopping at lightning speed for eight days and nights does not sound very

great but I tell you it gives one some idea of the distance. I did not see any buffaloes or as many wild animals as I expected yet we saw a good many antelopes and prairie dogs, chickens, etc. The railroad has drove (sic) the game back north and south.[8]

The expansive corn and wheat fields of Iowa and the snow in the Rocky Mountains on the trip west impressed him. San Francisco was uncomfortably cold when he arrived.

But I shall not suffer long from the cold because they tell me that 'tis "hot as hell" where I am going (Arizona). By the way, I see by the papers the Indians are very troublesome there and I expect to have some fun with them if I am not hunted but can do the hunting myself. I hate them already. They are a mean and vicious set, I know by their looks they are not to be trusted.[9]

He reported to the general who commanded the Pacific Division of the army on July 6 and awaited orders impatiently.

While in San Francisco he purchased a large Smith & Wesson pistol, "the best six shooter. Will shoot accurate two hundred yards. No one thinks of going to Arizona without being well armed. Even the stage ride is dangerous."[10] In 1883, seven years after the battle of Little Bighorn, a group of surveyors found a six-shot .45 caliber Smith & Wesson revolver on the battlefield.[11] The gun is shown in a photograph "courtesy of the Smithsonian Institution, Washington, D.C." Cavalrymen were issued Colt revolvers but "some soldiers chose to buy their own." Could this have been Porter's and lost in the mad scramble for safety? He testified under oath before the court at the Reno Inquiry that he was unarmed. Of course, any of the soldiers could have lost the weapon, but it is interesting to speculate.

On July 31 he was ordered to report to Angel Island in San Francisco Bay to accompany troops to Fort Yuma by steamship. He sailed from San Francisco on the *Newbern*, a wooden-hulled coal powered steamer, on August 3 down the coast of California and the Baja California Peninsula and then up the Gulf of California to the mouth of the Colorado River to Yuma. On August 31 he was in Ehrenburg, Arizona Territory, and from there he crossed the Arizona desert with four companies of troops to reach Mullins Station where he was left by the troops when he became sick, possibly from the alkaline water that acted as a strong purgative. Sickness for Porter was an uncommon event, but newcomers to the West were commonly afflicted by violent diarrhea due to the bitter drinking water.

Already he was beginning to have second thoughts about his adventure. On September 10 he wrote:

You have no idea what a poor miserable country this is. If I had had, I never would have been fool enough to come here. 'Tis a vast desert, no water—nothing but mountains, sand and Indians and heat—so hot. Well I thought that I had seen and experienced hot weather in Washington — but it was nothing. Here the thermometer has been standing at 100 and 102 and the breeze we get feels like the hot air from a furnace. I can't see any use in the government sending troops here to protect so miserable a country at such enormous expense — better let the Indians have it. I may like it better after I get to a Post, but now I am thoroughly disgusted and if I had money enough, would return tomorrow.[12]

There was a shortage of water, further demoralizing Porter as he wrote from the isolated outpost of Mullins Station. Only he and three soldiers were there. At the time the nearest civilization was thirty miles away and the small detail feared that an Indian attack might overwhelm them. "We have our arms loaded and are ready if they give us a call."[13]

By the 19th of September he was at Fort Whipple, Arizona Territory, two miles northeast of Prescott, with orders to travel another forty miles northwest to Camp Hualpai (near present-day Paulden, Arizona) with the 5th Cavalry to accompany General George Crook's expedition against the Apache Indians.[14] He commented in a letter to his parents that this was the roughest life that he had ever seen and that as soon as he could get out of it, he would. Actually, he was just at the beginning of a way of life he would grow to love.

Two days later he rode out of Camp Hualpai (now called Juniper, Arizona) on Walnut Creek with three companies of the 5th Cavalry and ninety Hualpai Indian scouts under the command of Colonel Julius W. Mason to hunt Apache Indians. After going fifteen miles they camped for the night. Porter complained that after lying on the ground with a blanket over him, he awoke the next morning "damp and chilled through, eyes swollen, legs stiff and pains in the back and bad cold."[15] They traveled like this for three days through rough country, canyons and mountains until they encountered a band of Apaches that they routed at Muchos Canyon, a point where five canyons converged to form the Santa Maria.[16] Porter told that about forty Apaches were killed and one squaw and her infant murdered by one of the Hualpai scouts.[17] He summed up his feelings of regret and remorse on the 28th of September after returning to Camp Hualpai in a letter to his mother:

> I have always had a desire to see frontier life, to see the great west — to see the Indians and the Indian fights. I have seen the West and all the frontier life I care to see ... I am heartily sick of Arizona and homesick as I have never been before. I have no chance to read and improve my medical knowledge and I wish I had never seen Arizona. I have often been discouraged and had the blues but never so bad as now ... I ought not to write so discouraging a letter but I write just as I feel and am free to confess that I made one great mistake when I came to Arizona.[18]

Between expeditions there was the boredom of camp life made worse by the discomforts of sleeping on the ground. As winter approached the cold weather added to their misery.

3. Western Adventures

On the 19th of October Porter accompanied another expedition. This time the Apaches were aware of the attackers and fought well from a mountaintop. All but ten Indians escaped.[19]

On November 4 while camping near Camp Hualpai, there was a cold rainstorm during the night that drenched the troops and covered the mountaintops on either side with snow. A bear prowled and growled around Porter's tent. He wrote, "The old fellow came near enough so that I could hear his footsteps."[20]

Porter began to gain confidence and informed his mother that he was beginning to enjoy the life of the military surgeon and had discovered that he could ride fifty miles or walk fifteen miles a day over some of the roughest country just as well as the soldiers. "The more I see of Army life, the more I like scouting and think I'd rather scout than be at a post after all. In fact, the Doctor at Hualpai wants to go on the next scout and wants to exchange with me but I'm not going to exchange. Sometimes I think I've traveled about enough, then again think as I have been a quarter around the world I may as well [have] made the other three-quarters before I stop."[21]

General Crook's campaign against the Apaches began when he marched out of Fort Whipple on November 15. Three companies of Fifth Cavalry troops under Colonel Julius W. Mason, to which Porter was attached, rode out from Camp Hualpai on November 16 as part of the same operation. Of the three companies one was to go north of Bill Williams Mountain (thirty

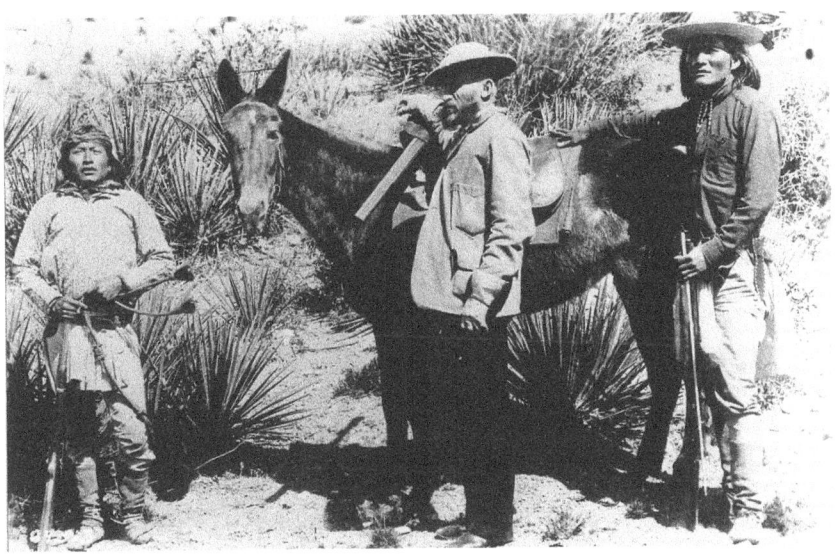

Gen. George Crook in Arizona Territory with his favorite riding mule, Apache, and two Apache scouts (National Archives [89513]).

miles west of Flagstaff), another company followed behind that company, and the third company, B Company, with Porter, was to ride south of the mountain. Water was scarce and the search for it critical. The Indian scouts walked and became exceedingly thirsty. The three hundred horses and mules suffered greatly, as did the soldiers until they finally found water.

Porter's unit arrived near Camp Verde, an army post forty-five miles east of Prescott, on December 1. To this point one company had killed eleven Apaches, another nine, and his own B Company killed two and captured one. Porter had the scalp of one Apache and he later mailed it home to his father.[22]

Porter found Arizona a "lonely sort of country" and fit only for Indians. "The few white people who live here (citizens) are as a general thing cutthroats, or thieves who have escaped from the states in order to escape the law ... I wish I had a good farm in the west, I believe it would suit me better than medicine. If you [his father] had not sold your farm in Minnesota, I should be tempted to go there and try my fortune."[23] He wished his family a Merry Christmas and regretted that he would not be with the family to enjoy his mother's "famous apple dumplings or plum puddings." His comments further demonstrated his continued lack of interest in the practice of medicine as noted before. He would, in fact, later own a farm near Bismarck, North Dakota, and make a fortune in real estate and business just as he had dreamed of while in the barren Arizona Territory.

Captain John G. Bourke described what Porter was encountering:

> At Camp Verde we found assembled nearly all of the Crook's command and a dirtier, greasier, more uncouth-looking set of officers and men it would be hard to encounter anywhere. Dust, soot, rain, and grease had made their impress upon the canvas suits and beards growing with straggling growth all over the face.... [24]

Bourke also mentions Porter by name in his *On the Border with Crook* as a member of "one class of officers who were entitled to all the praise they received and much more besides, and that class was the surgeons, who never flagged in their attentions to sick and wounded, whether soldier or officer, American, Mexican, or Apache captive, by night or day."[25]

The eastern press reported on December 15 that General Crook was "prosecuting the campaign vigorously against the hostile Apaches in the northern part of the [Arizona] Territory" and that his policy was "to follow the Indians constantly and hunt them down in every direction."[26]

From Camp Verde Porter's company rode out on the 21st or 22nd of December down the Verde River to Camp McDowell northeast of Phoenix (near present-day Fountain Hills), which they reached on January 5, 1873, a distance of slightly over a hundred miles through some "very rough and mountainous country." The press reported:

3. Western Adventures

General Crook's scouts have taken the field from [Camp] Date Creek, Camp Whipple, Camp Verde, Apache Camp, Camp McDowell, and Camp Grant are moving towards the Country occupied by the Tonto and Pinal Apaches. The scouts are assisted by Pah Ute, Apache, and Yuma Indians. The hostile Apaches of the Upper Verde River are retreating to the mountains. It is generally believed that the hostile tribes will be brought to terms during this Winter's Campaign.[27]

From Camp McDowell his troop scouted through the Superstition Mountains where Apaches were suspected of hiding.

Some of the letters to his parents reached newspapers back East. Porter wrote on February 1, "Your letter that I received at McDowell contained the extracts cut from the [Utica] *Herald* and of course I was pleased. I never expected to see any of my letters in print and these gave me more newspaper notoriety than I ever expected...."[28] This foreshadows later letters of his sent from abroad to newspapers while on his travels around the world. His complete letters from the Arizona Territory can be found in *Montana: the Magazine of Western History*, June 1958.[29]

Of note, Porter found the southern portion of the Arizona Territory quite unhealthy with large numbers of troops developing fevers that were unrelenting and which failed to respond to quinine.[30]

The cuttings from one such letter appeared in the Utica *Herald* as abridgements of his letters to his parents during the campaign. Edited out are some of the more gory details as well as all personal notes to the family. Also, removed are all references to "bucks" which are replaced with the words "warriors" or "Indians." Otherwise, when compared with the complete letters edited by Gressly in the magazine, *Montana*, the words are Porter's.

Under the heading "Facts and Fancies in Arizona, From an Oneida County Boy," the editor states, "We are permitted to make further extracts from letters received from the seat of the Apache War from Dr. H.R. Porter, late of New York Mills."

> We are now encamped about two miles from Camp Hualpai and waiting the return of our Indian Scouts who have gone to Beale Springs to have an Indian dance and pow wow before they start out with us again. There are two companies of cavalry here and a third will soon join us, we expect. Where we will go or when is very uncertain. General Crook is very quiet and secret in his movements and we know nothing about them until a day before we are ordered off. The last scout (my first) was considered a great success and has been the absorbing topic of conversation for the people of Arizona ever since. Tis thought now that scouting parties will be sent out from different points and the Apaches followed so closely that they will be obliged to sue for peace and remain on their reservations. As long as they stay on their reservations, they are not hunted but on the contrary are clothed and fed by the government the same as a soldier.
>
> This Territory cost the Government an immense sum every year — millions and millions, all to protect about two thousand people a great many of whom

are miserable vagabonds who have come here to escape from the hands of Justice. I do not know how much it cost the Government to keep a regiment of cavalry here a year but you can readily see that it would be no small amount when hay is 40 dollars a ton and grain 10 cents a pound. Everything is high here. I will give you the prices of a few of the necessary articles, butter $1.50 a pound; bacon 50 cents; all vegetables, such as onions, beets, etc., range from 10 to 20 cents; potatoes 8 cents; eggs $1.50 a dozen and salt 18 cents a pound.

Arizona is a poor place to live — anyone that has ever been here can testify and everyone seems to be looking forward to the time when they will leave. Tis as out of the way and as far from a railroad and civilization as a person can get in the United States.

We are camping in a valley surrounded on either side by mountains two thousand feet high. The horses have to be taken three miles in order to graze and guarded by soldiers in order to keep the Apaches from stealing them. The weather here is much cooler than almost any part of the Territory. Camp Hualpai is the most northern and the thermometer varies here very much. We have hot days and cool nights. Frost at night and at noon thermometer at 90 degrees. I hope we will get through with our scouting operations soon as the nights are too cold for sleeping on the ground. The Soldiers or officers don't seem to mind it but it don't suit my fancy altogether. I much prefer a feather bed.

Our duties in the field are light. Nothing to do except attend to the few medical cases I have and pass away the time the best way I can. I find the cavalry soldiers are not so apt to get sick as the Infantry.

We started out on the 19th of the last month on another scout. The Apaches were not to be caught sleeping this time, consequently the expedition was not so successful (that is as a killing expedition). This time only ten Apaches were killed. We saw quite a number but they saw us first and built signal fires which first attracted our attention. They were on the top of a mountain where they could watch our movements. When we first saw them they were a mile away with a deep canyon between us. As we advanced they ran and only ten were caught. They fought well until they were killed. Their arrows passed through our men's pants, hats, etc. One of our own Indians was shot and killed by a soldier who mistook him for an Apache. The Indians instead of burying him, as we would have done, burned him together with his clothing, beads, horse and carbine, the latter belonging the government. Thus they sent him to the happy hunting grounds fully armed and equipped at the expense of Uncle Sam.

We expect to leave here tomorrow or next day to have a long scout this time and I think my chances are good for being in the field all winter. However, I like it better than I did and find that I can ride fifty miles or walk fifteen, over mountains and through canyons, as well as any of the old soldiers. The 31st of December we were about 40 or 50 miles from Camp McDowell, we lay down as usual on the ground in our blankets. About midnight it commenced raining and rained for two days and two nights. We arrived at McDowell the 6th.... I think, and were ordered out again in a day or two with 20 days rations. To scout through the Superstition Mountains, where there was supposed to be plenty of Indians. After being out 5 days our Indian scouts found where they were came back and told us and we started on foot out at 4 o'clock P.M. and marched until daylight the next day, when we attacked the Apaches killing two or three besides, capturing the same number besides capturing nine squaws and papooses. Other Indians were near who got away but after they found their houses had been burned, they gave themselves up and were taken to Camp Grant.

Most all of the Indians paint themselves and they are dressed in every conceivable manner, some wear nothing but a pair of drawers that some soldier has cast off, others nothing but a vest or a hat and buck cloth, some of the wildest of them are naked all the year. Our horses have been a long time now without grain and they are giving out fast, all they get to eat is the grass they can pick. The last 80 miles out of ninety we have lost 20, some gave out so completely that we killed them, other were left on the trail. More were so weak that they had to be led along and could not be rode. I saved mine by walking one-half the distance.

On account of our horses giving out, we did not arrive at this place until four or five days after we expected to, consequently we had to live on half rations for 3 days. We had to live on beans and bread.

Tomorrow we start out again on a thirty day scout with nearly (sic) a whole regiment of cavalry besides quite a number of Indian Scouts. This is the largest command that has been out hunting Indians in this Territory since the rebellion.

I send you with this letter, an Apache scalp as you express a desire to see one. The one I send was taken from a young warrior age about 25. We were scouting around and near Bill Williams Mountain, November 20th, 1872, when we ran on to a small party of Indians who were out hunting. They scattered very quick and all escaped except two. This is the scalp of one that did not escape though. The other was a very old Indian we captured him. The old Indian tried very hard to get away. He ran and jumped over the rocks like a deer and when caught his legs were bloody and skinned. On the whole it was a good thing for us that he did not get killed as he guided us to water when we had been thirty-six hours without it.

I expect this large command was gotten together in order to go and clean out old Cochise, but Gen. Howard has been here and made peace with him, he will not be disturbed and we will scout in another direction. This old chief has a large band of brave warriors and they are nearly all mounted and have never been whipped, but on the contrary have always whipped the white man. This new Camp Grant or Camp Mt. Graham is a new post just started. Old Camp Grant and Camp Crittenden have been abandoned because they were both unhealthy Posts. Lieutenant Hall tells me that he had forty-three men there and forty-two of them were sick with the fever. The southern portion of the Territory is very unhealthy in the summer and the Arizona fever is very peculiar. It sticks to its victim. Quinine don't seem to have much influence over it [see note above].

If you could see us as we are sitting around our Camp fire at night, you would see a motley crew. You would see in our circle, officers–Mexicans–half-breeds–Negroes and Indians. We have quite a number of Indian scouts with us now. Some of them are sick all the time and make up some terrible faces when they take the medicine I have to give them. They have considerable faith in the "white medicine man" and are first rate to swallow pills. The other day I extracted a tooth for one of them an Apache. He did not like the looks of the instruments and wanted me to tie a string around it so to please him I did so but the tooth did not move. I then took hold of it with the instrument and it came out very quick and with it an Apache yell, and he looked as if he would like to take my scalp.

By the way, I have had two rather narrow escapes lately, the first was on the last scout as I was riding at the head of the Company next to the Captain. A deer ran across our trail and I pulled my pistol to shoot, but the Captain wanted to shoot first. He dismounted and as he did so, I saw that his horse was going to run so I spurred my horse to catch his and as I reached over to get hold of the reins, my pistol went off and the ball just grazed across the palm of my hand, did not hurt, only blackened the skin. The other happened day before yesterday. Lieutenant Sampson [*sic* Walter S. Schuyler] and myself were lying in our tents, were just talking about getting up, when a ball came whizzing through the tent just ten inches about my head, passing out past the front portion of the tent.

By the end of March 1873 Crook's campaign was over. On April 9, 1873, from the Headquarters Department of Arizona, Prescott (Arizona Territory), General Order Number 14 was issued from the department commander. The preamble describes some of the conditions that the campaigners met.

The operations of the troops in this Department, in the late campaigns against the Apaches, entitle them to a reputation second to none in the annals of Indian warfare. In the face of obstacles heretofore considered insurmountable, encountering vigorous cold in the mountains, followed in quick succession by the intense heat and arid waste of the desert, not infrequently at dire extremities for want of water to quench their prolonged thirst; and when their animals were stricken with pestilence or the country became too rough to be traversed by them, they left them and carrying on their own backs such meager supplies as they might, they persistently followed on, and plunging unexpectedly into chosen positions in lava beds, caves and canyons, they have ambushed and beaten the wiliest foes with slight loss, comparatively, to themselves, and finally closed an Indian War that has been waged since the days of Cortez.[31]

Acting assistant surgeon Dr. Henry R. Porter was cited for gallantry at the engagement in Superstition Mountains, Arizona Territory, January 16, 1873. He was again cited in the orders, "For conspicuous services and in the different engagements, in the closing campaign against the Tonto Apaches, in February and March 1873," along with thirteen officers and another acting assistant surgeon, Dr. H.M. Matthews.[32]

After April 25 Porter was assigned as post surgeon at the new Camp Grant (not where the Camp Grant Massacre of April 30, 1871, took place), near the foot of Mount Graham, in the Pinaleno Mountains in the southeastern part of the territory near the present town of Safford. He remained there until July 27 when he returned to San Francisco to have his contract annulled on August 25 at his request.[33]

He returned to Washington and New York Mills for visits to his sister and parents after an arduous year as contract surgeon in the Apache War. In spite of some close brushes with danger, he was ready for more.

From his sister's home in Washington, he applied to the surgeon general of the army on October 2, 1873, less than six weeks after leaving San Francisco, for another contract. In a typically formal letter of the time he wrote:

> Sir:
> I have the honor to make application for a position as Contract Surgeon, U.S.A. I desire to call your attention to the fact that I have served one year in Arizona and during that time I experienced the hardest kind of service.
> Hoping you will give my application a favorable consideration.
>
> I am very respectfully
> Your Obt. Servt.
> H.R. Porter[34]

Assistant Surgeon General of the Army Charles H. Crane responded on the 6th that no additional acting assistant surgeons were needed and that his "application had been placed on file for future consideration." But on October 16 he received orders to proceed without delay to St. Paul, Minnesota, to report to the Medical Director Headquarters, Department of Dakota, for assignment.[35]

An item from this time in an upstate New York newspaper, the *Citizen*, refers to "Another Lee-ite in Arizona," stating:

> ... Peace having perched on their banners, and having witnessed the unconditional surrender and submission of two of the most formidable bands of Apaches, his engagements were canceled with the government, and he has returned on a flying visit to his friends. After spending a few weeks with his sister in Washington, he renewed his application for another appointment, and received the same position he formerly occupied, but is now assigned to the Territory of Dacota [sic]. His destination is Fort [sic] Hancock, near Bismarck, at the terminus of the Northern Pacific Railroad, Dacota [sic] T. He visited his parents at N.Y. Mills en route, and is before this time at his post. He is looking well and has enjoyed excellent health in his absence. The toils and hardships of scouting have seemed to be no detriment to his physique, but has seemed rather to develope [sic] it. It is expected that after another year's experience, he will settle down in the more staid and less exciting business of a practitioner of the "healing art."[36]

He was now headed to Camp Hancock in the new frontier town of Bismarck, Dakota Territory, as contract surgeon for the post. This was not to be a field operation but an army post at the end of the Northern Pacific Railroad where it stopped on the banks of the Missouri River. Now he was a veteran of Indian fighting. In the Arizona Territory he had proved himself steady under fire and showed that he had the courage and endurance to meet the hardships and the dangers of battle. Here he would care for the more routine medical and surgical needs of garrisoned army troops.

Chapter 4

Bismarck, on the Frontier

Porter arrived at Camp Hancock in Bismarck on October 31, 1873, with orders to replace Dr. Benjamin Franklin Slaughter as post surgeon on November 5.[1] Slaughter had tendered his resignation in August 1872 and it was accepted. Not wishing to return to field service with the army, he was happy to be released and become Bismarck's first full-time physician.[2] He had, of necessity, already begun a busy and lucrative practice, as described by his wife, Linda, as new settlers of all sorts arrived daily into Bismarck seeking medical attention. While serving at Hancock, Slaughter had been the only doctor in the vicinity except for an army doctor, J.V.D. Middleton, at Fort Abraham Lincoln, across the river.

At this time six to seven hundred rugged citizens lived in the frontier town of Bismarck with ungraded, unpaved, dusty streets just as they had been laid out, a handful of buildings, and a few businesses. People lived in log cabins or shacks constructed of warped cottonwood boards, daubed with mud for insulation. The only available water came from the Missouri River at twenty-five cents per barrel to be used for all purposes including drinking water.

The town had been named Bismarck, for Germany's Iron Chancellor, in July of that year with the hope that German capitalists might financially assist the expansion of the railroad. "An immense map was prepared and sent to Vienna on which Bismarck, D.T., was pictured as being in the exact center of the universe with railroads diverging in all directions."[3] But this ploy failed to attract money. Before it was Bismarck, it was called Edwinton, named for Edwin F. Johnson, chief engineer of the Northern Pacific Railroad. The first train had pulled into town June 5, 1873, not quite five months before Porter arrived there on his new assignment. Burleigh County had been organized July 9, 1873.[4]

Bismarck, of course, owed its existence to the railroad line, which in 1873 ended there. A bill signed July 2, 1864, by President Abraham Lincoln committed the government to the largest land grant ever, ultimately 60 million acres, in establishing the Northern Pacific Railroad.[5] As construction advanced across the country, the railroad would be given alternate sections, twenty miles on each side of the tracks in the states and forty miles in the territories. The railroad was given an odd number of sections of townships and an indemnity area of land, often referred to as lieu land, for lands already owned by individuals or companies. It was incumbent upon the railroad to begin work within two years, complete no less than fifty miles per year after the second year and finish construction to the West Coast by July 4, 1876. The government was to extinguish Indian titles to land in the area of the grants. Land was not granted outright, but was given only after construction was completed on each section of the line. Financing was to be accomplished by the sale of the granted land; mortgage or construction bonds were prohibited by charter. There were plans to cross the Missouri River at Bismarck and push westward. Prior to Bismarck and Edwinton, mail arrived there often addressed to "The Crossing, N.P.R.R [Northern Pacific Railroad] on Missouri River."[6]

Unfortunately for Bismarck and for the rest of the country, economic disruptions in Europe and an over-expansion of railroad construction in the United States led to the collapse of the financial house of Jay Cooke and Company in Philadelphia, the financier of the Northern Pacific Railroad, on September 18, 1873, that led to the bankruptcy of Northern Pacific Railroad. Shock waves went through the entire economy. Banks failed, many railroads went bankrupt, and the Panic of 1873 was underway. The New York Stock Exchange closed for the first time for ten days. Thousands of factories closed and workers lost their jobs. For example, Baldwin Locomotive Works in Philadelphia cut their work force from 2,800 full time employees to 1,400 three-quarter-time employees over the ensuing eight months.[7] Bismarck was devastated and according to the *Tribune*, "the failure of Jay Cooke ... knocked the bottom of the incipient boom [in Bismarck] and in 1874 it was as dead as Riley's cat and as dull as the jokes of London *Punch*."[8] It would be 1878 before there was full economic recovery. The last train left Bismarck November 17, 1873: "The tanks have been dismantled; the help discharged and the road closed for the winter."[9] The trains stopped running during the winters of 1873–74, 1874–75, and 1875–76. In the summers of these years the railroad was mainly used to move military supplies. Tracks were laid across the frozen Missouri River during the winters of 1878 and 1879, and on one occasion they almost lost a locomotive, according to Frank Vyzralek, North Dakota's first state archivist.[10] In the winter of 1879 Northern Pacific Railway built a wooden trestle over the ice that was swept away with the ice breakup. From the spring of 1879 until October 1882 during the ice-free months, locomotives and rolling stock were transferred across the river by steamboats. The railway bridge at Bismarck crossing the river was begun in 1880 and completed in October 1882. The first train crossed the Missouri River on the new bridge on October 18, 1882, engine No. 88 with twenty-five "empties."[11] Thus, it took six years for the railroad to reorganize and resume track construction.[12]

What began as Fort McKeen, an infantry post located across the river in June 1872, was renamed Fort Abraham Lincoln in the fall. Congress authorized $200,000 for a cavalry post there in 1873, and Custer arrived that year as first commander of the enlarged fort. Also, Camp Hancock, to which Porter was assigned, began under the name Camp Greeley (named for Horace Greeley), only to be renamed in 1873 shortly before Porter arrived.

One of the earliest settlers to the new town of Bismarck was a thirty-year-old Civil War hero and Minnesota journalist, Colonel Clement A. Lounsberry, who arrived May 11, 1873. His plans for starting the first newspaper were delayed until completion of the railroad for delivery of his "Washington hand press, fonts, and other supplies." These items arrived on the first train on June 5, and the first issue of the *Tribune* appeared July 6, 1873.[13] Porter received his first mention in the newspaper on November 5, 1873, regarding his arrival to relieve Dr. Slaughter as post surgeon at Camp Hancock.[14] He was now twenty-five years old, single, had traveled extensively, both in the United States and the British Isles, had served as acting assistant surgeon in the Arizona Territory, and had been cited there for valor as previously mentioned. He was no greenhorn or tenderfoot; he had been around. At Camp Hancock, he lived at first in the surgeon's quarters, a portion of the camp that still stands on Main Avenue in Bismarck.

Occasionally, he was mentioned in the *Tribune* as he carried out his duties. For instance, "A soldier accidentally shot himself last Monday afternoon. His wounds were dressed by Dr. Porter, after which he was sent over the river to his Post."[15]

In May 1874 George H. Fairchild, son of President James Harris Fairchild of Oberlin College, a prominent American educator and hero of the runaway slave case at Oberlin in 1858, moved from St. Paul to Bismarck, buying out A. Allen in the banking business of Raymond and Allen.[16] Fairchild had previously worked in Keokuk, Iowa, as an office clerk in the Kellogg, Birge Wholesale Grocery Company, co-owned by his uncle Charles A. Kellogg, and later in St. Paul.[17] Raymond had arrived the year before from Minnesota with a stock of clothing and general merchandise to open J.W. Raymond and Company and with Allen opened the Bank of Bismarck on July 3, 1873. This was a time when "a wire counter-screen, an iron safe and some money and the equipment was complete. There were no banking statutes to bother and impede, and no state supervision to meddle with the personal affairs or financial standing of those who chose to hold themselves out to the public as proper depositories for the safe keeping of other peoples' money."[18] This was the first and only bank in what was to become North Dakota for a period of time.

4. Bismarck, on the Frontier

Fairchild was described as "a young man of means and ability, respected by all who know him."[19] Fairchild's wife, Helen Josephine Viets, would later invite her younger sister, Charlotte, of Oberlin, Ohio, to visit, and she would marry Porter in 1877, making Fairchild and Porter brothers-in-law.

Helen Fairchild did not accompany her husband to Bismarck, although he was planning to build a home soon.[20] He maintained a lively correspondence with her in Oberlin, where she remained with her parents rather than endure the discomforts and dangers of the new frontier town of Bismarck. He usually wrote letters to her on Sundays trying to persuade her to come out to Bismarck.

The first of the letters that we have is as follows:

> Bismarck, Dakota
> June 21, 1874
>
> My Dear Dear Helen,
> I guess this is the hottest day of the year here. Mercury stood at 96 (in the shade at two o'clock) ... General Custer's Expedition to the Black Hills on Saturday morning [Custer's Expedition to the Black Hills while under preparation went into camp on June 19 to accustom the men to camp life and the horses to rope before leaving Fort Abraham Lincoln on July 2, 1874, to explore the Black Hills for gold[21]] ... went into camp a few miles from the fort. We have sold a good many goods to the soldiers and officers and also to settlers and citizens

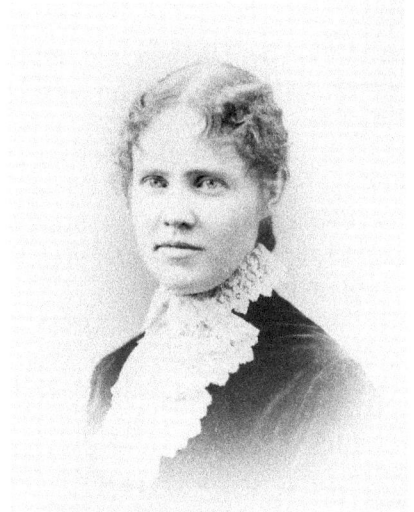 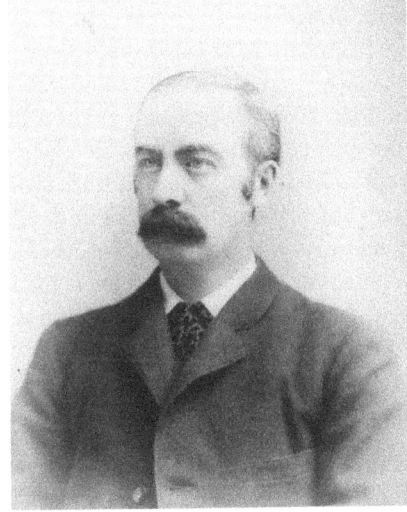

Left: *Helen Viets Fairchild (1846–1923), wife of George H. Fairchild and sister of Charlotte Viets Porter.* Right: *George Hornell Fairchild (1844–1894), Bismarck banker and brother-in-law of Dr. H.R. Porter (both photographs courtesy Wyman Family).*

who are going along [more than 1000 participated].[22] The saying is that these Black Hills are rich in gold deposits and that the Sioux have succeeded in keeping white men from there hitherto. Custer is determined to explore them. He expects to go there in two weeks. Spend a month in explorations and return here by the 1st of September. [he returned August 30].[23] There is a good deal of interest here in the result. Everyone says if Gold is found 'twill be the making of a *city here* [his emphasis], as this is the nearest point. I presume it will be more quiet here after the "Expedition" has gone.

Mrs. Gen. Custer was in the store yesterday. I simply saw her, was not introduced. She is a young lady rather pretty. *Very* nicely dressed in brown silk heavily trimmed with brown silk of another shade — Everyone seems to think a great deal of her. Her husband's bro. Col. Tom Custer comes over with her quite frequently — are driven over in a larger square closed carriage with four mules.[24]

In a letter to Helen that Fairchild probably wrote in July, he mentioned that the expedition to the Black Hills would be back in September and that J.W. Raymond would be back. Since August was likely to be a dull month, it would be September before Bismarck would become more active, especially with the fall trade up the river. Bismarck's population at the time stood at 600, according to him. "I think, Dearie, you will have to depend mostly upon me for society when you are here.... Are you intending to fix over your black silk before you come out here? I rather think you had better. And then if you should go to a party in Gen. Custer's new house a plan of which you will find on the back of the paper which has the store on, next winter you will have something to wear."[25]

On July 5, 1874, in his weekly letter to his wife, Fairchild told of his headache and his health in general. He wrote, "Raymond writes his friends that he is very happy and pleased in his new partner. Has shown me some letters of congratulations which he received ... Friday eve Mr. Douglas[s], Dr. Porter, Mrs. Douglas[s] and her sister were out horseback riding. They said they had a splendid ride. Next day I saw two other couples. I am told they sometimes get eight or ten together and go over the prairies full tilt. Oh we'll have some sport here."[26] This is his first mention of Porter.

At this time Porter was eating at a boarding house run by a huge woman of African-American descent known as Aunt Sally who had acquired property in Bismarck and claimed to have cooked on the first boat that ever went up the Missouri River.[27] According to the *Tribune*:

> Eight young men of Bismarck went to mess in a club; they engaged the services of Aunt Sally, and put up five dollars per week, or as much more as may be necessary, to pay expenses. They live on the top shelf, have all that heart can wish, and have just the nicest boarding place in town; and get it at cost. The parties are Capt. McCosh, Dr. Porter, W.S. Brown, J.B. Bowen [judge], [Josiah] Delamater and G.P. Flannery [lawyers], N.S. Wells, and John Carnahan [telegraph operator].[28]

4. Bismarck, on the Frontier

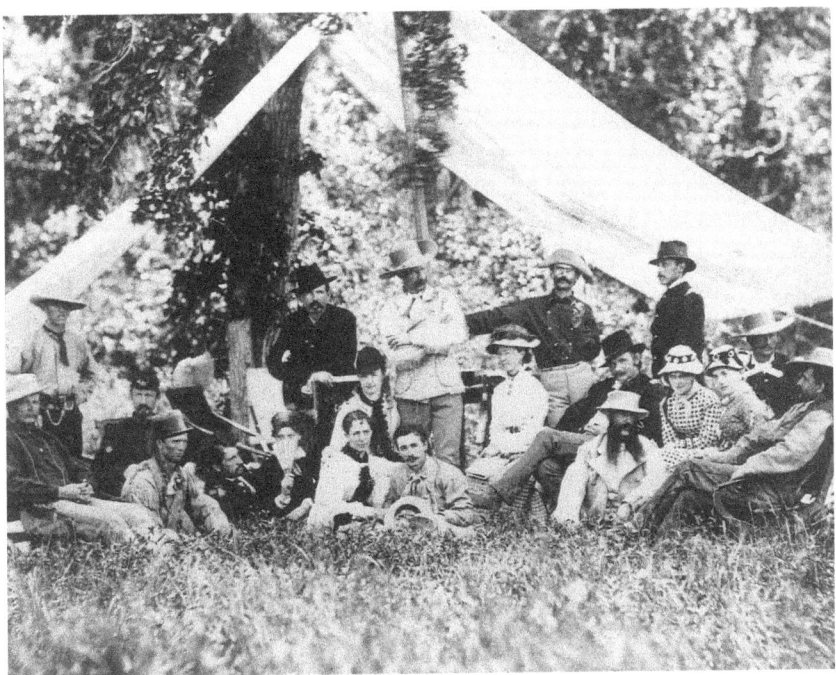

*Colonel George Armstrong Custer and party at Little Heart River near Fort Abraham Lincoln, July 1875. Those in **bold print** died at Little Bighorn. From left to right, **Lt. James Calhoun**, Leonard Herbert "Berty" Swett (son of Illinois lawyer and politician), Capt. Stephen Baker, **Boston Custer**, Lt. Winfield Scott Edgerly, Emily Watson, **Capt. Myles W. Keogh**, Margaret Custer Calhoun, Elizabeth Custer, Dr. Holmes O. Paulding, **Col. Custer**, Nellie Smith, **Dr. George Lord**, Capt. Thomas B. Weir, **Lt. William W. Cooke**, Lt. Richard E. Thompson, Nellie Wadsworth, Emma Wadsworth, **Capt. Thomas Custer**, and **Lt. Algernon E. Smith**. Photograph by O.S. Goff. (National Archives [83991])*

Porter posted in his scrapbook three clippings that mention the Reverend I.O. Sloan, founder of the First Presbyterian Church, Bismarck.[29] But Porter's affiliation with the congregation was limited. Records show that while his wife, Lottie, was admitted to membership September 18, 1878, Porter did not join.[30] Both Helen and George Fairchild were quite active in the First Presbyterian Church. He served as director of elders and was a member of the building committee when the church decided to build "a larger and more attractive edifice" in 1884.[31] Early on, Sloan formed a Bible Society that included a number of Porter's friends and future business partners, J.S. Mann, W.B. Shaw, W.S. Brown, Henry F. Douglass, and Josiah Delamater, but not Porter.[32] From a very religious upbringing as attested by his letters back from Scotland and England, Porter became a life-long non-participant in church activities.

Dr. Fannie Dunn Quain wrote that the Presbyterian Church and the Catholic Church came to Bismarck about the same time, the former being organized June 15, 1873, in a tent on Main Street near Third that was otherwise used for gambling.[33] Saloons on either side closed during services, and when the hat was passed many poker chips were dropped in that were exchanged by a faro dealer for cash to go into the treasury of the first church organization in North Dakota. On Sunday afternoons, services were held at Fort Lincoln and once were partially disrupted by an attempted robbery of cattle in which one Indian was killed. The first [Presbyterian] church building was described as an "elegant little church costing about $4,000" in September 1873. The Reverend Mr. I.O. Sloan preached the first sermon.[34]

In his letter of July 26, 1874, George Fairchild after complaining of problems with diarrhea wrote, "General [George Brown] Dandy and wife came over here. Mrs. Dandy is a beautiful little woman. Raymond [Fairchild's business partner] says she is as nice as she is pretty. The Gen. is cousin to Raymond."[35]

On August 2, 1874, he expressed disappointment that the issue of a house had not been settled. There were delays over Raymond's wife's problems with a sick son.[36]

On August 9, 1874, "Sunday morning," he wrote Helen, who was sick in Oberlin, wishing her well and wishing that she were with him to plan for a home in Bismarck.

> I think Dear that Mr. [J.W.] Raymond will stop a day at Oberlin about the middle of next week—he wants to see Father and Professor [James] Monroe and get letters from them to the Rev. Geo. Whiffle in New York and others.... He will not stay long in O. but I want him to have a pleasant time if there is any such thing. Any impressions he may get will help him like us. Ask him all about his wife and boy.
>
> Since writing the last sentence R. says only *in certain event* he will stop at Oberlin. It depends on whether we hear and what we hear from Washington.
>
> Note:
>
> A 'Hop' will be given by the officers of Fort A. Lincoln at their Post on Thursday evening next. Yourself and the ladies of your family are respectfully invited to attend. Dancing at 8. Supper at 12.
>
> M.A. Reno
Maj. 7th Cavalry[37]

On Sunday afternoon, August 16, 1874, in addition to many expressions of love and longing, he wrote:

> When people talk to you about the *Indians* and the dreariness of life in Bismarck, just tell them they are talking about what they *know not a thing*. The Indians are no more trouble here than they are in Oberlin. And life here will never be so dreary as in *that* little *burgh* ... I will never take you *anywhere* unless

I know I can make you comfortable and happy there. So comfort your dear self about all *that*. The rooms of the house that you live in here will be just as pleasant as you could get in *Oberlin*. You can take your ponies and get three friends in a wagon and ride over splendid drives *anytime*. Ride horseback over the hills anywhere up on bluffs two or three hundred feet high where you have beautiful views ahead out before you for 10 or 20 miles. The air is *clear*, bracing and dry all the time. No damp dews at night, no *east winds* with their damp chilliness and the most beautiful sunsets God ever made, *very often indeed*. I have not said much about the country before because I don't want you to be disappointed when you get here. The longer I stay here the more I think of the place, the climate, the soil, the prospects for the future. It is just what I have always felt was the thing for us to do if we want to get wealth. Commencing house keeping *will* be pleasant.... Am glad Lottie is Ended with Mr. R. Better never to be married by all odds. I know you could not begin to tell her all R. said that time in the store, neither could I, but surely it was uncomplimentary to the women. No harm in telling her.[38]

Lottie [Charlotte Viets], Helen's sister, thus had just broken up with a "Mr. R." She would be married to Porter three years later.

In his letter of Sunday, August 23, 1874, Fairchild commented on plans Helen sent for their house and wrote:

You needn't believe any body's *fearful* stories about Bismarck. I'd rather live here than in Oberlin and so I think you will.... Then there is a pretty general impression that the Black Hills Gold Excitement will do a big thing for Bismarck.[39] No one can tell how it will be. I had a long talk with Charley Reynolds ["Lonesome Charley Reynolds"], the most famous Scout and hunter of the northwest who went out with the Expedition and came back by way of Omaha.[40] He says there is gold there and that he is going out as soon as any party goes. He is a modest, bashful young fellow who never glows or says a thing that is not strictly true and is very careful what he says always.... You will improve in health right off when you get here. The air is so clear, dry and exhilarating.[41]

The letter of September 6, 1874, is the last of the year suggesting that Helen went to Bismarck shortly afterwards. He wrote, "Everything is bustle and excitement in Bismarck. Steamboat[s] coming in and going out. The trains seem to bring more passengers than usual. The soldiers have been paid off. Army officers dashing about on horseback in gay uniforms and white pants with orderlies following behind."[42]

On December 1, 1874, Porter requested and had granted the cancellation of his army contract allowing him to enter private practice as the second physician in Bismarck and partner in the second drugstore in Bismarck. J.P. Dunn, the first druggist, had arrived in May 1872 a year before it became Bismarck, and set up business in a tent with a small stock of drugs and goods.[43] He built a small building (18 × 30 feet) out of cottonwood, the only wood available then, in the fall of the same year. When it dried the lumber warped and shrank leaving cracks in the construction. He kept a red-hot stove in the center of the building, slept on a buffalo robe on the floor, but still had snow drifts accumulate in the room overnight that first winter of 1872–73.[44] He twice expanded it by May of 1874 when the *Tribune* reported that "they now carry a large and full stock, embracing also glass, paint, putty, etc., and notions. They have sold a large amount of garden seeds this spring, to one man ten bushels of seed corn."[45] It would later become the Pioneer Drugstore.

O. Nicholson and Porter opened another drugstore on December 2, 1874, just as Porter was released from his army contract at Camp Hancock. The account of their opening in the *Tribune* stated that they had a fine stock of drugs, a variety of stationery and fancy goods, cigars, and "some of the finest liquors for medicinal purposes."[46] They leased a new building from Colonel Robert Wilson said to be "the best finished house in Bismarck." With a "large glass front and the arrangements inside the store present[ed] a very creditable appearance." Nicholson was said to be an "old hand at the drug business" and a man who "thoroughly understands it." They were soon advertising coal oil [kerosene] for fifty cents per gallon and a medicated breast protector to keep from catching cold.[47] For unknown reasons, the business partnership was dissolved March 29, 1875, after only four months, and O. Nicholson departed Bismarck for Deadwood, Dakota Territory, where a gold rush in the Black Hills was underway. A correspondent from the Deadwood *Champion* reported to the *Tribune* two years later that O. Nicholson was the first there "to open out with a stock of goods."[48]

In the same notice of dissolution of Nicholson and Porter, a new firm, Wilson and Porter, was announced, "who were authorized to settle up the old firm's business."[49]

A description of the new business in May called it an "elegant establishment."

> Merchants Wilson and Porter continued improving the appearance of their drug store, having recently added another coat of paint, put in circular counters, and otherwise improved the interior appearance, until there is no drug store in the west more elegant or convenient. They carry a full line of stationery, notions, etc., not to speak of a fine and full assortment of drugs, and are now putting in a full line of paints, oils, etc. Col. [Robert] Wilson, the senior member of the firm is well known as a public-spirited citizen and high-toned gentleman, and Dr. Porter, the junior member, as an excellent gentleman and successful physician.[50]

On July 14, 1875, the *Tribune* noted their "well displayed advertisement. They have all the things enumerated there (drugs, medicines, paints, oils, stationery, blank books, fine imported liquors and wines, choicest brands of tobacco and cigars, a full line of perfumery, and confectionery, choice and fresh) and much more, and in addition one of the neatest and best arranged drug stores west of Chicago."[51]

4. Bismarck, on the Frontier

The business, however, was short-lived; the co-partnership was dissolved October 18, 1875, so that Porter could devote more time to his practice. This had not been a good time to start a business as the country was in the midst of a serious economic depression, and Bismarck was especially vulnerable to its effects. Also, Bismarck probably could not support two drugstores. Porter had an office building under construction by Wells and Winston Lumber Company on Main Street opposite the Tribune Building, and he was in it in November.[52] While he was in the drugstore business, Porter had been seeing his patients at the store.

His early practice was of the most general sort as illustrated by the following anecdote.

> A day of two since we heard of a party rushing into Dr. Porter's presence, holding on to his jaws with both hands—the cause was evident, an aching tooth—he sat down, the Doctor applied an instrument to a molar that had been several times yanked at, gave a couple of good strong pulls, out pops the obstinate ivory, up jumps the sufferer with a "whoop-e-e" and an exclamation of "you have got it by G-eorge, and what's to pay?" "One dollar—one dollar, take two"—handing over the sugar and then departed the happiest man in Bismarck.[53]

Another of his procedures that was publicized was the following account of a paracentesis, probably the first one done in the territory, which he accomplished by piercing the abdominal cavity with a large needle or tube to drain off the fluid.[54] Dropsy, or free fluid within the abdomen, was commonly caused by heart failure or cirrhosis of the liver, less often by a large ovarian cyst.

> Dr. Porter performed an operation yesterday on a lady living in Apple Creek, who was suffering from dropsy. The operation is called "tapping" and consists in puncturing the abdomen and inserting a small silver tube for the fluid to run out. In this case the amount of water was enormous, twenty-four pints escaping in a short time, much to the relief of the patient, who before the operation could hardly breathe.[55]

By the end of 1875 Bismarck boasted a population of about 900, and the *Tribune* claimed that no city within 450 miles claimed to be its rival.[56] It reported that "two or three houses of prostitution could be found without difficulty, but the club rooms and dance halls were long since closed." Thirteen saloon owners were listed.

Porter's practice must have been slow to develop and his venture into the drugstore business unsatisfactory, because he resumed duty [part-time] at Camp Hancock under contract for sixty dollars a month on November 1, 1875.[57] He would work there until May 14, 1876, when he entered into a new contract to join the well-publicized Custer Expedition that was forming at Fort Abraham Lincoln to drive the Indians off the plains and back to their reservations. His love of the open country, horses, guns, and the camaraderie of the campfire, including all the attendant hardships to be encountered, and danger, lured him back once again to a military campaign. He was paid $125 a month for duty beginning on May 14, 1876, and for the adventure of his life.[58]

Dr. E. J. Clark, another acting assistant surgeon, originally engineered Porter's involvement in the expedition by getting him to take his place. Clark was sent anyway along with the troops at Porter's former pay of sixty dollars a month, and he missed the battle at Little Bighorn by being assigned to the supply depot at the Powder River.[59]

Meanwhile, Custer had become such a celebrity that the *Bismarck Tribune* in 1874 and 1875 offered a free 19 × 25 inch chromolithograph portrait of him with any yearly subscription to the newspaper.[60]

Custer was commander of the fort and was already widely known by the citizens of Bismarck for his daring and bravado. He already was an attractive, dashing military hero based on his Civil War exploits and his recent expedition to the Black Hills.

When Dr. James W. DeWolf arrived in Bismarck on April 14, 1876, as acting assistant surgeon, prior to assignment to the Terry-Custer Expedition, he wrote his wife:

> Bismarck is squalid dunghill sort of place, all wooden buildings, broken board walks on the front street. It is on prairie ground on the margin of a bluff. The flats of Missouri extend back about one mile to this bluff. [Camp] Hancock is on the bluff and we are camped immediately under this bluff on the Missouri flats. It is dry and nice, sleep in tent — board up town at the Capital [Hotel] — nothing nice but tolerable — called on Dr. Porter who attends Camp Hancock.[61]

Dr. DeWolf had been "kindly received" by Porter and had met Colonel Clement A. Lounsberry, editor of the *Tribune*. When Dr. DeWolf reached Fort Lincoln he was surprised to find what he called "the mania" for gambling among the officers of the 7th Cavalry but found them otherwise good fellows.

After the Terry-Custer Expedition left on May 17, 1876, there was a sense of increased anxiety as reflected in a letter that Samantha Viets of Oberlin sent the Fairchilds in Bismarck. Little did she know that her daughter's future husband, Dr. H.R. Porter, was headed into battle.

Oberlin, May 27, 1876

My Darling Children,
    ... Our hearts were thrown into a *flutter* this A.M. by the news that a dispatch had been sent to Washington "for troops to guard Bismarck" as they were threatened by *Indians*. I do hope and pray that you may not be in danger from that source. But still our hearts are disquieted within us knowing which [*sic*] a

treacherous force the Indians is to the white man and when so many troops were ordered away on the Expedition I was fearful less the Indians might embrace that opportunity for a raid on your little town. If an attack is eminent [*sic*], Helen will probably leave at once for home as your father says that Geo. can take better care of himself if his wife is away. If any dreadful thing should befall you — or you are obliged to take flight for safety, this letter may never reach you but the writing of it will be a little relief to me. Mr. Battle imparted his news to your father and he understood that it was taken from telegraph wires on the way to Washington. We have no different ideas about the matter. But not withstanding our very hearts *stand still lest harm* should come to our dear ones so far away. But it is a great consolation to commend them to the guardian care of our Heavenly Father who is able to shield them from harm and danger....

Lovingly,

Your Mother[62]

It is true that Bismarck was left lightly guarded by the movement west of over a thousand soldiers and, indeed, there were rumors of Indians about to attack, but the feared Plains Indians, no longer on reservations, were gathering near the Rosebud River and moving toward the valley of the Little Bighorn, several hundred miles away. They posed no threat to Bismarck.

Chapter 5

The Road to Little Bighorn

In May 1875 General Philip H. Sheridan at Headquarters, Military Division of the Missouri in Chicago, ordered Colonels James W. Forsyth and Frederick D. Grant, oldest son of President Ulysses S. Grant, to explore by steamer the upper reaches of the Yellowstone River. "I want a careful examination made of the south bank of the Yellowstone and the mouths and immediate valleys of the rivers coming in from the Black Hills, and especially those of Tongue River, Rosebud, and Big Horn, and if you go higher up the Yellowstone, the Big Rosebud, giving an account of the timber, soil, and geological formations, also the depth of the water in a general way, and the character of any rapids passed over above the mouth of Powder River.... It may be necessary, at some time in the immediate future, to occupy by a military force the country in and about the mouths of Tongue River and Big Horn."[1]

The two colonels met in Bismarck, reaching it by Northern Pacific Railroad, and boarded the *Josephine* on May 23 for the intelligence gathering mission. Protected by 100 troops on board and armed with a Gatling gun, the steamer under Captain Grant Marsh carried them up the Yellowstone. They found the Bighorn to be the practical head of navigation on the Yellowstone. The water was muddy and at the mouth it was 150 yards wide.

The *Josephine* returned early on June 12. Forsyth and Grant departed on the 7:15 A.M. train the same morning for Chicago, apparently closed-mouthed about their findings. The *Bismarck Tribune* reported, "Gen. Forsyth and Col. Fred Grant arrived on the *Josephine* Saturday morning and went east on the morning train. No interviewers need apply."[2] Travel by rail in those days provokes no envy. It took eleven hours and fifteen minutes to reach Fargo, a 193 mile journey, which averages to about seventeen miles an hour. They still had another 650 miles to travel before reaching Chicago.

An enterprising reporter from the *Tribune* was able to get information from some of the other participants, very possibly Captain Marsh Grant, about the exploration and filed an interesting report, some of which refers to the Lewis and Clark Expedition.

5. The Road to Little Bighorn

On May 23rd the steamer *Josephine*, Grant Marsh, Master, chartered by the Government, departed from Bismarck with Gen. Forsyth and Col. Fred Grant on Board, on a tour of inspection up the Yellowstone river. Last Saturday, at 4 o'clock A.M., the steamer and party landed at Bismarck, having been twenty days out. As a result of the trip we have gleaned the following information: The steamer succeeded in reaching a point within ten miles of Clark's Fork of the Yellowstone, a distance by river of five hundred miles from Bismarck. From the mouth of the Yellowstone to Pompey's Pillar, a distance of nearly two hundred miles, good river was found, the stream narrow, not very crooked, and deep, above that point to the uppermost point reached, the stream was found narrow, swifter shoaler [sic], and more difficult of navigation, yet not presenting any serious difficulty to navigation. When the party reached the mouth of the Big Horn river, the route was changed temporarily, and a distance of fifteen miles was run up that stream without meeting with obstacle. From the Indians—the Crow tribe—it was learned that snow on the peaks of the mountain region of that section was perpetual. En route immense herds of buffalo, elk, antelope and deer were seen, while numerous bands of wolves and many black bear were surprised into sight by the approach of the steamer. At Pryor's river a band of Crows, numbering three thousand, were found encamped. Gen. Forsyth had a brief "talk" with them, the character of which was of a general nature. They were well clad, had an abundance of food, were well armed, and showed no disposition of hostilities towards the whites, or any antipathy against civilization upon their domain. At the mouth of Tongue river there was seen a fresh camp of a large party of Sioux, but none of the scalp lifters were seen. At Pompey's Pillar, cut in the solid rock, was found perfectly distinguishable, the name of William Clark, bearing date of 1806. There were other names carved in the Pillar dated 1844. This point has seemed to be a natural camping spot for surveyors, adventurers and scientists for many years. The valley of the Yellowstone is represented as being very beautiful; being of a prairie formation, ranging in width form two to five miles, and from ten to twenty-five miles in length, presenting a luxuriant grass and flower covered surface that, at this season of the year makes the western prairies so peculiarly fascinating and beautiful.

The brook trout streams region were [sic] reached, but the time of the party was so limited that none were taken. Above the mouth of the Big Horn river the waters of the Yellowstone are clear, cold and limpid, possessing a gravelly and pebbly bottom.

As the trip was made especially for military purposes, but little can be known of the future action of the Government until an official communication shall be made; yet enough has leaked out to show that the intention of the government is to establish a post either at the mouth of the Powder river or Big Horn river during this season. At all events Gen. Forsyth's report can do no less than develop the fact of an exceedingly fertile and desirable section for settlement and improvement, all of which is directly tributary to Bismarck....[3]

The military now had information regarding the geography and navigability of the Yellowstone, even water levels for May and June for the first time, a year before the ill-fated Custer expedition. Forsyth and Grant presented their findings to Sheridan June 22 and 23, 1875, and these were published by the Government Printing Office the same year.

Custer testified in Washington at the Belknap hearings in 1876 much to the displeasure of President Grant. Secretary of War Belknap had been accused of conspiring with post traders. He resigned on March 2 admitting no guilt. Custer testified before the Clymer Committee on March 29 that Secretary Belknap had appointed one Robert T. Sipe as trader at Fort Abraham Lincoln on July 1, 1874. Thereafter, charges for goods at the post became so exorbitant that officers at times would go to rival traders five miles away. Sipe then complained about this and threatened those officers that he had enough influence with the secretary to have them removed. Belknap sent down an order that, in effect, drove out the other traders and forced the officers to buy at the inflated prices from Sipe. Custer testified that Sipe would even stop and search officers' wagons coming on the post to see if Belknap's orders had been violated. Custer advised Belknap of the practice but got no reply. Custer stated before the committee, "I sent for Sipe and asked him what he had been paying to hold his post; he said he estimated his profits at $15,000 annually, one-third of which he paid to General Hedrick of Iowa, and one-third to General Rice; out of his profits of $15,000 he only received $2,500; he said but he did not know, but he understood a portion of it went to the Secretary of War." Custer added that Belknap had visited the frontier "to perfect arrangements whereby whiskey could be brought across the border at a reduced rate and increased advantages given to post traders."[4] Grant's brother, Orvil, was also implicated in the scandal. Whether his motive was from moral indignation or as a Democratic Party partisan, Custer had involved himself in the dangerous and risky political arena. Grant immediately removed Custer from his command of the 7th Cavalry just prior to a proposed military operation against the Sioux Indians. Belknap went on to impeachment by the House of Representatives but acquittal by the Senate, where a two-thirds majority could not be mustered.

After having been given an ultimatum to return to the reservations and their failure to accede, the Plains Indians were to be subjected to a three-pronged attack from Fort Abraham Lincoln in the east, Fort Ellis in the west, and Fort Fetterman in the south. Generals Sherman, Sheridan, and Terry asked the president to reconsider and allow Custer, the most experienced and the one perceived to be the best Indian fighter in the West, to lead the 7th Cavalry from Fort Lincoln. Grant ordered Custer to command the 7th Cavalry, but put him under the leadership of General Alfred Terry as a spiteful compromise.

The *Chicago Tribune* commented that "the country will very generally endorse the action of the President in assigning Custer to the command of his regiment, from which he had been relieved, and ordering him to join the

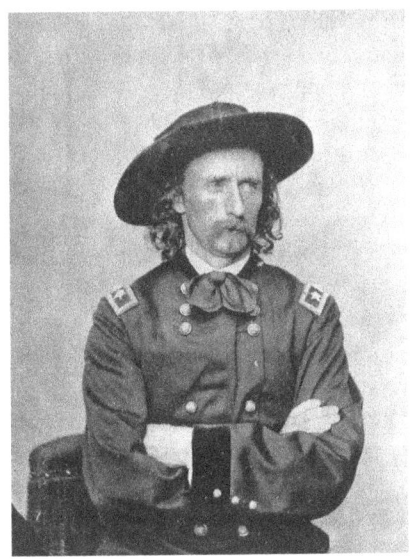 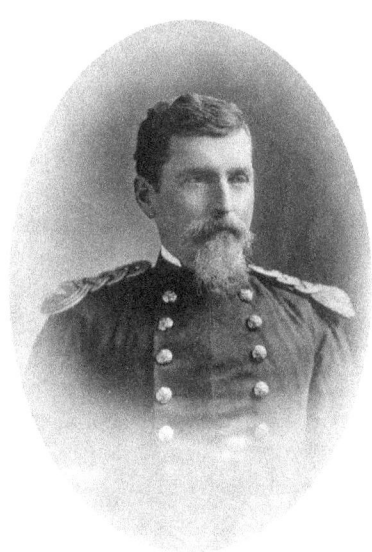

Left: *General George A. Custer at the end of the Civil War, May 1865. Brady Collection. (National Archives [B-5931])* Right: *Colonel John Gibbon, commander of the District of Montana and of the column from the west that began at Fort Ellis. Brady Collection. (National Archives [BA7])*

expedition which is now moving against the Indians." It chided, "General Custer, although he is a very garrulous man, and talks too much for his own good, is a gallant officer, whose past record ought to have spared him the humiliation from which he so narrowly escaped.

It should prove a warning to him, however, of the danger of being such a swift and willing witness in partisan investigations, especially when it eventuates that he has nothing to say of any value."[5]

Colonel John Gibbon passed through Helena on March 24 on his way to Fort Ellis, Montana Territory, where he would command 450 men from the 2nd Cavalry and 7th Infantry.[6] Elements would leave on March 30 and Gibbon on April 3 to join Terry and Custer at the mouth of the Powder River. Gibbon, who was born in Pennsylvania but grew up in Charlotte, North Carolina, had served heroically in the Civil War on the Union side and had been severely wounded at Gettysburg. There was only one doctor along to support the group, Dr. Holmes O. Paulding, a twenty-four-year-old post surgeon of Fort Ellis. The fort had been built near Bozeman in 1867 to protect travelers along the Bozeman Trail from the Indians. Soon after departure, the troops faced severe snowstorms and nearly impassible roads as they crossed the Crazy Mountains, a formidable mountain chain lying on the western edge of the great Montana prairie. Some peaks are over 10,000 feet high. Indians killed and mutilated three of the soldiers on the march who had gone out from the expedition to hunt. By April 23 the command had reached Old Fort Sarpy on the Yellowstone, an abandoned American Fur Company trading post. A wagon train was sent back to Fort Ellis for more supplies.

Although the men were bone-tired, they had a long march ahead, and they were sanguine about their prospects. A correspondent from the Helena *Independent* wrote, "If we had [Sitting Bull] here, there is no question but what we could give him a terrible thrashing and teach him good manners for all time to come."[7] This speaks to the overconfidence that prevailed before Little Bighorn. No less than 1,000 and as many as 3,000 armed warriors were anticipated, yet the army expected to give them a "terrible thrashing." Gibbon's command met Terry's on the Yellowstone on June 9.

General George Crook would leave Fort Fetterman, Wyoming, on May 29 and proceed north with fifteen companies of the 2nd and 3rd Cavalries and five companies of the 4th and 9th Infantries for a total of forty-seven officers and 1,002 men, a pack train of 320 mules and 106 mule teams with 115 packers and teamsters, all armed.[8] The medical team was led by Captain Albert Hartsuff, formerly Fort Laramie post surgeon. There also were Captain Julius H. Patzki, Dr. Junius Powell, and Dr. Richard H. Stevens. Little is known about surgeon Stevens; however, Vaughn records his presence based on Bourke's diary.[9] Of the three commands converging, Crook's was the strongest and Gibbon's the weakest.

Across the river from Bismarck, Custer's 7th Cavalry under Terry's overall command passed in review on the parade ground at seven A.M. on May 17th before moving out from Fort Lincoln with fifty-four officers, 1,026 enlisted men, and 130 packers, scouts, support personnel, and teamsters. The band played "Garryowen" at the review and "The Girl I Left Behind Me" on departure. Custer led with one troop of the advance guard.

Porter, one of five doctors, was assigned at first to the Head-

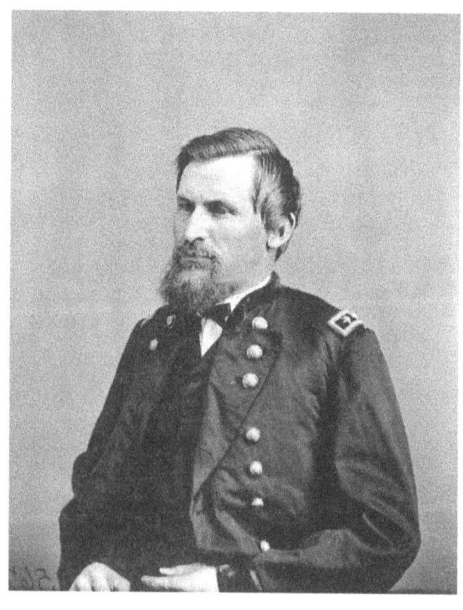

General George Crook, commander of the Department of the Platt and of the column from the south that began at Fort Fetterman. Brady Collection. (National Archives [B2196])

quarters and Battery sections. Dr. J.W. Williams of the regular army headed the entire medical group. Dr. James DeWolf attended the Right Wing, which included six companies of cavalry and scouts under Major Reno, and Dr. E.J. Clark supported the Left Wing, which included six cavalry companies under Captain Benteen. Dr. Isaiah H. Ashton provided medical coverage for two infantry companies.

There had been no attempt to keep troop movements secret. In fact, the campaign had been widely publicized about three months earlier in the press across the country. The only change of plans from newspaper accounts was to delay implementation due to the weather and to revise upwardly the number of Indian warriors. The *New York Times* had reported February 21 that an Indian War was anticipated.[10]

> An Indian War, the dimensions of which are entirely a matter of speculation, seems to be near at hand. Reports coming from the West, with much reiteration are that Sitting Bull of the North is behaving in a very unhandsome manner, and some suggestions are made that the mining camp in the Black Hills is to be attacked by his warriors.... Sitting Bull of the North is a young and hostile Chief, and has caused the white inhabitants within a few hundred miles of him considerable uneasiness. General Custer is understood to have with him six companies [sic] of the Third Cavalry [sic]. Custer starts west from Fort Lincoln on the 25th inst. [sic], and Crook has already started from Fort Laramie and will go north. They will join their forces and attack Sitting Bull in the Powder River Country, which is west of the Black Hills, and about one hundred and fifty miles east of the Big Horn Mountains. Sitting Bull is supposed to have from six hundred to one thousand warriors, and if the cavalry force is found not to be sufficient for the attack reinforcements of infantry will be taken from other forts.

The following appeared a few days later on March 2, 1876, in an Iowa newspaper and presumably in many others.

> Information has been received at the war department that General Crook has started with a force from Ft. Laramie and Gen. Custer with troops from Ft. Lincoln, to be joined by a detachment from Montana, to move against Sitting Bull, near the Powder River in the Yellowstone country. Sitting Bull has fifteen hundred warriors, and sets at defiance the treaty which requires his people to remain on their reservation. The number of United States troops in the expedition is about two thousand.[11]

Within five or six hundred troops on either side, this is an accurate plan for the proposed attack. It is known that a number of warriors left the reservations in the months leading up to the Little Bighorn battle; consequently, there were more warriors than were mentioned in this second account.

Progress of the Terry-Custer column was slow. The trail westward from Fort Lincoln was, for the first nine days, not far from the present day Interstate 94 and the Burlington Northern Santa Fe Railroad tracks. By the eve-

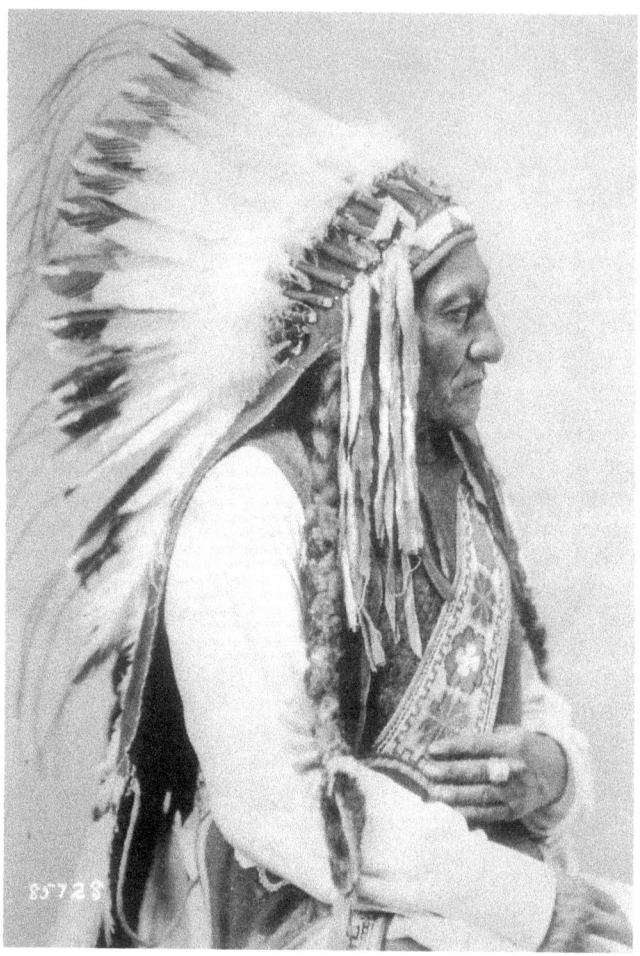

Sitting Bull, Hunkpapa Sioux chief and medicine man. Photograph by David F. Barry, ca. 1885. (National Archives [85728])

ning of May 25 the command had crossed the Heart River and over the hot, open Dakota plains before halting. Dr. DeWolf complained in a letter to his wife of pain from his sunburned ears.

> We expect to reach the Little Missouri [River] day after tomorrow. Dr. Porter has been out from the command today and killed an antelope. I should like to try but dear I am a little lazy and do not want to have my scalp lifted yet — though I do not think there is any danger yet but I am going to be on the safe side and stay with the command. I guess you will have some trouble reading this for I have wrote it in all shapes and the band plays now and every evening and marching out of camp every morning.[12]

5. The Road to Little Bighorn

Porter's willingness to risk danger by hunting game outside the protection of camp contrasts with DeWolf's caution. Yet DeWolf was the one to be killed one month later to the day at Little Bighorn. Porter would survive.

As the column moved westward, Custer suggested to General Terry that he be allowed to lead a scouting party up the river to look for large bodies of Indians, which had been suspected of camping in the Little Missouri River Badlands. On May 30 Custer led four companies of 7th Cavalry (C,D,F,M) on a ten-hour, fifty-mile scout through the rugged river valley but saw no Indians. Dr. James DeWolf accompanied the troops. Porter remained behind with the stationary camp but could not hunt in spite of plentiful game nearby for fear that gunfire might alert Indians who might be nearby.

On the morning of June 1 with the expedition camped west of the Little Missouri, reporter Mark Kellogg of the *Bismarck Tribune* noted in his diary:[13]

> Jun 1st Reveille at 3 A.M. looked out found two inches on ground and snowing hard. Has snowed nearly all day. Have not moved. 7 P.M. Snowing harder than ever, wind blowing fr. N.W., growing colder. Stock feeling the storm. Very dull in camp, some card playing, no incident, wood plenty, and fires kept burning all around, but few Sibley stoves,[14] at Hd.Qrs. and 3 or 4 officers tent. Yesterday 8 miles W.L.camp. Saw a coal strata on fire, looked like whole side of mountain on fire vein about 4 ft thick. Lignite cropping out all along.

This became known as Snow Camp. No attempt was made to advance on either June 1 or 2. The wet and chilled troopers remained in camp until the morning of June 3. Of interest is that the same late season storm system punished Crook's column that was advancing north from Wyoming. Lieutenant John G. Bourke noted in his diary on June 1, "A cold miserable day; heavy clouds laden with rain hanging over us; snow and sleet falling during the morning."[15]

Dr. George Lord left Fort Buford on the steamer *Josephine* on May 14 along a battalion of the 6th Infantry, seven officers, 120 enlisted men, three scouts, and many supplies. The *Josephine*, said to be one of the best steamers on the Upper Missouri, was 180 feet long, measured 31 feet on the beam, and drew only 20 inches of water. It took them up the Yellowstone River to Stanley's Crossing near the mouth of Glendive Creek where they remained at month's end. Later Lord would reach the mouth of the Powder River to join Terry and Custer around June 11.

The expedition reached the Powder River on June 7 after traveling through some of the most desolate and unfriendly country that the troops had encountered.[16] General Terry, accompanied by the companies of Keogh [I] and Moylan [A], left camp the next morning and marched down river to the mouth of the Powder River at the Yellowstone. There they met with a party from General Gibbon's command aboard the *Far West* steamboat and moved up the Yellowstone River to the mouth of the Tongue with plans to meet Gibbon the next morning to plan strategy.[17] Here General Terry learned that there was evidence of increased Indian activity in the area of the Rosebud and Bighorn Valleys and hurriedly returned to the command. On June 10 he ordered Reno, with the 7th Cavalry, Right Wing, Companies B, C, E, F, I, and L, one Gatling gun, Arikara scouts, and 100 pack mules, to proceed up the Powder River to the mouth of the Little Powder, then cross the headwaters of Mizpah Creek, go downstream until it joins the Powder, then cross Pumpkin Creek and the Tongue River, and return to the junction of the Tongue and the Yellowstone.[18] Mitch Boyer, a half Indian guide and interpreter, eight Indian scouts, and Dr. Porter were ordered to accompany the troops.[19]

Porter, who had formerly attended Headquarters and Battery, was thus shifted to join Reno's scouting expedition to give additional medical support to Dr. DeWolf. On June 11 Custer's command under Terry arrived at the confluence of the Powder and the Yellowstone after a rugged march. The *Far West* under the command of Grant Marsh was already there and was loaded with provisions and forage. At this point a supply depot was established. All the wagons, several hundred mules, recruits without mounts and those on sick detail, along with three companies of the 6th Infantry were ordered to remain here under the command of Major Orlando Moore. A trader and purveyor of whiskey came on the *Far West* to operate in the vicinity to the delight of the thirsty troops. Lonesome Charley Reynolds was also at Powder River and came under the care of Dr. Porter for an infected left hand.[20] He healed sufficiently to go to battle two weeks later and die.

With six companies under Reno's command, the scouting force had left Powder River at 5 P.M. on June 10 and traveled up-river eight miles before camping. The next two days they rode another fifty miles in the same direction along the Powder until June 13 when they bent westward, then northward to Mizpah Creek. Scouts probed south to the fork of Little Powder and the Powder and northward along Mizpah Creek without encountering hostiles.[21] Reno, at this point, chose to deviate from General Terry's orders, which were to go downstream on Mizpah Creek to its junction with the Powder River. Instead, suspecting that he might find nothing there, he turned westward toward the Tongue, crossed Pumpkin Creek, and camped at the fork of Little Pumpkin and Pumpkin Creek for the night of June 14. The next day Reno's troops traveled twenty-five miles to the Tongue River. On the 16th they went down the Tongue River about eight miles where they found evidence of a large Indian campsite about one month old. Further violating Terry's orders, Reno led his scouting troops westward to Rosebud Creek where they found no Indians, but evidence of a camp used a month earlier. On the 17th they traveled first up Rosebud Creek and then looped back down the creek along which they camped for the night. On the 18th they advanced down the

Rosebud to the Yellowstone River where the streams met and camped just across the river from Gibbon's command. They communicated that no Indians had been found and told about the very large month-old campsite. This information was forwarded to General Terry. On the 19th Reno's troopers marched east down the Yellowstone River thirteen miles to a site eight miles from General Terry's command at the mouth of the Powder River. In all, Reno had traveled about 250 miles through the rugged country, not always in accordance with his orders from General Terry, but had found evidence that Indians had passed through the area in large numbers.

Unknown to Terry and Custer, General Crook had met stiff resistance in his approach from the south. After a fierce battle with Sioux and Cheyenne Indians at the Rosebud River in southern Montana on June 17, he turned back in defeat, although he never admitted it and called it a victory. The battle at Rosebud occurred just eight days before Custer's battle at Little Bighorn.[22] The fight was less than forty miles (Vaughn said twenty miles) from Reno's scouting expedition at its farthest probe.[23] Historians have speculated on the implications of the outcome of the battle. According to Vaughn, "What might have occurred had General Crook been able to defeat the Indians at Rosebud? History would read differently today had he been able to maintain his position and complete his role in the pincers movement. Without doubt, the disaster at the Little Big Horn would have been averted."[24]

The command was reunited on June 20 where Terry ordered troops under Custer to advance up the Yellowstone to Reno's campsite. When united Dr. DeWolf retained the Right Wing, and Dr. Porter assumed medical coverage for the Left Wing.[25]

On June 21 DeWolf wrote his wife, "I and Dr. Porter messed together and had a nice time.... Yesterday I went out with Dr. Porter, Lt. Harrington and Lt. Hodgson pistol shooting and came out second but, Porter was best so you can see some of the cavalry cannot shoot very well."[26] Of these four, only Porter would survive the battle and not because of his shooting ability.

On June 22 Custer now commanded the entire 7th Cavalry regiment. Dressed in a fringed yellow buckskin suit, wearing a felt hat, and armed with a Remington sporting rifle and two English pistols, Custer reviewed his cavalry troops with General Terry and Colonel Gibbon. At noon they marched out of camp four abreast to the tune of "Garryowen" played by trumpeters of the regiment.[27] Thus began the fateful march to the Little Bighorn. Three doctors rode out with the regiment. Only one would return.

Dr. George Edwin Lord, assistant surgeon, thirty years old, was the adopted son of a Congregational minister in West Auburn, Maine, north of Portland. He taught school and graduated from Bowdoin College in 1866. He carried a letter of personal reference as to character and worthiness in his military file from Joshua L. Chamberlain, former president of Bowdoin and governor of Maine and better known as the hero of Little Round Top at Gettysburg. He graduated from Chicago Medical School in 1870 after three years of study and clinical experience at Mercy Hospital in Chicago. After serving at Fort Randall and the Whetstone Agency in the Dakota Territory, surgeon for the Northern Boundary Survey, Fort Snelling and with the team aiding "grasshopper sufferers" in Minnesota all as an acting assistant surgeon, he passed the written examination and was certified for appointment by the Army Medical Board as assistant surgeon, U.S. Army, with the rank of first lieutenant on June 26, 1875.[28] In August of that year he became post surgeon at Fort Buford located at the confluence of the Missouri and Yellowstone rivers. He was noted to be physically frail and wore eyeglasses. On his army examination for an appointment as assistant surgeon on January, 11, 1875, which he passed, one question was to describe the antiseptic treatment of wounds and compare its results with other dressings. He answered, "The antiseptic treatment of wounds is based on the theory that certain agents called antiseptics have the power of destroying certain organic germs said to exist in the air and to be injurious to the process of healing—in my opinion it is injurious to freshly granulating surfaces."[29] This is an accurate reflection of the general medical understanding of the time regarding wound care based upon the work of the British surgeon, Joseph Lister. It would be another decade before aseptic wound care and steam sterilization would be advocated.

The second doctor, Dr. James Madison DeWolf, a thirty-three-year-old acting assistant surgeon, was a native of rural Pennsylvania. His ancestry can be traced back to the DeWolfs of Bristol, Rhode Island, the largest slave-trading family in the United States.[30] He had enlisted in the Civil War at age seventeen and sustained a gunshot wound to the arm at Bull Run on August 30, 1862. After discharge, partially disabled, he re-enlisted in September 1864 and served until June 1865. After the war, in October 1865, he enlisted in the infantry, but was appointed hospital steward the following year. After discharge, he re-enlisted in the Idaho Territory as hospital steward from 1868 until 1871 under the name James DeWall. He enlisted again in 1871 under the name James Madison DeWolf. While serving as a hospital steward at Watertown Arsenal, Massachusetts, he studied medicine at Harvard School of Medicine from which he graduated June 26, 1875, only a year before the Little Bighorn. Failing to pass the examination for assistant surgeon, he resigned as hospital steward to become a contract surgeon with the Department of Dakota in November 1875.[31] Though a seasoned veteran of combat and military life, having spent almost half his life attached to army units, he was an unseasoned and inexperienced doctor.

Dr. Henry Rinaldo Porter was the third. He went into battle with an amputation kit that was in a box 17 × 7 × 3¾ inches and made by J. Tiencken, New York. The wooden box had two latches for security and was labeled

"U.S.A. Hospl. Dept."[32] Contents included an amputation bow saw with an ebony handle, a trephine with antler handle, amputation knives, and a Pettit's tourniquet, now ragged from use and soiled with blood and dirt.[33] He had, also, a leather-covered minor surgical kit made by Brinkerhoff in New York with tortoise shell handles consistent with use in the days before steam sterilization.[34] Finally, he had access to a wooden chest that weighed over a hundred pounds and was carried by mule in the pack train. This metal-strapped U.S. Army Field Surgical Chest No. 2 contained six numbered drawers and a tray that held medications, surgical instruments, bandages, and distilled liquor.[35] For the catastrophe that would ensue, he was woefully ill prepared.

Chapter 6

The Battle as Seen by Porter

Custer left base camp with twelve companies of the 7th Cavalry, Indian scouts, guides, interpreters, packers, a reporter, and an eighteen-year-old nephew, Harry Armstrong Reed. Porter rode with the 647 men two miles up the banks of the Yellowstone, then forded Rosebud River to go along its west bank for another ten miles, and reached camp at 4 P.M. Not present were infantry troops or Gatling guns which had been left behind to expedite mobility. The pack mules struggled badly. Godfrey called them "badly used" up from the earlier Reno scouting party that Porter had accompanied.[1]

Each trooper carried a 7.5 pound Model 1873 Springfield "trapdoor" carbine that had an effective range of 500 to 600 yards and a Model 1873 Single Action Colt .45 Revolver known as the "peacemaker" or the "thumb buster," sighted for twenty-five yards. Each man carried a fifteen day ration of hardtack, coffee, and sugar and a ten day supply of bacon.[2]

The next morning they moved out to the south at 5 A.M. and soon observed signs of an earlier Indian migration through the area. Dr. Lord, who usually had ridden alongside Captain Benteen, was missed. Sometime after the evening meal had concluded and all had turned in for the night, Lord struggled into camp and told Benteen that "he had halted alone some miles back, being completely tired out, broken down, so much so that he had given up all hopes of getting into camp. He declined tea and wanted nothing to eat or drink." Benteen later regarded this as a significant early indicator of Lord's physical condition shown before going into the battle.[3] Porter was twenty-eight years old and in excellent physical condition as contrasted with Dr. Lord.

On the 24th, the day before the battle, they saw evidence of a sun dance camp including a soldier's scalp. At 7:45 P.M. they camped on the right bank of the Rosebud only to be summoned to resume marching during the night.[4]

Porter told how they had been "on the trail all that day and night. The night was very dark and we lost the trail once, but found it again by lighting matches."

"We proceeded until four o'clock, the morning of the 25th, when we

6. The Battle as Seen by Porter

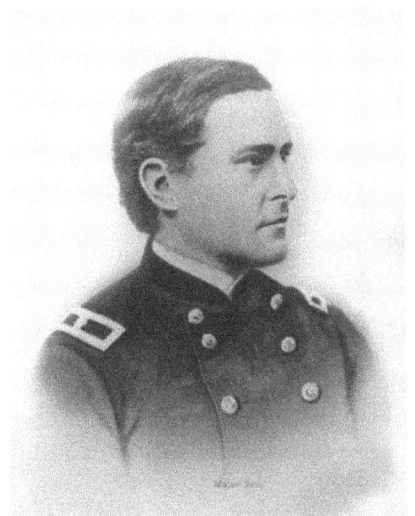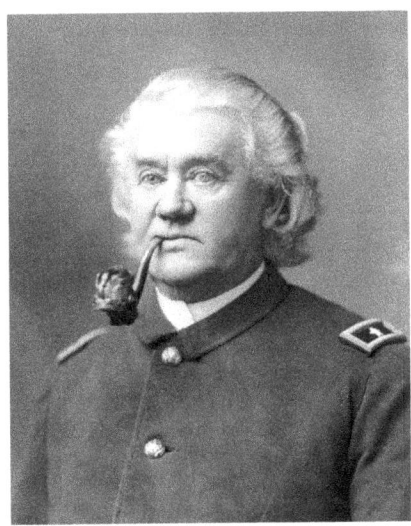

Left: *Major Marcus A. Reno, 7th Cavalry. Photograph by David F. Barry. (State Historical Society of North Dakota B0174)* Right: *Captain Frederick Benteen, 7th Cavalry (State Historical Society of North Dakota E0109).*

camped in a deep ravine where the Indians could not see us. We were not allowed to unsaddle or unpack. Being very tired after our long ride, we laid [*sic*] down and slept, each man holding his horse by the bridle reins. In about an hour the scouts reported a large camp of Indians ahead. The command was ordered to get ready for action. Custer came to me and said: 'Porter, there is a large camp of Indians ahead, and we are going to have a great killing.' At six o'clock (Chicago time) we started." Thus, Custer was completely aware of the large number of Indians ahead. What he did not anticipate was their aggressive fighting spirit. Much of this can be attributed to the leadership of Crazy Horse, who had already blocked General Crook's forces at the Rosebud on June 17.

Custer divided the command about 10 A.M. on Sunday morning, June 25, taking Companies C, E, F, I, and L with him to ride northward along the bluffs on the east bank of the Little Bighorn. He assigned Companies A, G, and M to Major Reno with orders to ford the river and charge to the north up the valley toward the Indian encampment. Captain Benteen with Companies D, H, and K was directed to scout to the southwest and block any Indians from escaping. At this point the Indians had no intention of escaping. Captain McDougall's Company B was to protect the pack train.

Porter recalled, "Just as we were ready to start, Custer came to me and said: 'Doctor, I would like to have you go with me, as you are younger and more robust and Dr. Lord, the chief surgeon is not feeling very well.' I replied, 'All right. I would much prefer going with you.' Custer then said: 'I will see Dr.

Lord and ask him to consent.' We rode over to where Dr. Lord was, and Custer spoke to him about the contemplated arrangement. The Doctor replied: 'Not much. I am going with you.' The poor fellow in those few words saved my life and sealed his own doom."[5] It is clear from Benteen's observation of Lord's condition on the 23rd that he was far from able to withstand the rigor of battle.

Porter then went with Reno's battalion and had only gone a short distance when Custer's adjutant, Captain William Cooke, came up to Reno and said, "The Indians are right ahead of you, and you are ordered to charge them as fast as possible."

As soon as they crossed the river they encountered ten or fifteen Indians who ran from them causing them to believe that all Indians would do the same. Reno's troopers charged up the valley as ordered and, to their dismay, encountered "terrific fire." He ordered them to dismount and form a skirmish line. Indians charged toward them, a few at first and then in great numbers. "The ground seemed to be fairly alive with them," said Porter. "They were all naked and their bodies were painted hideously. They all rode their ponies bareback."

As an acting assistant surgeon, Porter was not entitled to an army uniform and entered the battle wearing a linen duster. Chief guide "Lonesome Charley" Reynolds warned him that it was attracting attention, according to Joseph H. Taylor.[6] Reynolds said, "Look out Doctor, the Indians are shooting at you." These were Reynolds' last words before he was killed as the two stood near the timber.

Porter described the action:

> The fire finally became so hot that Reno ordered his men to mount, and led them under cover of the woods. Then the Indians closed in on us, shooting through the branches, killing some of our men. A soldier was shot in the little clump of trees where I was. I dismounted and found him mortally wounded. Reno ordered the troops to mount and "charge" [back across the river and up a steep bank to the hilltop now known as Reno's battle site]. A running fight ensued. My horse was rearing and plunging, and I had all I could do to hold him. The Indians, in their mad pursuit of our troops, did not notice me in the timber. They were passing within ten feet of where I was. I placed laudanum [opium tincture] on the wound of the soldier and bandaged it as best I could, and again mounted my frightened horse. As I was leaving the poor soldier said: 'For God's sake, Doctor, don't leave me to be tortured by those fiends." Bullets were flying thick and fast, and I turned my horse loose and caught up with our troops, who had gotten half a mile away. In that half-mile ride I think I was the target of a thousand rifles, but I escaped without a scratch.

Porter saw the Indians drag Lieutenant McIntosh from his horse and "riddle him with pistol shots as he lay at their feet." In his opinion, the Indian casualties were "insignificant" when compared with those of Reno.[7]

Throwing his arms around the neck of his horse, Porter scrambled frantically up the steep bluff as did the lucky ones in Reno's command. Dr. DeWolf was killed near Porter just as he reached the summit, leaving Porter as the only surgeon for the growing number of wounded. Dr. DeWolf's soldier orderly fell near him. Sergeant Kanipe said that had DeWolf gotten a few more feet he would have been saved.[8] The bodies of DeWolf, W.D. Meyer, Clair, and Gordon were so near the Reno hilltop command that they were not scalped. Porter retrieved DeWolf's bullet-ridden body the next day for burial and was able to save his diary and some personal items to send later to his widow.

Porter recalled,

> We took a stand on the top of a steep hill. A few minutes later Benteen, with his three companies came up, as did McDougall with the pack train. Benteen, after leaving us when the command was divided, had gone southwest to the river. Not seeing any Indians and hearing the firing he rushed back and joined us. We fought there the remainder of the day, surrounded by [an estimated] three thousand savages, while there were only three hundred of us, all told. The men dug rifle pits with their knives and tin cups. At dark the Indians stopped firing. Some of the men then crawled down to the river and secured water. We had been fighting in the broiling sun all day without a drop of water, and the wounded were begging for a drink. I had some brandy with me, but I told them that it would make them worse. They insisted on having it, anyway. Next morning the Indians again opened fire on us. Although Reno was the ranking officer, Colonel Benteen was really in command, and to his coolness and bravery those of us who were saved owe our lives. With the air thick with bullets and some of them piercing his clothing, he stood calmly directing the troops. [He also sustained wounds.] Occasionally a band of savages would dash up to within two or three hundred yards of us, and our men would then charge them. Several Indians were killed in these charges, and finally one of the soldiers killed and scalped an Indian in plain view of the others. This frightened them and they kept a safe distance away after that. A perfect storm of leaden hail was poured in on us all day the 26th until about four o'clock in the afternoon, when the firing gradually ceased. We were then frightened, as we thought the Indians were up to some bloodier mischief. Finally we saw them moving off in a body. That night most of the soldiers slept, and were much refreshed in the morning. After the Indians left we were able to procure water. We had all been nearly famished. During the morning of the 27th General Terry and his command came up. He said his staff were all crying, and General Terry said: "Custer and his whole command are killed. We thought you were, too."

> During the two days we were surrounded by the Indians the inquiry among our men for Custer was loud, and that General's court-martial was freely speculated upon. After separating from us Custer had gone through a rough country for a distance of four or five miles and attacked the Indians in the rear. As soon as we could several of the officers and myself went over to where Custer had fought, and found what General Terry had reported to be only too true. We found Custer's body stark naked, as white and clean as a baby's. He was shot in

the head and breast. The body of Captain Tom Custer, General Custer's brother, was horribly mutilated. He was disemboweled, and his head had been crushed in by a blow from a stone hammer used by the Indians. The only arrow wound I found was in his head. He had the Sioux mark of death, which was a cut from the hip to the knee, reaching to the bone. His heart was not cut out, as had been reported by Rain-in-the-face, one of the Sioux chiefs who took part in the fight. I cut a lock of hair from the head of each officer as he lay, and gave it to their families on my return home. The steamer *Far West* was moored at the mouth of the Little Big Horn. She was the supply boat of the expedition and had made her way up the Big Horn farther than any other boat.

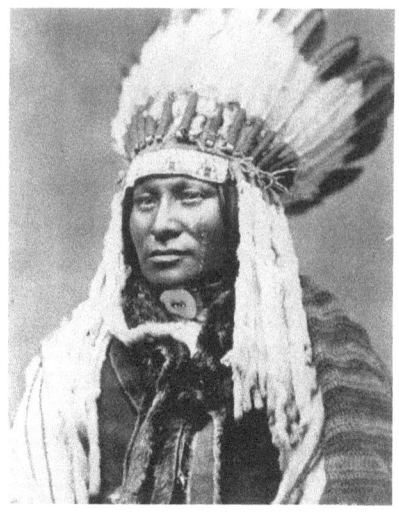

Rain-in-Face, Hunkpapa Sioux warrior (National Archives [111SC 85725]).

After burying the dead we took the wounded on litters ten or twelve miles to the boat, and I was detailed to go down to Fort Lincoln with them. Colonel Smith, Terry's adjutant general, was sent along with the official dispatches, and he had a traveling bag full of telegrams for the Bismarck office. Captain Grant Marsh, of Bismarck, was in command of the *Far West*, and the steamer performed a feat unequaled in western steamboating.[9] Marsh put everything in the most complete order and took a large supply of fuel. His orders were to reach Bismarck as soon as possible. The steamer never received the credit due her, nor did her gallant captain. The Big Horn is full of islands, and a successful passage is not an easy feat, but the boat made it without an accident, after a thrilling voyage. At Fort Buford and Fort Stevenson we stopped a minute to tell the news, and at Fort Berthold a wounded scout was put off. Two of the wounded died, and we went ashore to bury them. We approached home with something of that feeling that always moves the human heart. It was one mixed with sorrow and gladness. At eleven o'clock on the night of the 5th of July we reached Bismarck and Fort Lincoln, having made one thousand miles in fifty-four hours. Colonel Smith and myself hurried from the land up town, and called up Colonel Lounsberry, the editor of the *Tribune*, and the telegraph operator, J.M. Carnahan, who took his seat at the key and scarcely raised himself from his chair for twenty-two hours.

What he sent vibrating around the world is history."

Porter's care of the wounded included the amputation of Private Michael P. Madden's right leg below the knee early in the morning of June 27 with only whiskey to dull the pain.[10] Military medical doctrine since Napoleonic wars advocated amputation for open fractures of the limbs. Madden survived.

6. The Battle as Seen by Porter

Porter's field hospital was in the open air on a tarpaulin in a shallow depression near the center of the hill that was scantily protected. Captain Benteen later described it as follows: "The hospital was established at the upper rim [of a saucer-like depression] and was about as safe a place as there was around the vicinity, the blue canopy of heaven being the covering: the sage brushes, sand being the operating board; but the stout heart and nervy skillful hand of Dr. Porter was equal to the occasion."[11]

There were seventy-eight wounds in sixty-eight men under Porter's care. This does not include Privates Meador, Gebhart, and Voight who were killed outright in the hilltop fight. Also, some injuries were so minor as not to require attention. Of the sixty-eight wounded, six died for a mortality of 8.9 percent; of the six deaths, one died on the bluffs, three died on the steamship *Far West* while being evacuated, and two died later at Fort Abraham Lincoln hospital.[12]

The time required to get the wounded from the end of the battle on June 26 to Bismarck on July 5 has provoked some controversy. In spite of the fifty-four hour dash from 5 P.M. on July 3 until 11 P.M. on July 5 by Captain Marsh and the *Far West*, the question of July 1, July 2, and July 3 remain. The delay getting stretchers made and carrying the wounded to the straw and canvas covered decks of the *Far West* then at the mouth of the Little Bighorn by the early morning of June 30 seems reasonable.[13] General Gibbon's column and Reno's survivors from the 7th Cavalry left to march down the Bighorn to the Yellowstone about the same time that the *Far West* departed from the mouth of the Little Bighorn. The *Far West* reached the Yellowstone, fifty-three miles downstream by the end of the day (June 30). The *Far West* lay at the north bank of the Yellowstone July 1, July 2, and until 5 P.M. on July 3. "Waiting for the column" or as Hanson writes, "though every instinct of humanity demanded that the suffering wounded be taken to Fort Lincoln without delay, military necessity required the *Far West* to await Gibbon's troops at the mouth of the Big Horn, whence they were to be ferried across to the north bank of the Yellowstone for rest and refitting."[14] Was this delay necessary in light of seriously wounded soldiers awaiting hospitalization? As mentioned, there were three deaths aboard the steamship of Little Bighorn combatants.

William David Nugent, private, A Company, gives another opinion. His account is not always reliable. For example, in his memoirs written in 1933, he did not believe Porter was with Reno in the valley, which without doubt he was. In another place he errs regarding directions on the battlefield. But Nugent makes this comment about the delay:

> Why should this boat be held at the mouth of the Big Horn from the 29th to the evening of the 3rd of July with a load of wounded on her deck suffering with the intense heat, and the medical attention that could not be given on that boat? I may not be able to tell all the reasons for his boat being detained. One guess is

that it was a difficult problem to write a report that would suit the occasion. I am not surprised that it was ten days before the wounded reached Fort Lincoln as it took more time to manufacture a report that could be read in any way that it would to have reached Fort Lincoln. That boat left on the afternoon of July 3rd and reached Bismarck about 11 P.M. on the 5th sure in a hurry to get his report off. The wounded were taken to Fort Lincoln on the 6th. The report that went out, the official one, I have reference to, did not make a charge against anyone. No that was left to the press reports that went out with this boat....[15]

Of the many dozens of personal recollections of the Battle of Little Bighorn, Porter's favorite was General Edward Godfrey's as the one most accurate, according to what he told Dr. Fannie Dunn Quain of Bismarck.[16] Godfrey's account is far from unbiased with regard to Reno's role in the battle. His dislike of Reno is obvious.

Chapter 7

After the Battle

On July 4, 1876, the *Far West,* on its return toward Bismarck and Fort Lincoln with the wounded on deck, stopped at the supply camp on the Yellowstone near the mouth of the Powder River. Private Wilmot P. Sanford of Fort Buford, then stationed there, recorded the event in his diary:

> Tuesday July 4, 1876. Clear and hot. Boat came in this mourning [*sic*] and left for Bismarck. Had on B Co and 25 wounded men of the 7th cavalry. Fearful news. 5 Cos of the 7th Cav. and all the Custers and all the officers of the 5 Cos killed and Dr. Lord of [Fort] Buford.... Soldier of the 7th buried here today. Came down on the boat. Died on the way down.[1]

Another private recorded the July 4 stop at the supply depot, Jacob Horner of K Company 7th Cavalry who was detached from his company and missed the battle. He noted, "They lay on blankets on hay strewn over the deck. It was a sad day."[2]

The soldier buried at the camp at the mouth of the Powder River was Private William M. George, Company H.[3]

Porter wrote a letter to his family on the same day while aboard the *Far West,* his first since the battle. He told of the suffering and deaths and about the amputation that he had done.

> I established a hospital in the center of the mules and horses, where the wounded were brought in faster than I could attend them. Men and animals were killed all around me, and the horses fell over on my wounded men. Dr. DeWolf was killed near, just on my left, at the commencement of the fight, consequently all the duties fell to me. On the afternoon of the second day my wounded were suffering terribly for water—they needed it for their wounds as well as thirst. Some soldiers were ordered to get water, but some were killed and others wounded. No more were ordered. Volunteers were called to get it for the wounded. Plenty of brave men were found and enough was procured for a taste [of water] for each man. One man [Madden] who volunteered was shot through the leg, both bones crushed and the fleshy parts lacerated so that I had to amputate the leg below the knee.[4] He is doing well although the operation was performed under many difficulties.... I accompanied the party that buried the dead, on the third day after the fight. We buried over 200 bodies. They had undergone

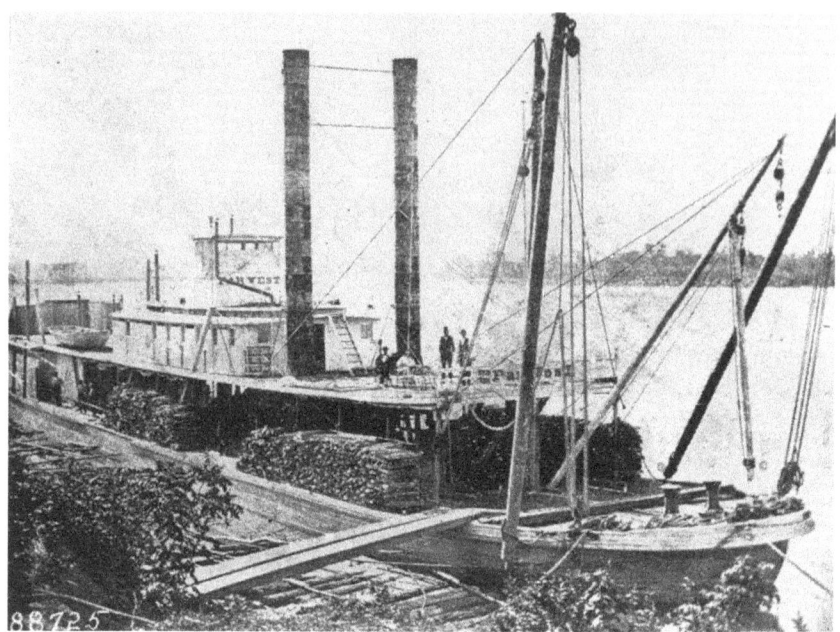

Far West, *steamboat on Yellowstone and Missouri rivers used to carry supplies for the Terry-Custer column, as headquarters for General Terry, and for evacuation of the wounded from the battle to Fort Abraham Lincoln (National Archives [88725]).*

rapid decomposition and some of them were fearfully mangled and cut. All were more or less stripped of their clothing. In one spot I counted 35 dead and recognized the following officers: General Custer; Colonel [Thomas W.] Custer, his brother; Colonel [William W.] Cooke; Captain [Algernon E.] Smith; Captain [George W.] Yates; Colonel [Myles W.] Keogh; Lieutenant [James E.] Porter; Lieutenant [William Van Wyck] Reily; Mr. Boston Custer, who was also the General's brother; Lieutenant [James] Calhoun; Lieutenant [James G.] Sturgis and others. Assistant Surgeon [George E.] Lord's remains were not fully identified, but there is no hope that he escaped. You see that the medical department suffered severely. Of the three doctors I am the only one living. I expect to arrive at Fort Abraham Lincoln tomorrow, where I get new medical supplies and return immediately, when a larger force will be put into the field, and I hope we will be able to punish the red devils, whom the government and Indian Department have so splendidly armed with improved rifles to kill United States troops with.

Yours, in haste
H.R. Porter[5]

As soon as the *Far West* tied up at the Government Warehouse in Bismarck about 2 A.M. on July 6 a sergeant bearing the news was ordered to Fort

Abraham Lincoln. Upon receiving the report the commanding officer, Captain William S. McCaskey, called the officers together and informed them of the disaster. Notification of the widows began shortly before 7 A.M. when McCaskey, Dr. J.V.D. Middleton, and Lieutenant Charles Gurley knocked on the back door of the Custer house waking up the housemaid who summoned Mrs. Custer, Mrs. Calhoun, and Miss Reed to the parlor. Mrs. Custer's first response was to ask why the early visit before learning the terrible news. It soon spread throughout the post.[6]

The wounded were transferred from the *Far West* to the Fort Abraham Lincoln Hospital during the early morning hours of July 6 accompanied by Drs. Porter and Ashton.[7] Later another soldier who was wounded and another who was sick were brought in on July 21 on the *Josephine* for a total of forty-two patients admitted from General Terry's expedition for the month of July according to the log of Dr. J.V.D. Middleton of Fort Abraham Lincoln.[8] One body, that of Private James C. Bennett, C Company, 7th Cavalry, was brought back for burial. He died on board the *Far West* on July 5 from a spinal injury and paraplegia.[9]

One of the wounded, Private David Cooney, with a gunshot wound to the right hip died at Fort Abraham Lincoln on July 20 of pyemia or blood stream infection.[10] Corporal William M. Smith, Company B, required resection of the right elbow joint on August 29 and drainage of an axillary abscess on September 5, but survived. Michael Madden, saddler, Company K, and who underwent the battlefield amputation of his right leg below the knee by Porter, recovered from surgery and was released from the hospital September 13. He was later admitted for domiciliary care to the U.S. Soldiers Home in St. Louis on August 15, 1877. Madden was last known to be living in St. Louis in 1883.[11]

Frank Braun, another of the wounded, was returned to Fort Abraham Lincoln by the *Far West* with wounds of the face and left thigh.[12] Surgeons drained his wound on September 13 under ether anesthetic after he worsened and removed foreign bodies, perhaps cloth from his uniform or bullet fragments. He died October 4, 1876, of his wounds at Fort Lincoln. His hip bone was removed by the surgeon and was sent to the Army Medical Museum, now the National Museum of Health and Medicine, Washington, DC, where it is held today. The hip shows evidence of the infection that proved fatal to him.[13] The museum holds two Little Bighorn specimens.

A Western Union telegram went out from Bismarck sometime on July 6 and reached Porter's parents at 8:45 A.M. July 7 in New York Mills.

To H.D. [*sic*] Porter
Henry arrived safe in charge of wounded men after a terrible battle.

P.T. Douglass[14]

George Fairchild wrote an account of how the news of the battle was received in Bismarck in a letter to his wife who was visiting in Oberlin.

> Bismarck, D.T. July 6th, 1876
> Thursday Evening
>
> My Darling Wife,
> Your letter written a week ago yesterday came tonight. Did not get any last mail. Well Darling we have sad, sad news today. 5 companies of the 7th Cavalry including all the Lincoln Officers that we know except Moylan and Baker (Captains) annihilated by the Indians. Gen. Custer, Col. Custer, Col. Keogh, Col. Yates, Col. Cooke, Capt. Smith, Capt. McIntosh, Lt. Calhoun, Lt. Hodgson, Lt. Riley, Lt. Porter, Lt. Sturgis, Lt. Crittenden, Lt. Harrington, Boston Custer, Surgeon Lord, Surg DeWolf, Mr. Reed (nephew of Gen. Custer) Charley Reynolds, M. H. Kellogg (reporter) and Companies C,E,I,F, and L were surrounded and so far as can be ascertained every man of them killed — Dr. Porter is here, Came down on *Far West* with 40 wounded — goes right back. He is said to have shown great coolness and bravery, even amputating a man's leg in good shape under sharp fire — He was with Reno and 3 companies that made a Charge and Retreated with great loss — This occurred 25 miles above the junction of Little Horn with the Big Horn rivers in the former — Dr. Porter was all over the battlefield and helped bury all these officers and men — they were terribly mutilated. They found Tom Custer with a TWC tattooed on his arm. Others were recognized by other means. Oh it is dreadful — dreadful — about fifteen Widows at Ft. Lincoln today including laundresses. Mrs. Raymond's housekeeper Mrs. Kelly [Pvt. John P. Kelly of Company F and Pvt. Patrick Kelly of Company I were both killed in the battle] lost her husband. The details are too sickening to relate. Reno's Command of Co.'s were surrounded for 36 hours nearly dying for water. Indians numbering about 4000 or 5000 — Mrs. Calhoun lost her husband, three brothers, and a nephew. You will see it in all the papers before this reaches you. We can hardly think of anything else and 'tis almost impossible to do any business and yet we have been rushed all day supplying 3 boats. It will be some time before we hear any more about it I presume — the *Far West* goes right back. Well Darling good night — cannot tell when I shall start. Shall try to be home a week before Commencement. A world of love to you and many kisses from your ever loving
>
> George[15]

Sometime shortly after his return, Porter and George Flannery gave a dinner attended by Captain Edward W. Smith, General Terry's adjutant; General John B. Sanborn of St Paul; J.W. Raymond; and George H. Fairchild.[16] Porter described for the group the advance on the Indian village and the apparent surprise as well as Reno's disorderly retreat "before there were any casualties [*sic*] and the disaster which followed in crossing the river and getting up to the high land where they rallied on Benteen's command."

Rachael Raymond, wife of J.W., turned her home over to the six widows of the officers until they could arrange to leave Bismarck and with them came

7. After the Battle

Mary Adams, Custer's faithful cook.[17] She kept house for Raymond for a time after the widows left.

Porter was not through with Indian fights. At the end of July he was back with General Terry's command along the Yellowstone and was involved this time with a combined force of the 5th and 22nd Infantry Regiments under the command of Major Orlando H. Moore, whose mission it was to retrieve forage stolen by the Indians. The grain was recovered but in the "skirmish at Powder River" of August 2, 1876, a scout, Wesley Brockmeyer, was shot in an ambush. Moore, who would in 1882 become commander of Fort Abraham Lincoln, reported, "the scout, mortally wounded, was cared for by the gallant Dr. [Henry] Porter."[18] George W. Morgan, another scout, killed the Indian who shot Brockmeyer. David Campbell, boat pilot who accompanied the two scouts, scalped the Indian. Porter "later sent the grisly trophy to Bismarck for display."[19]

Porter remained at the camp on the Yellowstone until the end of September when his contract was annulled on the 30th.

One can assume that by this time Porter, age 28, who had ridden all over the West with the army and had risked his life too many times to count, was ready to settle down. His love of adventure was not extinguished nor would it ever be, but he elected to pursue less dangerous activities in the future. At his request the army cancelled his status as contract surgeon on December 1, 1876, and he returned to Bismarck, Dakota Territory, to practice medicine and surgery. Nevertheless, he signed another contract on December 2 to take care of medical problems at Camp Hancock, Bismarck, for sixty dollars a month.[20]

Chapter 8

Recalling the Battle

In later years Porter would frequently comment about the battle both to his friends and to reporters. One issue invariably discussed was Reno. It was no secret, as he admitted in 1891, that he was no friend of Reno's, but he did feel that he "was an abused man" who, if he had not been so excited, "might have done a little better."[1] This comment to a reporter came after Reno was dead. He further stated:

> The night on the bluff I shall never forget until my dying day. It was awful. It was frightful; the frenzied Indians were howling about us on all sides and were firing at us all night. We could not get down the steep embankment for water, for the Sioux were on the alert and would shoot at the spot where a leaf rustled or a twig cracked. The groans of our men were something heartrending. Men crying and begging piteously for water to moisten their parched lips which were soon to close and stiffen in death. The blood from wounds that could not be properly washed, and the curses of the men anxious to kill the Indians, yet not daring to attack against such superior odds. All tending to make the night dreadfully long, full of anxiety and care, for at dawn we expected the Indians to make an attack and kill us all. There was just a third of the command killed or wounded that night. In the retreat out [of the valley] many more were killed. When Terry's command came to our relief, we came near having a fearful disaster, for as they came down the road, the dust flying, wind blowing, mounted on ponies, we, from our shelter thought them Indians, came quite near shooting at them. What might have resulted is hard to conceive, for they would have returned fire, and then a second fight would have occurred.

An account of the battle by Private John F. Donoughue of Company K was published in 1888 in the *Bismarck Daily Tribune* as a defense of Reno's actions. Donoughue (also spelled Donahue, Donoughe) was a 24-year-old native of Tipperary, Ireland, who had enlisted two years earlier in Boston. His company, K, was assigned to Benteen.[2] After the battle he worked as a ranch hand near Devils Lake, Dakota Territory, 180 miles northeast of Bismarck.

> The following communication received from John F. Donoughue, a private of the Seventh United States cavalry, who fought in the Custer battle and who is

8. Recalling the Battle 67

now in Bismarck is doubly interesting from the fact that it contradicts several points of history and gives a graphic account of the famous battle:

Editor Tribune:

In reading the article under the heading of "Whispers" in the [St. Paul] *Globe* of the 8th inst., all the incidents of what is known as "the Custer Massacre" or the battle of the Little Big Horn come back to me very forcibly; and having read the articles as published in regard to this memorable battle, find a great many inaccuracies in said published statements, and also find Major Reno charged with cowardice.

On the 17th day of May A.D. 1876, the seventh United States cavalry, left Fort Abraham Lincoln on a march into the interior and this is all the men knew at this time of our ultimate destination, always supposing, of course, that we were after Indians. We marched to the crossing of the Hart [*sic*] river and went into camp, Mrs. General George A. Custer accompanying the command on horseback, returning next day, and this is the last Mrs. Custer ever saw of her husband alive.

From this point nothing of any importance to the general reader occurred until reaching the camp on the Powder river, on which part of the command camped for several days, while Major Reno with the left wing was ordered to scour the headwaters of Tullock and O'Fallon creeks. The result of said scout was that Major Reno discovered a large Indian trail leading in the direction of the Rosebud river, which he was satisfied was the trail of the Indians we were after. Reno then went into camp on the Tongue river and sent a courier with dispatches back into headquarters at Powder river giving full particulars of what he had found and awaited further orders, which came in next day, which were for him to remain in camp until joined by headquarters and the balance of the regiment.

The next day at headquarters "Boots and Saddles" was sounded and troops marched to join Major Reno. (Will say here that the troops under Major Reno at this time were not the same as at the time of the fight on the Little Big Horn.)

At this camp something of great moment happened to myself, as any old soldier can say if he has ever been in such a position. We were ordered on retiring to be ready very early. When I retired it was too late to undress, so I laid [*sic*] down fully attired, spurs and all on. When the call sounded I jumped up quick and hurried to the parade ground, and being a little late could not wait to disengage my "pup" tent from my spur and so dragged the same with me. For this I was ordered to "carry a log."

Falling in, everything passed off as usual until we reached the Tongue river. Here we were kept busy drawing rations, forage, and ammunition for fifteen days and packing the mules. Now was the first full information the men had of their destination or objective point.

Major G...'s [Colonel John Gibbon] command lay on the opposite bank of the Yellowstone river.

All preparations being completed on the evening of the 22nd day of May [*sic*, 21st of June] we received orders to be in readiness to march on the following day. After being reviewed by General Terry and Gibbons [*sic*] (I being in the rear guard this morning) I heard each of the aforesaid generals speak in glowing terms of the appearance of the regiment.

In regard to the orders General Custer received General Terry asked General Custer if it would not be better for him (Custer) to take the artillery with him. He answered, "I do not need them and they will only be an incumbrance." When General Terry spoke of the infantry Custer thought they could not keep up with him and therefore would impede him. His orders were: "You are to strike the Indians on the 26th of June in conjunction with my command unless you think the Indians are liable to get away from you. Then, "use your own judgment." These may not be the exact words used by General Terry but he will not gainsay them, I think. Later, I propose to show that Custer tried to obey these orders to the letter.

On the night of the 24th of June we lost the trail, the night was intensely dark and one long to be remembered. General Custer and his adjutant, Colonel Cooke, could be seen lighting matches and candles in advance, trying to find the trail, which they succeeded in doing in a short time. About 4 o'clock in the morning on the 25th General Custer made camp and this is the first time in my life that I saw a lot of hungry men refuse vituals [sic]. The men were ordered to leave the horses saddled, mules packed, and they all lay down as they were, refusing food, all being too tired to eat on account of the forced marches they had undergone. About 6 o'clock in the morning we were again in the saddle leading our pack animals. From here General Custer sent scouts out to ascertain the strength and locality of the enemy.

About 10 o'clock A.M. a halt was ordered and General Custer and staff and his favorite scout, Bloody Knife, could be seen a short distance ahead riding over a small hill. When Custer and staff returned he ordered the saddle taken off his brown horse and put on his favorite sorrel. I turned to my companions and said, "Boys, we are going to have some fun as General Custer has had the saddle put on 'Dandy,' as I knew when Custer had any fight to do he always rode "Dandy," as he was a fighter too. At once I heard "officers' call" sounded and Custer was quite close to the group of men of which I was one. Officer Lieutenant L.R. Hare [Company K] (a brave soldier by the way) asked me to hold his horse while he attended to the call, this placing me in a position to hear the orders given by General Custer. General Custer was lying on the ground in a reclining position and other officers formed around him. He said, "My intentions were to give the Indians a daylight surprise on the morning of the 26th, but we have been discovered by an Indian who was fishing in the creek, and several of us saw the Indian ride at full speed towards the Sioux camp to give the alarm. Consequently we will be attacked and I would rather attack than be attacked. We will march on them at once." He then made three divisions of the regiment, himself taking the right, Major Reno the center and Captain Benteen the extreme left, an adjutant being appointed for each division.

These are the orders given by General Custer: "Major Reno, you will charge down the valley and sweep everything that will come to you; Captain Benteen will take the extreme left, I will take the extreme right with five companies" (naming the letter of the companies). General Custer here described the point that Major Reno should strike the camp supported by Captain Benteen and his three companies. "I will strike them on the opposite point and we will crush

8. Recalling the Battle

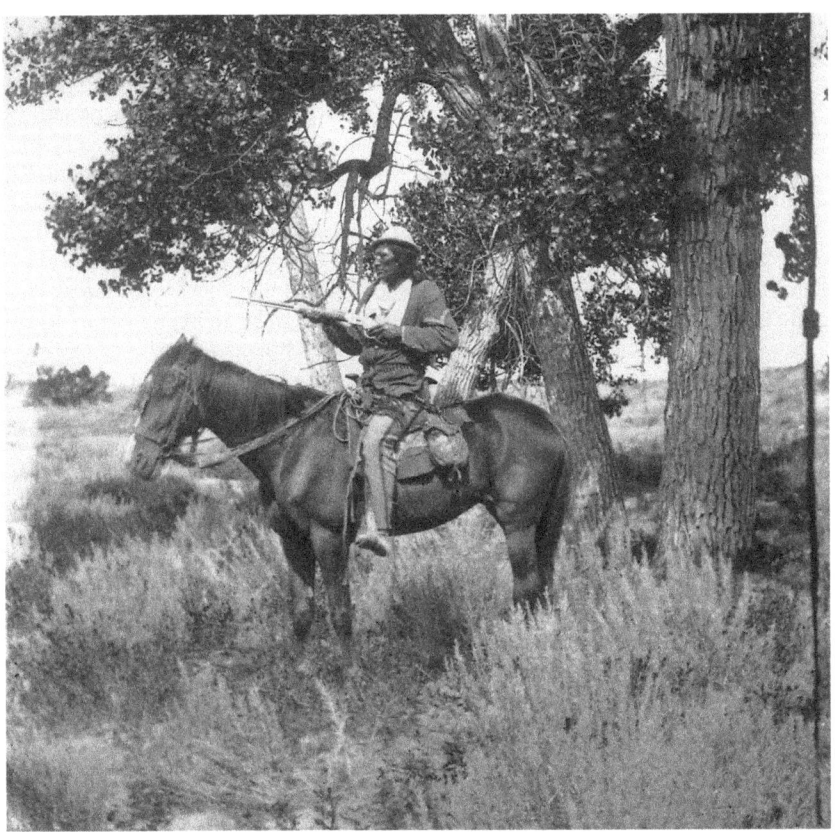

Bloody Knife, Custer's scout of Hunkpapa Sioux and Ree parentage, who was killed near Major Reno in the valley fight at Little Bighorn. Photograph by William R. Pywell, 1873 (National Archives [American Indian Select List 165]).

them between us," this leaving Reno with three companies. Captain McDougall being left to bring up the rear with the pack animals, the "forward" was sounded. After marching a short distance General Custer sent the adjutant back to each division with orders to march in separate trails as they were making so much dust that the Indians could tell too plainly the exact plans of our troops and govern themselves accordingly. We marched on for about two miles. General Custer away to the right in advance and Captain Benteen on our left rear, we were on the Indian trail which was quite fresh, and only a short distance ahead we saw a smoke, the men calling out "villages ahead." Our officers ahead raised their hands and gave the command "charge." Then came the throwing away of all surplus material, such as overcoats, haversacks, etc. to make themselves as light as possible and be in fighting trim. Reaching the place, where the smoke was seen it was found to come from a lone tepee which General Custer's command set fire to and destroyed.

Major Reno kept on at as quick a speed as his horses could stand and so far ahead of Benteen that we could not even hear his bugle calls. At last we sighted the village which was a grand sight—located on the Little Big Horn bottom and on the opposite side of the river from us. When we reached the river bank we found it very steep: so steep, in fact, that the horses slided [sic] and rolled down into the water. We charged down the bluff and across the river without a gun being fired and formed a "left front into line" directly in front of a clump of cottonwood trees. Just before we commenced firing we could see General Custer's battle flag on bluffs on the same side of the river we had left (I don't believe anyone else recorded observing this). Then Reno opened this fight by advancing on the Indians and firing on them. The Indians seemed to be giving way to us at first but they rallied and returned a most disastrous fire upon us killing a number of officers and men. Here Bloody Knife was killed directly by Major Reno's side, as were also Charley Reynolds, the famous scout, a colored interpreter "Isiah [sic]" [Dorman] and Lieutenants [Donald] McIntosh and [Benjamin H.] Hodgkinson [sic, Hodgson].

Now Major Reno gave order to "Dismount and fight on foot," fighting viciously as long as there was any "show" for his men and falling back in good order, fighting stubbornly, to the clump of trees in our rear. There he held on for a time but the Indians gaining ground he ordered a retreat and we re-crossed the river. At this point was a sight that a man can only see once in a lifetime, two and three men, one horse and others holding on to horses tails, climbing up the steep bank of the river; men being killed and wounded while in the river and more while climbing up the bluff. After reaching high ground Major Reno formed his men in line of defense and not knowing where Custer was located. Benteen having just come up, ordered "D" troop out, mounted, commanded by Lieutenant [Winfield Scott] Edgerly [Company D] with "K" troop dismounted covering them commanded by Lieutenant E.S. Godfrey [Company K](as brave an officer as ever entered the service). "D" troop got as far as the highest point between where Custer and Reno were, when they were met by a galling fire from the Indians and had to retreat which left Godfrey with his troop to face the enemy.... He ordered a slow retreat. He placed himself as centre skirmisher and ordered his men to dress on him, he having a carbine in hand and firing as often as any of his men and I am sure with good effect. The Indians were very close and the men retreated only far enough each time to enable them to reload their carbines and turn and fire. Whilst retreating Lieut. C.A. Varnum [Company A] came from Major Reno with orders to Lieutenant Godfrey to retreat slowly as their [Reno's] line would cover his retreat, and although there was very heavy firing by the Indians, Lieutenant Godfrey brought his men in with small loss.

Major Reno sent all the men he dared, only keeping enough men to protect the great number of wounded he had on the high ground. It was an utter impossibility for Major Reno to join General Custer or drive the Indians and I believe by this time General Custer's command had been annihilated.

Here is where the bravery of Major Reno comes in. He personally went along the whole line, encouraging his men, telling them how to use their ammunition most effectively, never looking for shelter, always where the fighting was hottest, and often when a shower of bullets would fall around him he would call out,

8. Recalling the Battle 71

"Shoot, goose, shoot," thus encouraging his men. Major Reno seeing the Indians closing in on his command, ordered several dismounted charges, each time driving the Indians, at the second of which his orderly Private [Patrick M.] Golden was killed in front of K troop lines, First Sergeant [Dewitt] Winney of K troop falling at the same time, one falling on each side of myself. This state of affairs continued until dark on the evening of the 25th when the Indians ceased firing and we were ordered to do the same.

Pickets being posted for the night, the remainder of the men were digging rifle pits using their knives and tin cups, the only instruments they had. As I was on the picket line, I saw fires made by the Indians at which they were burning prisoners alive, singing and dancing around their victims and yelling like demons. The men had very little rest, as the Indians opened fire at 2 A.M. with greater determination than ever doing their best to annihilate us. But every man was determined and held on. Colonel Benteen losing 19 in killed and wounded out of his company alone before 8 o'clock in the morning [2 killed and 21 wounded in Benteen's company in total].[3] The Indians kept up a terrible fire until about 2 P.M. when they began to withdraw, only firing an occasional shot and at 4 P.M. we held this bitterly contested battle field. We had with our [part of the] regiment two physicians Drs. DeWolf and H.R. Porter. Dr. DeWolf being killed early on the 25th, left the whole responsibility on Dr. Porter, and I must say I never saw or heard of a man who acted a braver part than this same Dr. Porter — at work incessantly, taking off a limb here, helping in other ways men otherwise wounded and never flinching. How he stood the strain, I cannot conceive. Being under his hands myself, I do not speak from hearsay when I say that he did all that a man can do. [There is no record of this author, John F. Donohue, being wounded at the battle. He may have been under Dr. Porter's treatment for something else or possibly not at all.] After the Indians had gone, Major Reno, fearing another attack, moved his command nearer to water, something his men and horses sorely needed — and for the first time in seven or eight nights a few of us were allowed to sleep. Having a good rest and no Indians in sight, five of us got permission to visit the place where we first engaged the Indians. Here I found the waistband of Sergeant [Robert H.] Hughes' [Company K] trousers, he having been the bearer of General Custer's battle flag, showing that he was taken alive [not necessarily] and brought here, and moreover his body was never found. Searching a little further on we saw three tepee poles with a thick object resting on top, which was a camp kettle and underneath on the ground was the heads of three soldiers of Major Reno's command, they having been cut off with some very sharp instrument as there was no torn flesh. These heads were placed facing each other. While here we were startled by the sound of bugle and hurried to camp. Looking in the direction of the bugle call we saw a large cloud of dust which we mistook for Indians, but it turned out to be Generals Terry and Gibbon's command. They came directly across the Custer battle ground. Of course we were overjoyed to see the stars and stripes floating over this body of men. When this command reached us we had the first news of General Custer's command and the complete annihilation of the same. This is the first we had seen of General Terry's troops after leaving them on the Yellowstone river about noon of 27th of June [sic, 22nd].

General Terry now having command we were ordered to bury the dead and what a sight. I do not believe, I cannot, that such sights were ever seen by human eyes. Pen cannot describe the inhumanities some of these soldiers had undergone. General Custer being the only one that had not been mutilated.

From the position of his men we found that his command had never crossed the river, also showing he never reached the point he intended to start in at, all the Custer family falling nearly together. After the burial of the dead, we were marched back to our camp where we were busy the next few days making litters for the wounded to transport them to the Big Horn river where a steamboat was in waiting to take them to Fort Abraham Lincoln. General Custer lived and died a brave soldier.

Major Reno I class with such cowards as Washington, Lafayette, Grant, McClellan, Napoleon, and Wellington. I know him to be as brave as any human being could be. I feel it my duty to say this of Major Reno as what I have said in this letter I know to be true. Nothing in this is hear say. I saw and heard all this myself and have read that he was charged with cowardice.

John F. Donoughe

Ex-member Co. K 7th U.S. Cavalry[4]

What is to be made of this letter to the *Bismarck Daily Tribune* by Donoughe? The editor was wary of it, stating that it "contradicts several points of history"; nevertheless, he published it on page one. After all, conflicting accounts of the battle by the various survivors was almost universal. There are several major discrepancies in this letter that are unresolved when compared with more reliable witnesses, but there is much that can also be corroborated.

To complicate matters there were two troopers with nearly identical names, John F. Donohue (also listed as Donahue and Donoughe), private, Company K, and John Donahoe (also Donahue, Donohue, and Donahue), saddler, Company M, born Galway, Ireland, in 1848. The former wrote the letter.

It is uncanny how Private Donohue of K Company happened to be situated so near as to overhear so much of his officers' conversation regarding plans for the troop movements and plans. In fact, some officers testified at the Reno inquiry about their doubts as to whether or not there was truly a coherent strategy for the battle. Further, he fails to describe Benteen's march to the left in spite of the fact that he was a member of Company K that went with Benteen, and he describes being in the battle in the valley with Reno. If he was with Reno, he must have been one of the troopers assigned to a unit other than his own.

His claim to have been "under the hand" of Dr. Porter implies some wound or injury although no evidence of this is available. He also claimed, unsuccessfully, that he was a water carrier.[5]

Perhaps his account has been dismissed as unreliable or possibly it has

8. Recalling the Battle

been overlooked and not commented upon. A most readable account of the battle, in fact, as has been already mentioned, Porter's favorite, was first published in *Century Magazine* January 1892 by Lieutenant Edward S. Godfrey, commanding officer of Company K.[6] In contrast to Donoughue, Godfrey held nothing but contempt for Reno as a leader. Porter was somewhat more charitable toward Reno, but as his testimony in the Reno inquiry and other published statements will reflect, he considered Reno an ineffective leader in battle.

George B. Herendeen, a white scout and survivor, was quite critical of Reno in a letter to the *New York Herald*. He believed that had Reno pressed forward in the valley, "Custer would not have been so roughly handled, as the Indians were contemplating retreat."[7] This seems completely unrealistic in light of the overwhelming forces that Reno met. Had Reno pressed forward or even persisted, his command would certainly have been totally eliminated.

Frederick Whittaker's *Life of Custer* was rushed to publication in 1876 months after the battle, and it impugned Reno's "incapacity" and Benteen's "disobedience." The *Bismarck Weekly Tribune* commented disdainfully:

> The book has been pretty generally read in this vicinity, and while it is as entertaining (to those not familiar with the facts) as one of Marryat's novels [Frederick Marryat (1792–1848) English sea captain and author of best-selling Victorian novels about the sea, many of which are still in print], it falls far short of satisfying Custer's friends while it provokes the hostility of many not recognized among his enemies, and is generally regarded as being entirely too sensational for a book aiming to give correctly the events worthy of note in the career of a man of unquestioned bravery, and undoubted ability, so organized, however, that disaster was certain to overtake him sooner or later.[8]

Elizabeth Custer, for as long as she lived, was a powerful force in protecting her husband's reputation versus Reno's. [She died April 4, 1933.) It is likely that some accounts of the battle were less objective or even distorted by the strong influence of Mrs. Custer and her allies.

Reno asked for, and was granted, a court of inquiry in the aftermath in an attempt to clear his name of cowardice, but it would not take place until January 1879. An account of Porter's testimony will follow.

The story of the battle has been told many times in articles, books, and film and is still a lively subject. Porter, as a participant, has appeared in Ernest Haycox's fictionalized *Bugles in the Afternoon* (1944) and in Dee Brown's *Showdown at Little Big Horn* (1964), a narrative of personal accounts of the battle supplied with dialogue "for dramatic effect."[9]

One of the interesting sidelights of the Little Bighorn is the story of Sergeant John Noonan, alias John McKinney, Company L, 7th Cavalry.[10] John rode out from Fort Abraham Lincoln with his company on May 17 with the

Terry-Custer column and continued across the plains and the Badlands. Upon reaching the Yellowstone Supply Depot, he was left behind to tend to the cattle herd. His company (L) went on to battle and their deaths, every man.

He returned to Fort Abraham Lincoln and was discharged as a sergeant when his term of service ended on January 14, 1877; he reenlisted on the same day as a private. His wife was a laundress at the fort and was known only as Mrs. Noonan. She had reportedly been married before to a man named Clifford in 1869 and to James Nash in 1871 before marrying Noonan in 1873.[11]

She had once been in the millinery business at Fort Leavenworth before coming to Fort Abraham Lincoln. The laundry work for her assigned company was done in a manner leading to "the best of satisfaction." It was said that she was as handy with a needle as any woman in the fort and had made fine shirts for several different soldiers. She served as a midwife, both on the post and as far away as twenty-five miles, always "giving good satisfaction." On the walls of her tidy house were beautiful pictures. When queried about her children, she would reply, "We were never blessed with any."

She became ill and, fearing the worst, asked for her priest, Father Chrysostrom of Bismarck, to be sent for to hear her confession, which he did on October 29, 1877.[12] Under the care of Dr. Wolveston, post surgeon, she lived until 5 A.M. the following morning. She left one request, that she be buried in the same clothes that she was wearing. This was disregarded. When her body was turned over to some of the women at the fort to prepare for a decent burial, it was found by them to their shock that Mrs. Noonan was a man. It was later determined that he was a Mexican who was familiar with all the towns and cities from the Missouri River to the Rio Grande.

When Sergeant John Noonan returned from the field with the 7th Cavalry under Colonel Joseph G. Tilford on November 22, he told a reporter from the *Bismarck Tribune* that he was convinced that she was a woman, and he would always believe so. "There is something dark and something terrible," he said. "Where will it end?"

His comrades had given him "a sort of cold shake" after their return from the Sioux chase, and he deserted from his unit not able to face the overwhelming shame and disgrace upon him. On November 30, he tragically shot himself dead through the heart with a pistol.[13] Soldiers found his body in the stables.

This had all been front page news in Bismarck, but the story does not end here. On the front page of the *Tribune* a month later on December 30, a headline proclaims, "From out the Depths of Hell the Spirit of Mrs. Noonan Re-Visits the Earth, and Through a Medium Relates her Sufferings in this World and the Next — her Name was Joseph Drummond and She was a Murderer — a Ghastly Narrative."[14] The article goes on to tell of a "trance medium" recently arriving in Bismarck who, with a "coterie of spiritualists," was able to communicate directly with the late Mrs. Noonan. She related a life of crime and mayhem to their curious ears. The world-wide fad of knocks, raps, and other communications with the dead had reached Bismarck at last.

From the beginning, public reaction had been a blend of amusement and consternation. In the initial newspaper account on November 4, the reporter speculated that Sergeant Noonan upon return "will probably swear when he hears the sad news. The deceased was in the habit of shaving every day, and in that way, kept down a heavy beard. He was a Mexican with course voice, and masculine looks all over. The secret of the unnatural union and apparel may be clothed in some dark mystery." [Pun?] Another account raised the question, "What could induce a man to live so long as Mrs. Noonan has, since 1873, with the garrison? It is a mystery." Finally in the ridiculous news story of the gifted medium on December 30, the reporter still refers to "the mystery that hung over the matter."

Reading the story over a century later, one would be less likely to see mystery than to see homosexuality in the 7th Cavalry, a topic that the public was not able to discuss at the time.

Chapter 9

Return to Bismarck

By the end of 1876 the Plains Indians had been almost completely subdued by the army. Many of them returned to reservations where they were relieved of their arms. Crazy Horse and his warriors would fight their last battle on January 8, 1877, in Montana, and he would be dead before the year's end. Sitting Bull, on the run, would lead a group of some 200 Indian lodges into Canada in May of 1877 to avoid annihilation.

After a year of perilous service, Porter left the army as contract surgeon in December 1876 and returned to Bismarck to resume practice as the town's second doctor. Dr. Slaughter was still there, and Dr. William A. Bentley would not arrive until July 1877.[1] Porter returned to what was, by then, home.

Bismarck was growing but still had a population of less than 2,000. During his first two and a half years in town, and before leaving for Little Bighorn, Porter had been unsuccessful in the drugstore business as co-owner and never returned to it. This did not deter him from other business ventures in the future. Times were hard and the Great Dakota Boom would not begin until 1878.[2]

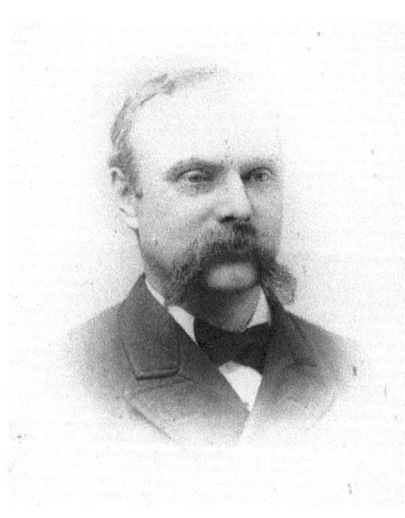

Dr. H.R. Porter. Photograph by D.F. Barry. (Courtesy Wyman Family)

Porter, twenty-eight years old, cut a handsome figure as he glided the Dakota snow in January in a "bran[d]-new cutter, a luxury that few in this vicinity care[d] to indulge as sleighing in the country is 'mighty onsartin,'" according to the *Tribune*.[3]

He opened his practice in March as physician and surgeon, with an office opposite the *Tribune* block on Main Street.[4] Bismarck's first major fire broke out the same month on the night of the 15th in the Arcade Saloon and destroyed the heart of the town. Wooden buildings like the Miners Hotel, Ostlund's Livery Stable, Joe Hare's Billiard Hall, Dunn's Drugstore, John Yegan's City Bakery, John Boyles's Saloon, the Western Hotel, and Sloan's Meat Market all went up in smoke.[5] The fire engine that the town had ordered had not yet arrived. There were no hooks and ladders, and precious little water. Fortunately, Porter's office was spared. Bismarck's buildings went up like tinder in several very destructive fires that occurred during the 19th century.

Stagecoaches rambled from Bismarck to the Black Hills early in 1877. With stations at twenty-mile intervals and hundreds of teams available, the North Western Express State and Transportation Company carried passengers in Concord coaches and freight in canvas covered wagons from Bismarck to Deadwood. An early settler claimed that it was "a sight to see ten yoke of wild Montana cattle strung out hauling two and three canvas covered wagons loaded with freight."[6]

In the spring Porter met Charlotte Viets, a cultured young lady, twenty-three years old from Oberlin, Ohio, who had studied music in the conservatory at the college. She was in Bismarck to visit her sister, Helen, wife of Bismarck banker George Fairchild, and spent the winter of 1876–77 there.[7] She left Bismarck for Oberlin on April 18.[8] There is no evidence to suggest that Porter had met her before he left on the Custer expedition in May 1876. They were to be married later in the summer.

There were few opportunities for eligible bachelors to meet educated women such as Charlotte in the booming and brawling frontier town of Bismarck. Of interest is the fact that Dr. Slaughter's wife, Linda, was also a graduate of Oberlin College and was a most remarkable woman who concerned herself with education, temperance, and women's issues. She served as Bismarck's first postmistress, first superintendent of education, and first Sunday school teacher. She later wrote features and historical articles about early Bismarck for the newspapers.

Once she clashed with Custer over the mail sacks.[9] When the first weekly mail was delivered to her overland after the Northern Pacific Railroad ceased to run in 1873, it was brought by Custer's mail carrier first, by way of Fort Lincoln, rather than to her. Since it could not be unlocked without a key, Custer sent his orderly to Linda to request the key. She allowed him to have it with the stipulation that the Bismarck mail be sent back as soon as possible. The next day, the mail returned to her as "a hopeless jumble of letters" with every package untied and mail to the surrounding forts in complete disorder. She requested that her key be returned, which Custer at first refused, but then she made the case to him that it was only out of respect for his position that she had allowed him to have the key in the first place, since it was against mail service regulations. He returned the key.

When the next mail arrived, Custer ordered his sergeant to get the key; she refused unless Custer would send her a written guarantee that it would be returned promptly. The sergeant reported this to Custer who angrily ripped the sack open with his pocket knife. She considered this a criminal act and reported Custer to the postal authorities in Washington who in turn contacted General Phil Sheridan, his superior, a close friend and admirer of Custer dating back to the Civil War. As might be expected, Sheridan laughed it off as one of those exigencies of the service. Mrs. Slaughter was able to clear up her problem with the mail much later only with the aid of General Hazen.

Porter made plans to return to the Tongue River country in Montana on the first anniversary of the battle "to view, under more favorable circumstances, the scenes made familiar by last summer's operations."[10] I suspect that he was not returning just to mark the anniversary as he suggested, but very possibly went to assist the army in identifying the remains of the officers for reburial. He had been present at the original burials and had knowledge that would have been essential to assist in the exhumations planned for July. He never mentioned this to the press, and we have no evidence for this other than a strong suspicion.

Lieutenant Colonel Michael V. Sheridan and Captain Henry J. Nowlin returned to the battlefield July 2nd with a "small detachment" of troops and some Crow Indians to recover remains of the officers and clean up the widely scattered bones.[11] Porter returned down the Yellowstone and Missouri Rivers to Bismarck on the steamboat *J.G. Fletcher* on July 9 along with the remains of "thirteen gallant heroes" in pine boxes that included those of Colonel Custer, Captain Keogh, Captain Custer, Captain Yates, Lieutenant Cooke, Lieutenant Calhoun, Lieutenant Donald McIntosh, Lieutenant Reily, Lieutenant Hodgson, and Dr. DeWolf. General Phil Sheridan spent most of July 21, 1877, at the battlefield with his brother, Michael, and General Forsyth. He not only studied the battlefield but also, with Troop I, 7th Cavalry, inspected where Michael had re-interred many of the bodies and had the field again searched for exposed remains. He recommended that the site be designated a national cemetery, which was done in 1879.[12] General Sheridan and his staff returned down the Yellowstone and Missouri rivers on the steamboat *Silver City* to Bismarck on July 27, 1877.[13]

On the day Porter had announced his plans to return to the Tongue River country, word of new Indian trouble arising near the mouth of White Bird Creek in Idaho reached St. Paul and Bismarck. A band of Nez Perce Indians retaliated against the murder of one of their tribe by killing his murderer, a white man, and three others. Another twenty-nine whites were soon killed leading to the murder of Chief White Bird and his family in retribution. The 1st Cavalry and 150 citizens pursued a band of some 2,000 warriors. The whole country was said to be "wild with alarm."[14]

9. Return to Bismarck

The nation was thus informed that another Indian war had begun. Chief Joseph had "vigorously opposed a war with the whites, and had done everything to avoid it."[15] But young hot bloods had instigated what would lead to the flight of the Nez Perce under Chief Joseph's leadership across the Rocky Mountains into Montana and the Yellowstone country of Wyoming and back into Montana, and then north toward Canada. As will be seen, this war would later touch the life of Porter and the people of Bismarck.

In late July the *Tribune* reported:

> From Dr. Porter, who has just returned from the Big Horn country, we learn that the boat upon which he came down the river, brought to this place [Bismarck] the remains of thirteen of the gallant heroes who fell with Custer.[16] They were accompanied by friends, and started East over the Northern Pacific this morning. The remains of Dr. Lord, Lieutenants Sturgis and [James E.] Porter, were not found. From the same source we learn that they are producing plenty of good whitewood lumber at Post No. 2 on the Big Horn, and everything seems prospering finely. No reliable intelligence from the gold hunters who have gone into the mountains. The doctor had a little experience in that wonderful hail storm of which mention was made a few days ago. He counted one hundred and seventy five Indian ponies killed by hail, and floating down the river. Six hundred were killed in all.[17]

Bismarck had a new hotel, the Sheridan House. When built in 1877 by E.H. Bly, proprietor, and S. McKenzie, contractor, it was the largest building in the territory.[18] It opened in late July.

It was a three-story structure built on Main Street between 4th and 5th Streets alongside the tracks of the Northern Pacific Railroad at the site of the present depot. It could accommodate 150 guests.[19] The rooms were heated by individual stoves and lighted by kerosene lamps. A wide platform extended along the entire railroad front. On the first floor there was a Northern Pacific ticket office, two "elegant waiting rooms," a telegraph office, a billiard hall and bar, a barber shop, a spacious hall with a staircase leading to the two upper floors, the dining hall with a twelve-foot ceiling and five chandeliers, and a fine kitchen having a large pantry and store room as well as a vegetable cellar and a wine cellar. This was the finest hotel of its day in the entire area and the one where major social events took place and where important travelers stayed. Porter himself lived there before building a home.

On August 20, 1877, Porter left Bismarck for Oberlin, Ohio, to be married to Charlotte Viets on the evening of September 4, 1877, at her parents' home in Oberlin.[20]

Lottie was the daughter of Henry Viets and his second wife, Samantha Joslin Viets. Henry, a wealthy real estate developer whose philanthropy extended to Oberlin College and its students, had five children: three (Henry Shelton, Edward, and Sarah Elizabeth) by his first wife, Sarah Elizabeth Boise, who died in 1844, and two (Helen and Charlotte) by his second wife, Samantha. It is said that Samantha "played no favorites" and "reared all the children with equal concern and affection."[21] Samantha was a teacher who had enrolled in the literary course at Oberlin College, the first coeducational college in America, studying there from 1844 until 1846.

Helen Josephine Viets, Samantha's first child, was born in 1846, educated at Oberlin College, and married in 1866 to George Hornell Fairchild, one of Bismarck's earliest and most prominent settlers, of whom more is to be heard.

Charlotte Jane Viets, "Lottie," was born July 1, 1853, in Huntington, Lorain County, Ohio, before the family moved to Oberlin. She was enrolled in the preparatory department at Oberlin College from 1868 to 1872, the conservatory of music from 1868 to 1872, the college from 1872 to 1874, and the conservatory of music again from 1874 to 1877.[22] She was a woman of education and culture with musical talent. The wedding was an elaborate home affair held on the evening of September 4. Large vases of white lilies with trailing vines were brought in from Cleveland to decorate the parlor. The bride wore a gown with no hoops, a long train, a wreath of white flowers around her neck and body, and orange blossoms in her hair. "The Dr. looked nicely too," according to the mother of the bride. She said, "I was surprised at myself for feeling like giving up Lottie to his kind care and protection with no misgivings."[23] Lottie's half-sister, Sarah, said, "I liked Dr. Porter very much indeed — he improves with acquaintance [a statement lifted directly from Jane Austen's *Pride and Prejudice*]. I feel from what I have seen of him that he has just the disposition suited to Lottie and will be so kind to her. I think he has a great deal of charity for everyone which is one of the best of qualities." George and Helen Fairchild were in Bismarck unable to attend the wedding due to George's illness, a bilious fever. His father, President James Fairchild of Oberlin, was present as were many family members and friends.

The couple left for New York Mills, New York, to allow the groom to introduce Lottie to his family and to show her by carriage "the familiar

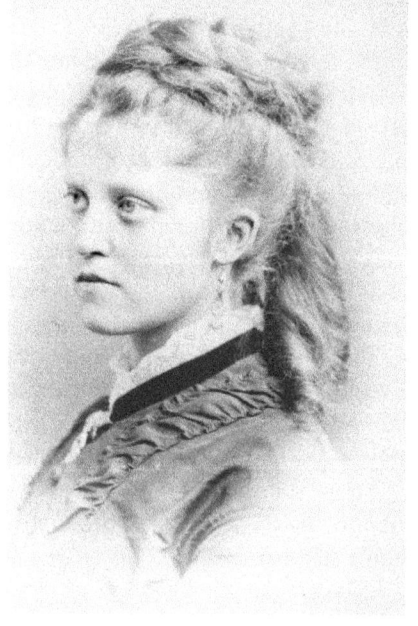

Charlotte Viets Porter, wife of Dr. H.R. Porter (courtesy Wyman Family).

9. Return to Bismarck

places of his childhood and early youth." They returned by ship from Buffalo, New York, through the Great Lakes to Duluth.

Back in Bismarck from their "wedding tour" on September 20, they moved into the Sheridan House.[24] Porter returned to his medical practice and to his ever-growing involvement in real estate and business dealings. It was clear to him that Bismarck had all the ingredients for growth, a new railroad connection, a vital port on the Missouri River, an army base, Fort Abraham Lincoln just across the river in Mandan, and an agricultural center on the frontier of the Dakota Territory. Porter shrewdly capitalized on this by taking larger and larger stakes in Bismarck's economy. The *Bismarck Tribune* documented his accumulation of wealth over the next quarter of a century.

Items such as the following appeared the month after his marriage: "Dr. Porter has contracted with Joe Pennell to break [plow] his seventy five acres near the cemetery next spring."[25] In the following month: "Dr. Porter has sold ten acres on the old W.S. Brown homestead to Geo. A. Jay at twenty-five dollars an acre. The Doctor will retain the balance and improve it from year to year."[26]

In publicity sent back East, Bismarck boosters described its merchants as sober and industrious and claimed that, as of 1877, there had never been a failure or bankruptcy on the court record.[27] The town's sphere of commercial interest extended west to the heart of Montana and south to Yankton and southwest to the Black Hills. A multitude of mules and oxen, both individually owned and company owned by the Northwestern Stage Company, plied the territory. Thirty-seven steamers on the river called at Bismarck. As for merchants, J.W. Raymond & Company stood at the top, carried a stock of one hundred thousand dollars, and made a lot of money for a small town. "Of no small importance, Mr. Fairchild conducts the banking business, and is a thorough-going and industrious gentleman." There were twenty-eight merchants and five hotels (Sheridan, Capital, Merchants, Custer, and Western), "all keeping busy [with] no time to inquire whether Gentile or Jew, but to use a western phrase, 'take in their chuck, pay their bills and go.'"

The *Bismarck Tri-Weekly Tribune* caught some of the expectations and shamelessly promoted the struggling town.

> Bismarck grows daily, almost, in size, and the public spirit of its inhabitants is as rampant as ever. New buildings are going up, and the town is assuming a substantial air. Officers and surveyors of the Northern Pacific [Rail] road are now preparing to push on the work of finishing the road to the Montana borders. The surveyors only await a proper military escort, which our skeleton army cannot provide now, every post near here being so lightly garrisoned that not a man can be spared. Brave exiles of Erin, with pick and shovel, stand ready to toss up the clods, and in the limitless future to pound in the golden spike of the last tie between Lake Superior and the Pacific.[28]

In truth, the railroad was in receivership and would not be able to resume construction westward until it could be reorganized. Bismarck would not fully recover, as a boomtown, for another five years, but there was plenty of hope for the future.

Chapter 10

Hail to the Chief

The Nez Perce War had just been concluded in October 1877 with Chief Joseph's surrender of his ragtag band at Bear Paw in northern Montana to Colonel (Brevet Major General) Nelson Miles as they tried to escape into Canada. Joseph made his famous speech that concluded with the following words:

> It is cold and we have no blankets. The little children are freezing to death. My people, some of them, have run away to the hills, and have no blankets, no food. No one knows where they are—perhaps freezing to death. I want to have time to look for my children, and see how many of them I can find. Maybe I shall find them among the dead. Hear me, my chiefs. I am tired; my heart is sick and sad. From where the sun now stands I will fight no more forever.[1]

It is said that the officers present were affected by the power of his words. A sense of relief swept the battlefield. In the words of the historian Josephy, "the troops fraternized with the Indians, trying to show their friendship and respect for a brave and manly foe. Roaring fires were built, hot food and blankets were distributed, and the shivering and starving people were revived by the warmth and cheer in the soldiers' camp."[2]

Colonel Nelson Miles was impressed by the valor of Joseph and his people and attempted to ease their path, but he was possibly thwarted by the hostile attitudes of his army superiors, Generals Sheridan and Sherman, toward the Indians. The 1,700-mile retreat of the people began when Chief Joseph and the Nez Perce resisted a forced move to a reservation far from their native lands in Idaho. This led to violence and war.

After surrender, the Indians were considered as prisoners of war. The sick and wounded warriors and some women and children were sent downriver on flatboats, 32 × 8 feet, made of whipsawed lumber and caulked with pitch and tar.[3] They were given rations of hard tack, green coffee, flour, baking powder, rice, navy beans, and salt. The strong traveled on army wagons. They reached Fort Buford on the way to Bismarck and Fort Abraham Lincoln with the ultimate destination of Fort Leavenworth, Kansas. There was grave concern among the Indians that they would be hanged, especially the leaders.

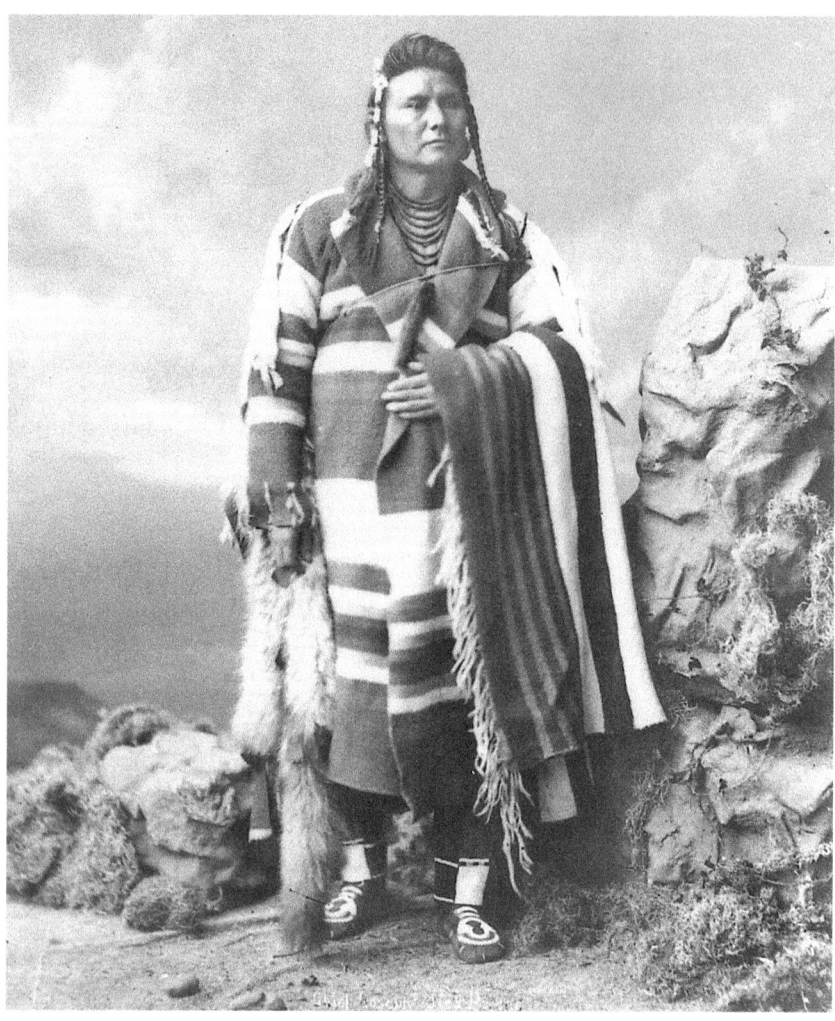

Chief Joseph, Nez Perce chief, before 1877. Photograph by William H. Jackson. (National Archives [American Indian Select List 102])

Joseph, his band, and their military escort arrived on Monday, November 19, 1877, one of the big events in the history of Bismarck. A military band from the fort was on hand. They arrived in wagons with mixed loads of "warriors, old men, women, brilliant forest maidens, and cute little papooses in the general muddle."[4] The whole town turned out to welcome the soldiers and "see their trophies." Five companies of the 7th Cavalry and two of the 1st Infantry led the battered wagons under the command of Colonel R.E. Johnston into Bismarck. It appeared to be a "strange and unusual review" to the onlookers. The wagon train had traveled 700 miles from the battlefield at Snake Creek. This was the first real halt for the soldiers and the Indians all summer. The last 250 miles from Fort Buford had taken nine days, a rapid march for a wagon train of that size.

The caravan entered town with General Miles and Chief Joseph on his left in advance.[5] Army troops surrounded the Indians forming a hollow square. Fred Bond, a flatboater who brought twenty-two Nez Perce Indians downriver, described a stampede at the corner of Main Avenue and 4th Street where women and children and some men "rushed the hollow square with all kinds of cooked food." He saw his restaurant waitress "beating her way through the hollow square with one half of a boiled ham." The command halted while the Nez Perce prisoners were supplied with "food of a good kind."[6]

Learning that Miles would be in Bismarck, a group of citizens hastily arranged a banquet to be held the evening of arrival in his honor at 9 P.M. at the Sheridan House, the fine new hotel. Some 150 guests attended. "A reference to the bill of fare will show that it was an elaborate one and would have done credit to any eastern city." After the supper, the 7th Cavalry Band from the fort entertained. Wine and speeches followed. Toasts to Miles were warm and felicitous, and in return he praised the energy and intelligence of the frontier people and recognized the progress made by Bismarck during the preceding fifteen months with every confidence in its future. Most important, he "alluded to [Chief] Joseph and the wrongs suffered by his people in a most feeling manner," sentiment rarely heard from a victorious commander about the losers. Much was made in the speeches of the value of the railroads, specifically of the Northern Pacific line to the army.

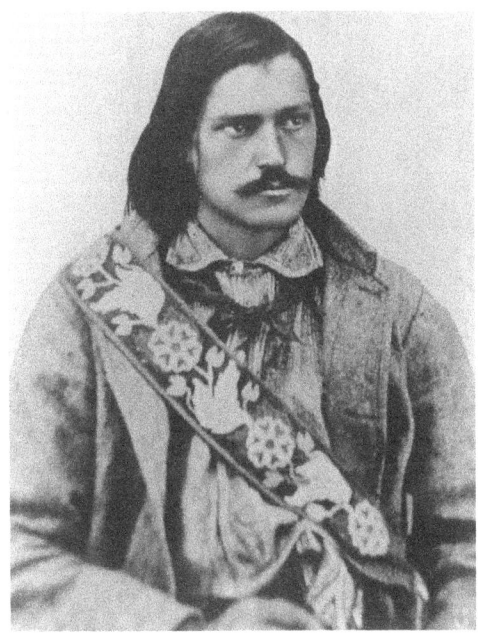

Luther Sage "Yellowstone" Kelly, famous scout who attended a banquet for Chief Joseph in Bismarck (National Archives [99670]).

The laconic Luther S. Kelly, known as Yellowstone Kelly and regarded by General

Miles as "the best, the truest and most resolute scout in the Army," had accompanied Miles to Bismarck and at the banquet was called upon to make some remarks.[7] He was regarded as a "strange, brave man" whose "quickness with the rifle" and many dead shots had led to the name of Man-who-never-lays-down His-Gun and the Lone-Wolf. He declined to speak of himself but said, "the home of the scout [is] on the prairie and in the mountains, surrounded by the broad expanse of nature, creating a feeling of quiet and repose which had become so instilled in his nature as to make it difficult to express himself, but his good right arm and his trusty rifle would ever be found in defense of his country and his friends."[8]

While in Bismarck Chief Joseph "expressed his confidence in Miles and evidenced his belief in the white chief's ability to help him return to his home in Idaho. He said he loved his country as he loved his mother."[9]

A local reporter noted that "most of them had never dreamed of as much civilization as they have seen in Bismarck. Yesterday [Tuesday, November 20, 1877] the more enterprising heads, squaws and their papooses waddled from sidewalk to street and took in the sights as modestly as captives would naturally be expected. They bought some things and in one instance at least, sold seven dollars worth of pure Idaho gold dust."[10]

Two days later there was another invitation. Through an interpreter the invitation was given to and accepted by Chief Joseph, Yellow Bull, Shaved Head, and Yellow Wolf as evidence of warm feelings from the people of Bismarck. Lavender calls this invitation "unique in the history of Indian warfare."[11]

> Bismarck, D.T. Nov. 21, 1877
> To Joseph, Head Chief of Nez Perces [sic]
> Sir: Desiring to show you our kind feelings and the admiration we have for your bravery and humanity, as exhibited in your recent conflict with the forces of the United States, we most cordially invite you to dine with us at the Sheridan House, in this city. The dinner to be given at 1½ P.M. today.
>
> Respectfully,
>
> Geo. W. Sweet
> H. R. Porter
> Wm. A. Bentley, Committee.[12]

At noon Joseph and the other chiefs were presented to a number of ladies of the house, probably including Mrs. Porter who, with her husband, was living in the Sheridan House at the time. The respect accorded the Indians was "on account of their humanity" to the U.S. soldiers taken as prisoners during the war. This was a most remarkable difference from that experienced with the Sioux Indians a year earlier.

The committee that extended the invitation was an impromptu affair not representing any organization. It included George W. Sweet, referred to as Colonel Sweet, a Bismarck lawyer and real estate broker, and two physicians, Porter and William A. Bentley.[13]

It was reported that the dinner was the "first square meal" that the Indians had enjoyed since they left Idaho five months earlier. Yellow Wolf asked if he might have salmon and when served he was "tickled." Joseph said it called to mind his own country. Observers noted that the Indian chiefs "handled knives and forks as if they were meant to eat with." Joseph was seen to use a napkin appropriately. The menu included potatoes, cabbage, beans, roast beef, salmon, pies and pudding, truly a feast for the malnourished Indians.

Arthur Chapman, a white man married to a Umatilla Indian and well known to the Nez Perce, interpreted all communication between the races.[14] Colonel Sweet, who had spoken on the importance of the railroad to Bismarck at the Miles banquet two days earlier, spoke to the chiefs:

> Friends, by that name I will address you. We have invited you to meet us, not to show a triumph over the vanquished, but in good will, and to show you that we harbor no hostility to you, but rather regret the circumstances that have placed you in your present condition. In ancient times, the successful warrior returning from war, exhibited his prisoners in chains, in order to heighten the splendor of his victory, and then condemned the poor prisoners to a life of slavery. Now all this changed; the white man has learned to be more generous to the conquered. He has learned that peace has greater victories than war. When the red man learns this lesson he will bury the hatchet, and seek those things which lead to peace and goodwill towards all men. It is to be hoped that he will yield to the changed condition of things, and live the friend and brother of the white man, as there is room enough for all of us, if we will only occupy the space that is necessary for us in which to procure the means of living. Allow me to repeat again, that we have no feeling of animosity toward your people, or race, but welcome you to our city and wish you health and happiness wherever you may go, and if we should never meet you again here we hope to greet you in the happy lands beyond the gates of death, where there will be no such struggle for existence.[15]

Sweet's conciliatory speech set the tone for the responses that followed from the chiefs. Neither Porter nor Bentley spoke, but it is likely that they had selected the silver-tongued lawyer and realtor to express their sentiments. Porter, not known as a public speaker, was at his best as a convivial conversationalist.

Shaved Head responded to Sweet after reflecting for a moment:

> Yes, today, my friends, I want to speak the sentiments I hold in my heart. I am thankful for the expressions I have heard the white chief make. I am thankful just as if I had shaken hands. Shaking hands and eating dinner together are both alike. They express the same sentiment of friendship. Inviting to dinner is making friends. I hope we will never be enemies but live in one house hereafter and

our children grow up together. I speak from the heart. Where the sun is today is the witness what I have said. [Shaved Head used the same formula as that pronounced by Chief Joseph at the end of hostilities, "where the sun is today."] That is all I have to say.[16]

Then Joseph rose, as if embarrassed, to speak and began somewhat tentatively:

My friends, as many are gathered here together, probably understand me and my heart. I always talk freely and plainly among my people and they understand me and obey. I always try to entertain good sentiments in my heart and I would now make you understand that I entertain them at this moment. Just as we plant a good tree to grow good fruit, I kept good sentiments to make a good man. All of us should have good sentiments and express them. If everybody did, there would be no trouble all the world over. Those who live with good sentiments never have trouble. I expect what I speak will be said throughout the land, and I only want to speak good.[17]

At this point Joseph, overcome by emotion, "broke down." The reporter concluded that "he was evidently affected by the kindness of his white brethren, and the latter were not a little taken in — willingly though." It is remarkable that a people living in a tough frontier town only four years old could suspend their anger and ill feelings toward Indians and embrace Joseph and his band in their captivity with such kindness and affection. Porter himself, who had known the savagery of Indian battles firsthand, must be credited with great strength of character to sponsor and attend the banquet for Joseph and the chiefs. It was easy for the citizens of Bismarck to entertain Colonel Miles; it was magnanimous to entertain Chief Joseph.

Bismarck gave a party that the Indians could never forget and the rest of the country could not understand.

The *Bismarck Tri-Weekly Tribune* editorialized:

As we suspected the first Eastern journal received containing a notice of Bismarck's banquet to Joseph would be puzzled to understand its meaning. The *Saint Paul [Minnesota] Pioneer Press* editorially comments as follows, and we have no doubt every other prominent journal in the country has followed suit: "A remote frontier outpost, within arm's length, so to speak, of the locality of Indian wars and Indian outrages, certainly near enough to form a rational and unclouded judgment of Indian character, is a curious place for the epidemic of sentimentalism in Indian affairs to breakout. The complaint has heretofore been confined to civilized points where Cooper's red man was the typical savage. The disposition to lionize Chief Joseph and his Nez Perce ... which is so apparent in Bismarck, must have some root not readily comprehensible at this distance. Certainly he has gained golden opinions from those worthy citizens during his short visit, which are altogether inexplicable upon the supposition that he is the average dirty, sullen, uninviting savage. He has been entertained like a prince, and his levees have been crowded with the elite of Bismarck society, men, women

10. Hail to the Chief

and children. It is possible that the noble red man is not a myth and that in Joseph we have a veritable latter day Uncas [chief of the Mohegan Indians who sided with the British in the Pequot War]? He and his braves will soon pass through St. Paul, and an opportunity to solve this knotty point will be afforded."[18]

The *Tribune* editorial answered the St. Paul newspaper's querulous comments forthrightly:

In the first place the banquet was only a "square meal." Joseph and his chiefs, however, considered it in light of a banquet or something in every respect its equivalent. All Bismarck wasn't there and all Bismarck didn't appoint "the committee" that extended the invitation, but we have yet to hear a single man take exception to the proceeding. On the contrary the universal opinion of those who have communicated with or observed Joseph's band is emphatic in its leanings that Joseph has been swindled, cheated and lied to, that he has been more sinned against than the public is aware of, and from the standpoint that he had a country of his own and was entitled to it, has been virtually driven into the position he now occupies. Bismarck people understand the swindling and cheating that have been at the bottom of the Indian troubles and are well advised that the Indian agent, who made in a short time $200,000 by close economy (as General Miles narrated in the speech at his banquet) is no myth but a veritable living animal. They believe Joseph is a decent Indian, that he thought he was doing right when he refused to leave his own Walla Walla [sic, Wallowa] and occupy a reservation that he never agreed to enter upon; that he did as Gen. Lee did, or as the average white man would under similar circumstances; that he means to do right and is not the treacherous red dog that many of Fenimore Cooper's typical savages are; that he is one of those products of primitive life whose word is better than our written law and who is absolutely ignorant of the deceits, guile, diplomacy and double-dealing of civilized life. He is, however, beginning to see there is a screw loose in our grand makeup, for he now asks this unanswerable question, "When will those white chiefs begin to tell the truth?" Joseph's band as it left here [Bismarck] has hardly a bad Indian in it and we believe they will make a quieter and more peaceable colony than Kansas [Fort Leavenworth] has received for a many a day. Their four days residence in Bismarck has shown them respectable guests. They have not been under strict surveillance but have been permitted to roam around as they saw fit. They have neither been thieves nor drunkards and their loafing has been strikingly respectable compared with some other people we could name. We don't take any stock in Sitting Bull, but we do believe Joseph is one of Cooper's good Indians.[19]

To cash in on the respect and good will of Bismarck and the celebrity in town, a photographer, J.B.C. Fouch, advertised portrait photographs of Chief Joseph in sizes from cartes de visite for fifty cents up to 11 × 14 inch prints for four dollars.[20]

Joseph and his band of 400 left Bismarck for St. Paul on eleven rail coaches on Friday afternoon, November 23. Many had never seen a train before. They had liked Bismarck for a good reason; the people had been good to them.

The city of Bismarck has received neither sufficient recognition for its hospitality to Joseph and his people nor the understanding that the dinner was an attempt to right a wrong visited upon the Nez Perce by the white man. The kindness shown has come close to becoming only a footnote in Chief Joseph's story and is only scarcely recalled.[21] Miles' attempt to gain mercy for them failed when his superiors balked, but his attitude was crucial in leading Bismarck to respond as it did.

Porter's involvement as one of three signers of the invitation to Chief Joseph to the banquet is one of the bright spots of his entire life. He was willing to risk criticism in order to stand up for his beliefs and lead the people of Bismarck in showing kindness to a woefully mistreated tribe of Indians.

Chapter 11

Early Business Ventures

Porter was not content just to practice medicine. He actively pursued opportunities to make money. One of the first of these after Little Bighorn was to develop a new railroad, despite it being a poor time to raise money for such a project. Nevertheless, articles of association were filed with the district court on November 21, 1877, for the development of the Bismarck, Fort Lincoln and Black Hills Railroad, a narrow-gauge track proposed to go 240 miles and cost $2,400,000.[1] It would pass through Burleigh, Morton, Delano, and Lawrence counties and the Sioux Reservation and serve as a line to the Black Hills where a gold rush was underway. Signers were Porter, Sweet, and Bentley of the recent committee that entertained Chief Joseph, as well as J.W. Raymond, Edmund Hackett, Colonel C.A. Lounsberry, William Thompson, John A. McLean, Thomas J. Mitchell, C.M. Cushman, John P. Dunn, John A. Stoyell, and John Rea.

J.W. Raymond went to Chicago in March 1878 to promote the venture and there told investors that $250,000, of the needed capital stock of $1,800,000, had already been pledged. Porter was a member of the board of directors. "The officers think they see their way clear to raise the whole amount necessary," Raymond told a reporter.[2] He indicated that the shortest survey showed it to be 225 miles from Bismarck to Deadwood and that "the route proposed traverses a region of country only slightly undulating and presenting no problem at all." The Northern Pacific Railroad had agreed to assist by offering discounted rates in moving construction materials for the new line, since it was anticipated that it would serve as a feeder for the Northern Pacific. Unfortunately the railroad was never built. The corporation was dissolved February 7, 1880.[3]

On December 18, 1877, a prairie fire "got away" and engulfed George Fairchild's house on his homestead a mile and a half north of town. All was lost except for the front door and a window, the only items salvageable by Porter and Fairchild when they arrived. Loss was estimated at one hundred dollars.[4] Fortunately, Fairchild's home was in town.

The surgeon general of the Army offered Porter another contract for a position as acting assistant surgeon on December 29, 1877; however, Porter respectfully declined by saying, "I appreciate fully and thank you for the honor thus conferred."[5] He had begun to enter very aggressively into the private practice of medicine and the business world of Bismarck and had no interest in the modest income of an army surgeon.

Not all was bad news for Porter's brother-in-law. Early in 1878, George Fairchild founded the Merchants Bank of Bismarck, "a financial institution that any city in the northwest might be proud of."[6] He dissolved his partnership with J.W. Raymond in the Bank of Bismarck. It continued to operate under Raymond until 1882 when he organized Bismarck National Bank and served as president, turning the assets of Bismarck Bank over to the new institution. This bank, Merchants, was later voluntarily liquidated with the assets turned over to the Bismarck bank headed by T.C. Power and I.P. Baker. Raymond would go on to serve as treasurer of the Dakota Territory, then move to Minneapolis to a distinguished banking career as president of the National Bank of Commerce and president of the Northwestern National Bank. The *Tribune* reported that, concerning Merchant's, Fairchild had given assurances "it will be universally recognized as 'safe' and abundantly able to negotiate all legitimate loans." The editor concluded, "George H. is entitled to a *banque*."[7] The bank opened with temporary quarters in Dr. Porter's building on Main Street near 2nd. It was said to occupy a neat and well lighted room and have a solid fire- and burglary-proof safe.[8]

Burleigh County commissioners elected Porter the county physician for the first time in January 1878, a post he would hold until 1890. He would care for indigent patients along with his private practice.[9]

In January Porter bought fourteen lots from George P. Flannery, a local lawyer, to make a significant beginning to his real estate dealings.[10] His timing was perfect. The Great Boom had begun.

In mid–March the *Tribune* reported that although the ice in the Missouri alongside Bismarck had melted and no ice was floating, the stagecoaches from Fort Buford and the Black Hills could not get to Bismarck because of snow.[11] The same issue of the *Tribune* announced that the Porters, who had been living at the Sheridan House, had "taken up their residence on Dr.'s handsome pre-emption claim overlooking the city." Under the Pre-emption Act settlers were allowed to claim a quarter section, 160 acres, improve it, and after six months buy it for $1.25 an acre.[12] On his 160 acres Porter planned to fence it, having already built a "neat little house and stable," and "planted a number of trees."[13] He rented the land with plans to sow eighty acres of oats the following spring. The *Tribune* commented, "It is a beauty too, and commands a fine view of the city and surrounding country."

Porter's business ventures continued apace along with his growing medical practice. He attended eleven cases of scarlet fever in April.[14] On March 25, Porter, along with ten associates, attempted to organize another railroad, the Bismarck and Lake Kampeska Railroad Company, an extension of the Chicago and Northwestern Railroad from its terminus at Lake Kampeska (near present-day Watertown, South Dakota) to Bismarck.[15] Several of the incorporators were associated with Porter's other railroad venture: Sweet, Mitchell, Lounsberry, and Thompson. Nothing came of their plans.

Little Bighorn was not forgotten. In August 1878, two years after the battle, the U.S. Court of Claims allowed Porter one hundred twenty-five dollars for a horse lost in the campaign.[16] It will be recalled that the horse saved Porter's life as he clung fast to its neck and ascended the bluffs where a defensive perimeter was established. The battle was *the* defining experience in his life. He would return to it or to the subject of it many times in the future. Porter was far from unique. The other participants did the same, attended reunions, told their stories, and published their memoirs.

Porter returned to Square Butte, not far from Medora, with Judge (of Probate) John Bowen and express agent Reed in mid–October 1878 on a hunting trip. There they found "plenty of [prairie] chickens but little big game that they could get at."[17] Porter had spent three nights in the same area two years earlier (May 31, June 1, June 2, 1876) at what was known as Custer's Snow Camp on the trail to Little Bighorn. Square Butte rises to an altitude of 3,345 feet in the rugged Badlands of North Dakota, not far from where Theodore Roosevelt would come as a rancher in 1883.

On another such trip an extraordinary runaway occurred. Porter and Judge Bowen "broke for the chicken grounds" in a fine new buggy behind a "high mettled steed" with their breech loaders and plenty of ammunition only to have the horse light out. "You ought to see that buggy and harness! Words are inadequate to the situation," said the newspaper. "The Doctor has not told us how he sat down and the Judge

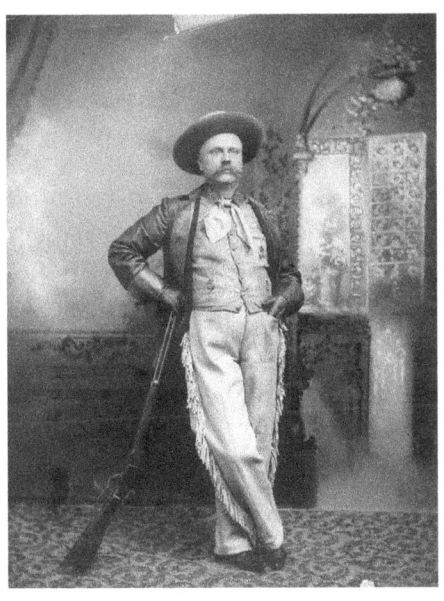

Dr. H.R. Porter in hunting attire, June 28, 1898 (State Historical Society of North Dakota 0264–27).

won't — so as they returned with a duck, horseless, buggyless, and right near bootless, we won't be harsh on the 'boys' this time."[18]

For hunting Porter wore a broad-brim felt hat, leather jacket, large leather gloves with gauntlets that flared half-way up the arm, a kerchief knotted at the collar of his shirt, a vest of fabric with embroidered flowers over the pockets, fringed buckskin pants, and pointed, well-polished cowboy boots.[19] The outfit was not dissimilar to that described by Theodore Roosevelt in his Dakota experience in *Hunting Trips of a Ranchman*.[20] Roosevelt described cowboy's dress as "a broad felt hat, a flannel shirt, with a bright silk handkerchief loosely knotted at the neck, trousers tucked into high-heeled boots, and a pair of leather 'shaps' [chaperajos] or heavy riding overalls." For hunting white-tail deer he found that "no dress is so good as a buckskin suit and moccasins. The moccasins enable one to tread softly and noiselessly, while the buckskin suit is of a most inconspicuous color, and makes less rustling than any other material when passing among projecting twigs."[21]

The Democrats nominated Porter for coroner in county convention on October 12, 1878, but he was defeated in the general election.[22] The Republicans were to nominate him for the same post in 1880 and he would lose again.[23] He was never thereafter active in partisan politics but was registered as a Republican.

Near the end of 1878 Bismarck boasted of over one hundred buildings growing from what had been a "collection of tents" to a population of 2,500. At the last election 626 voters voted.[24] "Bismarck prospers," the *Tribune* fairly shouted. Idlers were said to have been a thing of the past since anyone willing to work could find it. Nine first class steamers wintered at Bismarck that year allowing them to commence operations in the spring at least three weeks earlier than if they had been in St. Louis.

The Northern Pacific, recovering from adversity, was now planning another two hundred miles of track construction westward, but it would be some time before it could begin and service could be reestablished. Settlers were flocking in to within ten to twenty miles in all directions from Bismarck, and farming was becoming so successful that there was no further need to ship in oats or corn.

Bismarck was "in direct telegraphic communication with Deadwood, Fort Keogh [near the junction of the Yellowstone River and mouth of the Tongue River] and all points in central Montana." Service was available by stagecoach on the Fort Keogh line, Standing Rock line, Fort Buford line, and the Black Hills line.

Of the construction for improvements during the previous year, Porter spent two hundred dollars for a tenement and four hundred dollars for a dwelling and stable. The total value of construction in Bismarck came to nearly $100,000. There were now eight hotels, eight general merchandise stores, two banks, five dry goods and clothing stores, and seven restaurants as well as many small businesses and tradesmen. There were eleven lawyers; four physicians— B.F. Slaughter, H.R. Porter, W.A. Bentley, and Andrew Hogg; one dentist, A.T. Bigelow; and one pharmacy–Pioneer Drugstore, J.P. Dunn, owner.

Chapter 12

The Reno Inquiry

Even while shots were still being fired at Little Bighorn, troopers were blaming Custer for the terrible disaster. Fingers were soon being pointed at just about anyone in authority. Custer was only the first target. Reno and Benteen came next. Custer defenders were quick to accuse Reno of dereliction of duty. He had few personal friends to rush to his defense. Reno, in turn, blamed Gibbon for lack of support.[1] He also criticized Custer who, he believed, was "whipped because he was rash." The controversy soon spilled over into the newspapers.

After being attacked in print and having undergone an embarrassing, but unrelated, court-martial, Reno sought to be cleared of charges of cowardice relating to the battle. He had recently been found guilty of "conduct unbecoming an officer and a gentleman" that related to his interactions with Emily Bell, a captain's wife at Fort Abercrombie, Dakota Territory. While under suspension from rank and pay for two years, he requested a court of inquiry be convened to clear him of charges of cowardice at Little Bighorn.[2]

This was granted and summonses were issued. Porter was subpoenaed in late December 1878 to be at the court as a witness of Reno's conduct at Little Bighorn. The *Tribune* stated, "It has been the standing charge that Reno neglected or refused to go to the assistance of General Custer. Porter was an intelligent eye-witness of the scene. He is out of the army and his testimony will be free from all possible bias. He is nobody's friend, except history's."[3] Porter's integrity was unchallenged.

When asked en route to Chicago by a reporter of the St. Paul *Globe* about the case, Porter was reluctant to assign blame. He said that undoubtedly there was jealousy between Custer and Reno before the battle and that Custer and Benteen were not on friendly terms. "How did it come that Benteen was the leader [on the hilltop] when Reno ranked him in command?" the reporter asked. He answered, "Well the soldiers recognized the stronger mind and followed it. It will always be thus." Reporter: "Then I conclude that Reno did not cut much of a figure in the regiment?" Porter: "Reno was not a man to lead a regiment in such a time. Benteen took command naturally — just as strong men always do. It was not surprising." Benteen had no reticence in telling the same reporter that he believed Reno innocent of the charge of cowardice. The reporter then asked if he thought that the "massacre was due to the action of the lamented Custer himself?" to which he answered, "Most assuredly. In my opinion, it was the result of Custer's own actions, and it is an injustice to attribute the blame to someone else."[4]

Dr. and Mrs. Porter left Bismarck the week of January 6, 1879, with plans for Porter to accompany Lottie as far as Chicago; from there she would go to Ohio to visit her parents in Oberlin while he was testifying in the Reno inquiry.[5]

Before testifying, he made a brief trip to visit his parents in New York State. A local newspaper reported his visit:

> Dr. H. R. Porter having been called to Chicago as a witness in the Reno inquiry, quite unexpectedly to his friends here, made a short stop at N.Y. Mills. He stayed only one night, as he was obliged to return in time to reach Chicago yesterday [Thursday]. His opinion of the investigation is, that it will not amount to much; perhaps a censor at most. Dr. H. R. Porter was on the witness stand two days, and the reporter of the *Chicago Times* gives him this description: "Dr. Porter is a pronounced blond with a golden mustache, and like most other parties connected with the investigation looks out on nature out of a pair of blue eyes. Taking him for all in all, he appears to be a very agreeable sort of physician, one who would make it almost a pleasure to have a leg carved off through his instrumentality.[6]

The court of inquiry into the accusation of cowardice on the part of Major Marcus Reno convened at the Palmer House in Chicago, January 13, 1879. It was not until January 23 that Porter was called to testify and was sworn in as the fifth witness.

Colonel John H. King, 9th Infantry, served as president of the court. A reporter described him as "about five feet eight in height, his corners rounded off, and there is a perpetual smile on his face. His hair and his whiskers, which he wears in the English fashion, are a silvery color."[7]

Colonel Wesley Merritt, 5th Cavalry, another member, "had seen his fortieth summer [without] the slightest tinge of gray in his hair [and wore] a dark brown, coarse mustache with a comfortable Jeff Davis beard of the same color." Lieutenant Colonel W. B. Royall, 3rd Cavalry, the third member, was "a soldier of a scholastic and philosophical type [who did] not say much, but [thought] a great deal." First Lieutenant Jessie M. Lee, 9th Infantry, served as recorder. All appeared in dress uniforms as did Major Reno.[8]

Lyman D. Gilbert of Harrisburg, Pennsylvania, represented Reno. He would later serve as president of the Pennsylvania Bar Association. If his role was deflecting criticism from Reno, he acquitted himself well.

On the stand, Porter identified himself as a Bismarck surgeon who had served as an acting assistant surgeon under contract with the government on June 25 and 26 in Reno's command at Little Bighorn. As a contract surgeon he was a civilian, not active duty or a commissioned army officer, an important distinction. After the Civil War the Army Medical Corps declined to a very small but prestigious group with broad and difficult examinations required for entry. Contract surgeons were hired to meet needs for care on expeditions and the scattered frontier outposts. Only those in good health and of good character and graduates of the best medical schools of the time were hired. As civilians they served without rank or uniform and were considered to be equivalent to a second lieutenant in social standing. Of course, they were considered below surgeons in the regular army.

Testimony elicited from Porter indicated that he had heard an order given to Reno by Custer's adjutant about 1 P.M. on June 25 near the first tepee that contained dead Indians that directed Reno to charge the Indians just ahead. The adjutant advised Reno that Custer would support him. After this Reno's battalion went down to the river and crossed it but halted on the other side (the left bank).[9]

Porter stated that he carried no weapons into the battle. The horses, he said, were "high spirited and wanted to run." Reno offered Porter a gun but he declined it. The horses loped or trotted down to the woods without any opposition. Indians appeared to be driving their ponies down to the river. When the troopers got to the woods, they dismounted to form a skirmish line. At first Porter watched the fight behind the line, then he led his horse into the woods while searching for his orderly, who carried bandages and medicine. Shortly thereafter Porter learned that a man had been shot and briefly attended him. Not much later he heard Reno say that we would have to get out of there and that we would have to charge them. Men were coming from all directions searching for their horses. In the melee, the soldiers and the Indians were running toward the river.

Porter stated, "There were a few Indians between the command and me and I went out expecting to find the command charging the Indians, but instead of that, I found the Indians charging the command [Laughter]." He added, "They were all on the run. I got on my horse and let him go as fast as he could run and I passed some Indians and got to the edge of the river and my horse jumped in and crossed over with the rest of them."

Upon reaching the bluffs he first saw Lieutenant Varnum who said, "For God's sake men, don't run. There are a good many officers and men killed and wounded and we have to go back and get them." When he encountered Reno, Porter said, "Major, the men were pretty well demoralized, weren't they?" To which Reno replied, "No, that was a charge, sir." Porter differed and thought that the men were demoralized thinking that "they had been whipped."

After a few minutes the men on the bluff cheered, thinking Custer was arriving, but it turned out to be Benteen and his battalion. Safety in numbers fortified the morale of the surrounded troopers, at least for the moment. When asked what he was doing after Reno and Benteen merged forces, Porter told the court that they all went farther back upriver and found a little hollow for the hospital. He also told of Captain Weir going downstream a quarter or half mile.

Sharp firing from the Indians continued until dark, then ceased. Meanwhile, Porter was busy as the wounded were continually brought in. No troopers were brought up out of the bottom but seven or eight wounded, when reaching the bluff, "dropped off their horses."

Porter was critical of Reno. He testified, "I knew Major Reno was the actual commanding officer, but I thought that [Brevet] Colonel Benteen was the actual commanding officer. That was my impression." He then answered a series of questions relating to times and distances as well as various geographical points and features as well as the number of Indians engaged in the battle.

At this point the court adjourned on Thursday, January 23, to meet again on Friday, January 24, at 11 A.M. with Porter still in the witness chair. The *New York Times* reported:

> Dr. R. H. Porter [sic], who was Acting Assistant Surgeon under Custer, and was with Reno's battalion, was next put on the stand [after Lieutenant Varnum].
> From his testimony it seems that he understood that Custer was expected to support Reno. The adjutant had told Reno that Custer was coming along when Benteen was seen approaching after Reno had got to the hill. The men supposed at first that it was Custer coming to their relief.[10]

This is misleading. It should have been punctuated to read: "The adjutant had told Reno that Custer was coming along [to support him in the valley]. When Benteen was seen approaching after Reno had got to the hill, the men supposed at first that it was Custer coming to their relief." The information had been relayed by telegraph and incorrectly edited. Punctuation does matter.

The adjutant, Lieutenant William W. Cooke, nicknamed "Handsome Man" by the troops, had probably already been killed with Custer by the time Benteen's command arrived on the hilltop.

The *Chicago Times* reported that on the morning of January 24 the stenographer's transcript was reviewed and that "by the time Recorder Lee was ready to tackle Dr. Porter again the court room was comfortably full. The blonde Doctor gave his evidence in a straightforward fashion, and was not ashamed to admit, on cross examination, that he was a trifle excited when he started out of the woods to follow the command on its retreat to the hill."[11]

Lee asked further questions about the village and features of the terrain such as distances of points on the battlefield. Porter described the mortally wounded soldier whom he treated before the race to the bluffs. "I was just unbuttoning his blouse and saw he was wounded in the left chest. He was able to talk but I went out of the woods and did not see him again."

When asked about what he saw when he left the woods to reach his column, he replied, "I led my horse at about the same place where we went down. I saw the Indians running by. The command was also running. I had pretty hard work to mount my horse, but I finally got on. When I got out there were some Indians between the command and myself, and they were running and firing at the troops. I passed some Indians and quite a number of men. When I got to the river, there were, I should think a dozen cavalry men in the river, and some mounted Indians on the right of the bank, firing at those crossing. There were Indians riding behind too."

Q. When you came out and saw that condition of affairs, did you observe any officer attempting to do any thing to cover that retreat or prevent those Indians from riding down the column?
A. No, sir; I did not. I could not see the head of the column. I started at the tail end. I do not remember having seen any officer until I crossed the river.
Q. In what order was the tail end of this column?
A. It was in no order at all. Every man seemed to be running on his own hook (Laughter)....
Q. State your opinion, if you have any, in regard to the conduct of Major Reno in that timber — whether it was that of an officer manifesting courage, coolness and efficiency, such as would tend to inspire the command with confidence and fearlessness, or the reverse? [Reno's attorney, Lyman Gilbert, objected to the question because Porter was a doctor and not a military man, making him unable to render an expert opinion. Gilbert was overruled.]
A. I didn't see anything in his conduct particularly heroic, or anything that was the reverse. I thought he seemed a little embarrassed and a little flurried. The parties were coming in there pretty fast. I thought he didn't hardly know whether to stay there or to leave. That was my impression at that time.

Mr. Gilbert next cross-examined Porter, attempting to discredit his testimony by depicting him as a medical man without military experience or knowledge, but this was doomed to failure. Porter had more combat experience than many of the troopers in the expedition and was an intelligent and cagey witness.

"What kind of gun did Major Reno carry?" asked Gilbert.
"I think it was a carbine," Porter replied. "The same as the cavalrymen

carried?" "I don't know. I am not sure. I do not remember the gun particularly," Porter said.

Gilbert next tried to question Porter's ability to recall information while he was under battle conditions. "Were you so cool during the engagement that you perfectly observed the matters that were being transacted on all sides?"

A. I do not suppose I could take in every thing.
Q. Were you cool during the entire fight in the timber?
A. I was moderately cool. I expect I was a little excited, most of them were. (Laughter)
Q. Were you not so excited that you were unable to see and estimate a good many things that were being done?
A. I do not think my judgment was very much out of the way. I was not so flurried as all that.
Q. Did you ever say to any body that you were so frightened and so badly scared that you didn't see a great many things?
A. When I was on the run I was frightened; after I let my horse go [at maximum speed] I was frightened.
Q. Did you say you were frightened at any other part of the battle?
A. I guess so. I know I was. (Laughter)
Q. Have you not said you were so badly frightened that you were unable to see a great many things?
A. No, sir; I don't know that I have.
Q. Have you not used words that bear about the same meaning?
A. I do not know that I have. I never said I was not frightened. I have always said that I was.
Q. Did you never make a remark to that effect to Lieut. Maguire?
A. I perhaps made the remark that I was badly frightened going out of the woods for the river.
Q. Was that the only point at which you confessed to being flurried, or frightened?
A. No. I was probably frightened some on the hill. (Laughter)
Q. In point of fact you were, not being a military man, so badly frightened that you did not observe what was being done by Major Reno or any of the military officers?
A. No, sir; I observed every thing that was going on that came under my observation, every thing in my immediate vicinity.
Q. And at no point was your judgment obscured in respect to these matters by your fear?
A. No, sir; I do not think it was....

At this point the *Chicago Times* reporter commented:

Mr. Gilbert relinquished the witness at this point and Recorder Lee propounded a few more questions to him. Witness in answer thereto said the charge down the stream he spoke of referred to when they were riding down to meet the Indians. At the time the command was halted it was opposed or confronted by a force of Indians. A few shots were being fired at that time. He did not see any Indians in the timber. There was no firing in the timber as if hostile Indians were there. He did not know whether Major Reno saw the wounded man he attended in the timber. When he left the timber he did not suppose there were any men left in there. With regard to his excitement he stated that he was not particularly flurried until he came out of the woods and saw they were in a pretty bad fix. He did not want to go back to the wood. The Indians were between him and the command and seemed to be driving the troops. He had no arms with him and he struck spurs to his horse and let him go.

Recorder Lee — Indians have a fondness for medicine men.(Laughter)

At this point, Porter stated that he saw the Indian village moving away on the 26th of June. There was a large body of ponies and it seemed to him that the procession was about two miles long. He judged that there were about four or five thousand people in the village, including warriors, women, and children. He believed that the whole camp was on the move. The width of the village at parts was about one-sixteenth or a quarter of a mile and it was about two miles away from where he was standing. Returning to the *Chicago Times* report:

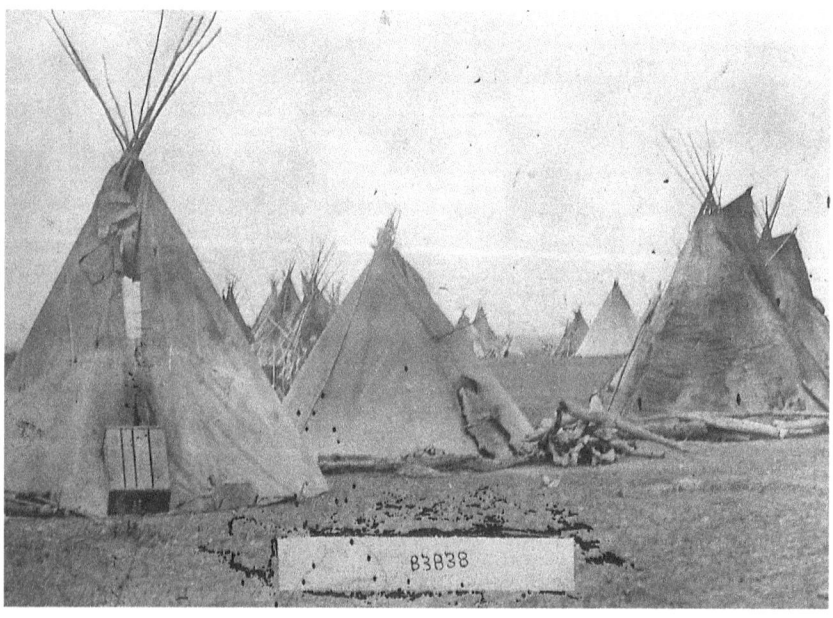

Sitting Bull's Camp (National Archives [83838]).

12. The Reno Inquiry

Q. [Mr. Gilbert] Are you accustomed to estimate the number of men moving in a body?
A. No, sir; I am not. I said several thousand. There might have been seven or eight thousand.
Q. If there were several thousand, what number of fighting men would there have been in the village?
A. I do not know, but I understood that one buck represents three, four, or five persons.
Q. Then if there were several thousand there would be about five hundred fighting Indians?
A. Well, I don't know about that.
Q. That would not be a formidable number of Indians for any command.
A. It seemed to prove pretty formidable for ours. (Laughter)
Q. Did you report that wounded man that had been left in the timber to Major Reno?
A. I do not know whether I did or not. I do not think I did.
Q. Was it not your duty to do so?
A. I do not know that it was my duty to report that. I think Major Reno knew about that man being wounded back there. I never thought about reporting him. It might have been my duty; but if it was, I neglected it.
A. Are you sure that Major Reno saw that wounded man?
Q. No sir; I am not. Everybody knew that there had been officers and men killed during the stampede. He knew it as well as I did.

The reporter concluded, "This wound up Dr. Porter, and he left the room with the admonition to come up and hear his evidence read over this morning."[12]

Unlike the official report, the *Chicago Times*' version is unedited by the witness and is informed by comments concerning the proceedings, such as "Laughter," or descriptions of Porter. The official report on a line-by-line comparison is less alive, as might be expected of the work of a court stenographer.

Porter proved to be a challenging witness for Reno's lawyer to discredit. His answers were precise and appropriately ironic. He refused to be led into making misstatements or unsupportable comments. Clearly, he had no admiration for Reno, who during the testimony tried to confuse him "by getting close to him and staring at him," but Porter was "imperturbable."[13]

The court of inquiry acquitted Reno after a hearing of twenty-six days and concluded "the conduct of the officers throughout was excellent and while subordinates in some instances did more for the safety of the command by brilliant displays of courage than did Major Reno, there was nothing in his conduct which requires animadversion from this court."[14]

In his analysis of the testimony, Pohanka points out that the strongest doubts about Reno's leadership came from the civilian witnesses, Porter, interpreter Girard, scout Herendeen, and mule packers B.F. Churchill and John Frett. It did not come from the professional military men.[15] Could officers be hesitant to criticize other officers publicly? This has been suggested but is probably wrong in this case. Benteen's forthright defense of Reno is no coverup for a fellow officer, especially one that he did not even like.

In August 1891 after Reno was dead, Porter made the following comment to a reporter in St. Paul:

> When we left Custer our hearts were light and we all felt that in a short time the hostiles would be ours. Little did we dream of what a bloody, sickening, disastrous fight would result and when we came on the village we saw that we were out numbered ten to one. Reno lost his head partly, and was unable to direct his men yet I think that he did all that he could and not have had his whole command massacred with Custer's. I was no friend of Reno's, but I wish to give the devil his due — not calling him a devil — and believe that he was an abused man. He was excited — who was not? — and might have done a little better had he not been so excited.[16]

Frank Anders, a historian of the battle who was born at Fort Abraham Lincoln in 1875, the son of a soldier, was of the opinion that "Reno saved the command on June 25th because he used common horse sense in getting out of the bottom. When he did, of course, he was aided by Benteen and others, but the responsibility was his and his alone. My father [Co. G, 17th Infantry] and mother knew Reno very well indeed. They never had anything to say except in his favor."[17] This seems to make a lot of sense. In the confusion of the battle, Reno's decision to return his troops from the valley to the bluffs to establish a defensible perimeter, in my opinion, probably saved the majority of his and Benteen's troops from the fate of Custer's.

Chapter 13

Banking on Bismarck

After the Reno court, Porter returned at the end of January 1879 to Bismarck to resume his practice. He added space to his office at 37 Main Street and acquired a horse for his rig that locals said "wouldn't take dust from anybody." He was again appointed county physician in 1879.[1] Along with lawyer John A. Stoyell, he was appointed commissioner of the insane of Burleigh County.[2]

In April 1879 Lottie Porter's prosperous father gave her a piece of valuable property in Oberlin.[3] Her wealth and Porter's seemed to rise in tandem. Seeing future economic growth in Bismarck, St. Paul businessmen were considering forming a new bank. Porter's brother-in-law, George Fairchild, already in the banking business, saw an opportunity for the whole family to participate. In a letter to his sister Mary (1846–1897) in March, he made her aware of the potential bank and suggested that it would be a worthwhile investment.[4] "My St. Paul Capitalists are seriously talking of organizing a First National Bank here July 1. I think it will be done. If any of you have money to invest in bank stock, it would be a good opportunity. I do not *see* how it can fail to pay good interest."

The First National Bank of Bismarck was organized in the offices of the Merchants Bank of Bismarck on August 6, 1879. The Porter and Fairchild families were among the major stockholders.[5] Walter Mann of St.Paul was elected president and George Fairchild cashier.[6] Porter, Fairchild, Dan Eisenberg, Asa Fisher, and Walter Mann were elected directors. Both Eisenburg, owner of a clothing store, and Fisher, a wholesale liquor dealer, were some of Bismarck's earliest settlers. Dr. Fannie Dunn Quain, daughter of pioneer druggist John P. Dunn, recalled the latter two in 1946, "Daniel Eisenburg came to Bismarck with 'a pack on his back' and lived here to be manager of a large department store in the Dakota Block and build a home — the second house north from Thayer on Fourth," and "Asa Fisher operated a liquor store and had banking interests. He built the home on the corner of Ave B. and Fourth which he sold to the State for the Governor's Mansion."[7]

Later that month Porter sold ten acres of his farm to J.F. Wallace for two hundred dollars and leased the rest of it for a number of years. Wallace had plans to grow small fruit — strawberries, currants, and raspberries — on the ten acres.⁸

With the recovery of the railroad, the first train to cross the Missouri River was an engine and flat car on a track laid across on ice three feet thick.⁹ This was on February 12, 1879. The following summer Porter was invited to ride on the Frank Thompson palace car on an excursion Sunday, August 31, 1879, to the end of the newly laid track. Track had already been laid westward from Mandan before the Missouri River was bridged. Frank Thompson, of Philadelphia, manager of the Pennsylvania Railroad, had sent his car to Bismarck to meet him and take him back East after an extended tour of Yellowstone Park. He did not arrive in time for the excursion on the new extension but invited a party of Bismarck men to ride in his car across the river to Mandan and the Coal Banks (Warnton), twenty-six miles away. Those less well connected rode on flat cars "having been arranged with seats for the occasion."¹⁰

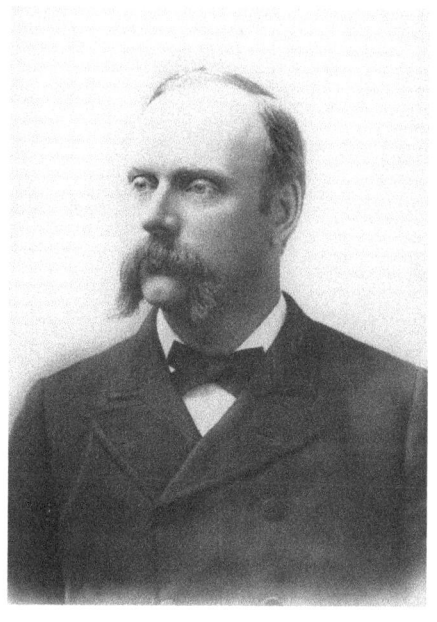

Dr. H.R. Porter. Photograph by B.F. Barry. (State Historical Society of North Dakota 00222-H-0021)

From Mandan a special engine took the cars to track's end. For those in Thompson's car such as Porter, "lunch and dinner were had on the car, and two better meals were never more relished than by this famished outfit. The car [was] fitted out with electric bells, and a waiter pops up in every direction at the request of any passenger. The car [was] lit by gas and heated by steam, contains a large library of railroad statistics, maps, etc., and its chairs suggest comfort and content."

The route taken by the excursionists carried them past Mandan through the beautiful stock-growing Heart River Valley that had "nutritious green grass" on the bottom levels and bluffs on either side. It was speculated that the coal banks at the end would be valuable someday. The place took the name of Warnton from its postmaster, John Warn.

In September Porter announced in the newspaper that he had been appointed U.S. examining surgeon for pension evaluations.¹¹ Examinations were done at his office at 37 Main Street, next to the *Tribune* building. His clientele were disabled veterans of the Civil and Indian wars who were eligible for small monthly pensions.[12]

As of the 12th of December, 1879, the First National Bank reported total resources of $130,717.16, with undivided profits of $1,600 as attested by its cashier, G.H. Fairchild.[13] The bank showed profitability from the start.

That winter Bismarck experienced brutally cold weather with temperatures dipping to twenty and forty degrees below zero for most of December. A fire in the downtown damaged several businesses but spared the First National Bank. It would not always be so fortunate.

Gentlemen in Bismarck celebrated the nineteenth century custom of formal calls upon ladies of their acquaintance on New Year's Day by stopping by for refreshments, wishing health and happiness during the New Year, and leaving their engraved calling cards. For New Year's Day 1880, Lottie received calls with her sister, Helen Fairchild, as well as Mrs. W.B. Shaw and Mrs. P.M. Eckford.[14] Helen had participated in the custom as early as 1875 when the *Tribune* noted that "in spite of frontier life and border civilization, Bismarck society did not permit the ushering in of a New Year without due observance of the customs long honored as belong to the season."[15] Among those listed as receiving their friends were Mrs. Fairchild and Mrs. W.B. Shaw. That particular day was said to be "severely cold, but the society men were resolved to do their duty, and there were no stragglers and none fell out by the wayside."

In M.H. Jewell's *First Annual Directory of Bismarck*, published in 1879, the population was now 2,800, of which 1,024 were men. The sheriff of Burleigh County at the time, Alexander McKenzie, was said to have "cleaned the city of the many crooks and blacklegs and established for Bismarck an enviable reputation for law and order."[16] (This assessment would be open to question later.) The Missouri River traffic was brisk. There were twenty-eight steamboats transporting goods and people between Bismarck and Pittsburgh, St. Louis, and Fort Benton. Wagon trains originating in Bismarck continued to carry tons of supplies to settlers in the Black Hills. Sitting Bull had not yet surrendered, as he would in 1881, and the Sioux Indians were still considered a threat to settlers. Therefore, Fort Abraham Lincoln, five miles away and across the river, was "one of the most important regimental military posts in the country." The Sheridan House Hotel was active and the most modern hotel in town. The *Tribune* was published at 41 Main Street, corner of Main and Second Street. The price at the time for a shave was twenty-five cents; a glass of beer was ten cents. The first man said to have reduced the price to five cents a glass was run out of town. In 1879 there were twenty-four saloons, six restaurants, eight hotels, 238 teamsters and stagecoach drivers, nine lawyers, four doctors, one dentist, and four bakers.[17]

For a small town, business activity in the late 1870s was at a fevered pitch. The Dakota Boom was underway. This provided the excitement that Porter thrived upon.

Business at the new bank was good; it was making money. A 6 percent dividend was anticipated and paid for July 1, 1880.[18] Another 6 percent was paid at the end of the year.[19]

Banker Fairchild saw many favorable opportunities to make money in Bismarck. He wrote to his father, "The town is filling up well this spring. The trains come in loaded every night and the boom for Bismarck seems about to begin." In addition to serving as cashier at the bank and running a small insurance agency, he was attempting to get a license as a trader at the Poplar River Indian Agency, about 600 miles up the river.[20] According to the *Tribune*, Porter had applied a new coat of paint to his office building in April 1880.[21] He also had a "fine, little store building for rent at 28 Main Street, next to Justus Bragg's meat market, "one of the neatest establishments in town."[22] (Bragg was Bismarck's mayor from 1885 to 1886.)

Porter was present when two silver spikes were driven in the track of the Northern Pacific Railroad at the junction of the Dakota and the Montana territories November 10, 1880.[23] A sleeper car and an observation car brought the railroad officials, army officers, newspaper men, and distinguished guests to the celebration where a large tent sheltered the participants. Colonel William Thompson, George P. Flannery, J.F. Wallace, Colonel C.A. Lounsberry, and M.H. Jewell, all of Bismarck, attended with Porter. Speakers praised the railroad's accomplishment of completing the Dakota section and looked forward to the eventual gold spike that would connect the railroad from both directions. After "a most excellent lunch in which the festive oyster figured conspicuously" and a supper and reception at Camp Huston on the return, they arrived back in Mandan about daybreak.

On May 23, 1881, a son named Henry Viets was born to the Porters. This, their only child, was announced in the *Tribune* by recalling that, "The fight of the Little Bighorn was a great event in the life of Dr. H.R. Porter, but it dwarfs into insignificance when compared with the event of Monday. His first child, a boy, weighing eight pounds, made its appearance, and the mother is as proud as the Doctor."[24]

George Fairchild wrote his sister Mary "to drop a line tonight to say that Lottie has the son she has been waiting for — born this morning 8 o'clock have not seen yet — say it is a very nice looking baby and Lottie is doing well and happy as can be. Dr. Porter telegraphed the Viets this morning but I thought you might not hear."[25]

Henry Viets was a delicate child and inclined in later years to music and travel. He was known as "Hallie" in childhood and "Hal" as he matured. The Porters were quite proud of their new baby.

Bismarck had a grand Fourth of July celebration that year. The planning committee was charged with arranging for a "proper recognition of our National Anniversary." Bismarck was "bound to outstrip all rivals," according to the *Tribune*.[26] Porter was a member of the Races Committee, an assignment in keeping with his love for horses.

A major event took place in Bismarck on Sunday, July 31, 1881, when Sitting Bull, after giving up his long fight, arrived by boat en route from Fort Buford to Standing Rock Agency.[27] A large crowd gathered at the levee to see the scantily dressed chief wearing smoked glass goggles. He was described as having jet black hair reaching below his shoulders hanging in three braids and wearing a pair of blue leggings, a blue blanket, a well-worn shirt ornamented on the sleeves with war paint, and moccasins. Much as Bismarck had done four years earlier when Chief Joseph was in town, it repeated with a reception at the plush Sheridan House and a dinner to follow at the Merchants Hotel held in honor of Sitting Bull. The following day the steamer *General Sherman* carried the chief and his party down to Fort Yates. Porter's friend H.F. Douglass, post trader at Fort Yates, headed up the group of travelers who accompanied Sitting Bull on the *Sherman* down to Standing Rock Reservation.[28]

In July Fairchild wrote his father, "Bismarck is improving this year a good deal — real estate is advancing all the time — 50 × 140 [building] corner of Main and 3rd St (the corner right down from our house and opposite Raymond's brick store) was sold yesterday for $10,000 cash by Sept. 1— The building [leases for] $215 per month."[29] Fairchild lived on the west side of Third Street north of Meigs where the Bismarck Theater was later situated.

The Fairchilds had a baby girl, their second, Katherine May, born in August 15, 1881, in Bismarck, and named for George's sister, Catherine, in Ohio. Their first child, Gertrude, born in 1869, had lived only fifteen months. Lottie said that her eyes were blue. She arrived slightly over two months after her first cousin Hal Porter. The two grew up together as close as any brother and sister and remained close throughout their entire lifetimes. Like Hal she was to be an only child.

Also in August, Porter was busy building a two story building on Third Street.[30] Plans were for it to be rented to the school board for a ward school.

In only five years since Little Bighorn, Porter's life had changed greatly. He was a prominent doctor, a family man with a wife and son, and was recognized as a respected citizen and businessman in a town on the cusp of an economic boom.

Chapter 14

A Capital Matter

In January 1882 George Fairchild thought that baby Katherine, now weighing twenty pounds, was the merriest baby he had ever seen.[1] His happiness was dampened, however, by his fear that some of the bank directors were trying to seize control of the First National Bank by buying up stock. Nevertheless, he felt the situation was under control since he and Porter had bought an additional fifty shares. They paid a fifteen per cent premium after the dividend to get them. He told his sister that the two of them had absolute control and that the others could never trouble them in this way again. But this was wishful thinking. The bank's major competitor, J.W. Raymond, Fairchild's old partner, was changing his bank into a competing national bank and opening it about April 1, 1882.

In Porter's practice of 1882 infectious diseases were common. In June a case of varioloid (a modified and mild form of smallpox) occurred on the steamer *General Meade*. As health officer for the port of Bismarck, Porter had the boat thoroughly disinfected and fumigated. He also vaccinated the crew of the famous steamer *Far West* before it left the night of June 1 for Fort Benton.[2]

Somewhat later the *Minneapolis Tribune* spread a rumor that there was a case of dreaded and widely feared Asiatic cholera (caused by *Vibrio comma*) in Bismarck. The paper presented the following account as copied by the *Bismarck Tribune*:

> It has leaked out here that the attending physician (Dr. Porter) would regard if he could trace any possibility of infection, as a genuine case of Asiatic cholera [that] has occurred in Bismarck, and that the patient is not yet out of danger. The sufferer is a prominent citizen [Henry Suttle] and it is understood that his symptoms are declared by Dr. Porter, who is one of the most eminent physicians of the state, and formerly surgeon in Custer's command, to be precisely like those of Asiatic cholera. The matter has been kept from the public to prevent alarm and the facts are secured only by an accidental revelation. There is some fear that the disease has been brought here by immigrants arriving from over the border and that in some way the gentleman attacked had been exposed without knowing it.[3]

Porter moved forcefully to squelch the false rumor by stating that one of his patients had sustained an aggravated attack of cholera morbus (once a popular name for gastroenteritis), not the dreaded Asiatic cholera. He had diagnosed it and said that there had been no attempt "to keep it quiet" and in referring to the article, called it a "lie" and attached to it an adjective that the newspaper said was "very, very expressive, indeed."

As surgeon for the Northern Pacific Railroad, Porter treated patients who had sustained major traumatic injuries. One such example was a workman struck in the neck by an iron rail that slipped off a moving freight train.[4] "One of the rails struck him on the back of the neck, cutting a fearful gash, and three other severe scalp wounds were made.... He was brought to Bismarck and treated by Dr. Porter." And there were lesser injuries. "Little Johnny Edick, while on his way to school yesterday fell and broke his wrist, or rather rebroke it, it having been broken before in the same place. Dr. Porter was the attending physician."[5]

Porter published a case report in a major medical journal of a fellow physician, Doctor S- (Slaughter) who fell off a sidewalk and sustained a clavicular (collar bone) fracture while making a night house call and who refused to let Porter splint it, yet who had a very good result healing with little displacement of the ends of the bone.[6] Porter stated, "I met the Doctor every day during the treatment of his fracture. He was very careful to walk on smooth ground, and the left arm received no unnecessary motion, and no treatment. The Doctor remarked that he had made worse jobs than that on other people, and I believe I have too."

Business in Bismarck was booming and had never been better than it was in 1882, and Porter was in the middle of it. He, Colonel William Thompson, and Orlando Scott Goff, owners of three Main Street lots on the north side at the corner of Second Street planned a three-story building with a seventy-five foot front and an eighty-five foot depth designed by Architect Carl Wirth to be completed before July 1, 1883.[7] They decided to call it Dakota Block and it was to be "first-class throughout."[8] Thompson owned the eastern section, Porter the center, and Goff the western. The building can be seen today on Main Avenue in downtown Bismarck (Main Street came to be Main Avenue over time). Fire destroyed the eastern section in the past, but the other two parts are still in use.

The First National Bank, now in its third year of business was paying dividends to its stockholders of 28 percent.[9] There was $8,725.25 of undivided profits. Bonds deposited to secure circulation were worth ten thousand dollars more than cost. George H. Fairchild was named president on January 26, 1882. Also, Porter's other business activities were paying off. He sold a lot in Mandan in October 1882 for twelve hundred dollars that had cost him one hundred fifty dollars two years earlier, and in addition he had

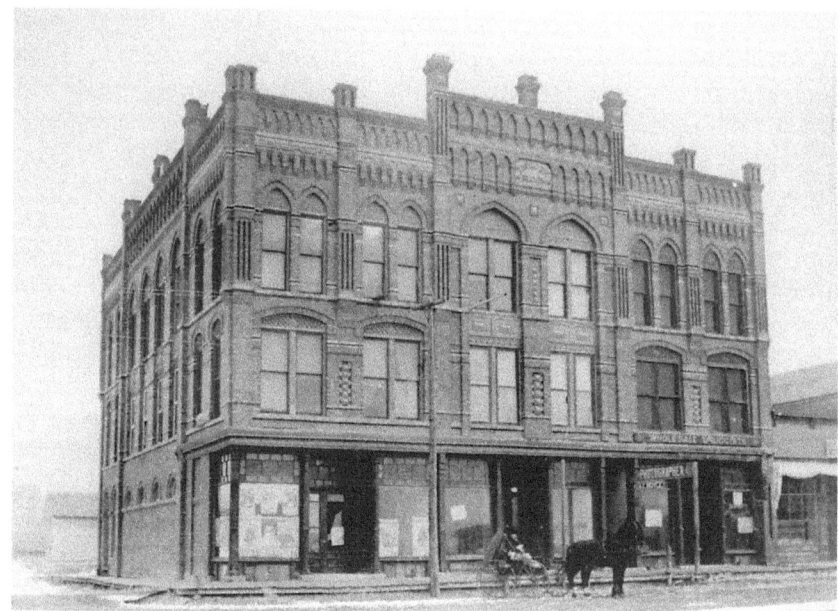

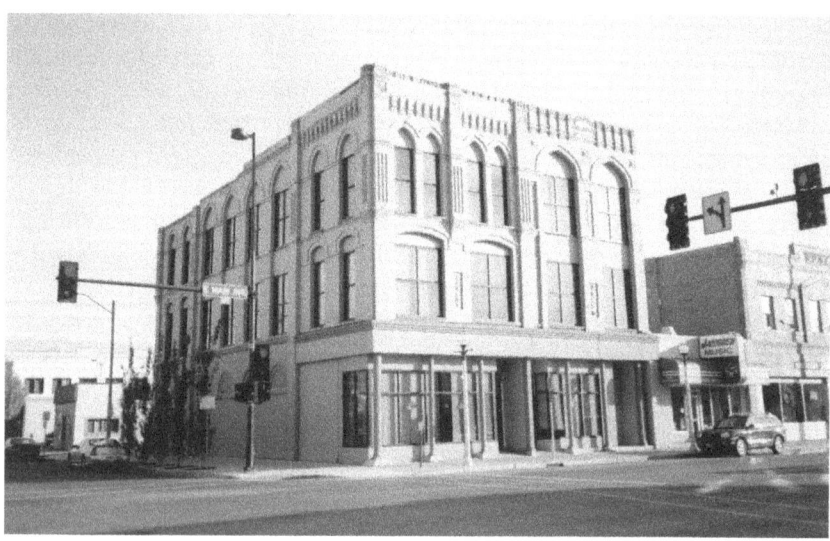

Top: *Dakota Block, Bismarck, North Dakota, late 19th Century (State Historical Society of North Dakota A-3438).* Bottom: *Dakota Block, Bismarck, North Dakota, 2003 (photograph owned by author).*

received ground rent of five dollars a month since its purchase.[10] He was renting two buildings on Third Street to the school board. The *Tribune* reported that he was having the roofs painted an aesthetic color.[11] Also, he had sold one hundred fifty acres of land adjoining the city on the north for six thousand dollars plus half of the profits from future sales of the lots. On November 16, 1882, he sold two houses and lots on Third Street.[12]

October 18, 1882, was a big day for the entire area. The million dollar railroad bridge across the dangerous and wide Missouri River at Bismarck, under construction since 1880, was first crossed. It was built sixty feet above the normal water level. This allowed "steamboats to pass under without removing or cutting off their smokestacks." The river was almost two-thirds of a mile wide at this location.[13] Prior to that cars had to be ferried across by boat, six at a time. Engine No. 88 of the Northern Pacific with twenty-five empties ran for twenty-five minutes to Mandan as a test. It returned with twenty-two half-loaded cars and completed the trip to a "great jubilee of whistles" at the bridge.[14] This was seen as connecting Bismarck more directly to "the great highway across the continent."

In November 1882 brother-in-law George Fairchild, who had been ill for some time, tried to reassure his mother by telling her that he was recovering and taking good care of himself, that his house was warm, and that his bank office was the most comfortable in Bismarck. Also, he was dressing very warmly wearing the thickest of flannels, and in addition to taking his medicines, he had drunk a half bottle of cod liver oil and a little Catawba wine. His diet was good, consisting of fine potatoes, sweet potatoes (Jerseys), squash, eggplant, pumpkins, beets, turnips and generous quantities of milk. By these measures he hoped to ward off rheumatism. He further reported that his wife, Helen, was fine, the baby was walking now, and that Lottie was visiting down at Fort Yates for several weeks.[15] She was probably visiting the Henry F. Douglass family who lived there.

On Christmas Day 1882 the Porters celebrated the day with dinner at the Fairchilds. "The two little tots look very nice together and had lots of Christmas toys," Fairchild wrote his brother James Thone Fairchild (1862–1947).[16]

Fairchild, after a recent trip, reported that Bismarck was being discussed by "line business men" as "likely to be a great city."[17] An editorial in the *Tribune* at the beginning of 1883 summed up its prospects:

> Great cities are built up not wholly by the exertions of its enterprising citizens but a combination of natural advantages and individual enterprise. Bismarck has natural advantages superior to any other town in the northwest, between Duluth and the Pacific coast; and this too, within a few years. Bismarck having the advantage of cheap transportation rates, contracts, absolutely, the trade of the Missouri slope and the northwest country as far, even, as Benton, twelve hun-

dred miles up the Missouri River, and west as far as Miles City on the Northern Pacific Railroad. The river makes a rate on freight to Bismarck from Chicago less than that from St. Paul to Fargo, two hundred miles east. Inside of two years the Chicago, Milwaukee and St. Paul and Northwestern railroads will be completed to this point and possibly another southeastern connection will be made. This will give Bismarck still greater advantages than she now enjoys in the way of rates. As the difference in cost of transportation makes the difference in towns, it will be seen that Bismarck has reason to expect much in the coming five years.

At Bismarck will now be found as large and as fine stocks as are carried in eastern towns of three times the population. It has two national banks and another about to start. A private banking institution is also promised for the early spring. Money commands from 10 to 12 percent, but if invested in real estate much more than that. Several brick blocks were built this year, the owners having rented rooms so that about 20 percent is realized over all expenses, for taxes, insurance, etc. The stores 25 × 85 bring from $100 to $135 per month rent, rented for a term of five years to responsible parties.

Bismarck is the headquarters of five lines of steamships plying on the Missouri river, not to speak of several independent boats. These boats run from Bismarck to Fort Benton, 1200 miles northwest, or up the Yellowstone to Miles City, Fort Keogh, and other points in Montana and south to Yankton, Omaha, St. Louis, and New Orleans. It is the headquarters of the northwestern division of the military telegraph line controlling over three thousand miles of wire, reaching from this central station all of the military posts, Indian agencies and principal cities of the northwest. Over 40,000,000 pounds of government and private freight was transported from Bismarck to points about this year. A United States quartermaster's depot which controls these shipments is located at Bismarck. Bismarck is the headquarters of the Bismarck land district which comprises the largest area of agricultural land now open to settlement in the world. The district is larger than the whole state of New York.

The population of Bismarck is now about 3,500 and increasing rapidly, even in the winter season when little travel would not [sic] be expected. Its people are thoroughly metropolitan and have all the refinement of the east.

It has five churches, viz. Methodist, Presbyterian, Episcopal, Baptist, and Catholic. The Lutheran Society has also purchased ground for a new church in the spring.

Bismarck has a graded system of schools under excellent management. The school board recently purchased one whole block in the central part of town and are [sic] now getting the plans for a $30,000 brick school building will be built as spring permits. The hotels are all that can be desired, and everyone that comes here is astonished at their excellence. There are several secret society organizations, the Odd Fellows and Masons having the finest halls in the territory. The climate at Bismarck is all that could be desired. The air is dry and invigorating and calculated to make people stout, active, and enterprising. The winters are not severe, the thermometer seldom reaching below zero, and when it does, one does not suffer half so much as he would in the east with the thermometer at freezing point. There are but few cloudy days in winter and but few bad storms. The snow fall is light, but of course, as in all prairie countries, blows from one place to another. The spring, summer, and fall seasons are delightful. In summer the nights are always cool and perfect in every respect. Malarial diseases are unknown, and Bismarck may be considered one of the healthiest places in the country.[18]

This summarizes the enthusiasm and boosterism of Bismarck of the early 1880s. It is obvious that citizens were especially sensitive about their weather. Overly enthusiastic promoters of the Northern Pacific, by their accounts of the wonderful weather, had led to jokes about "Jay Cooke's Banana Belt." In fact, the *Bismarck Tribune* was not above making jibes. On March 16, 1878, there were two such comments. In referring to the Buford Stagecoach arriving twenty-eight hours late due to a snowstorm, the sole passenger reported that it was the worst storm that he had ever encountered, but that 120 miles south of Bismarck he encountered the southern line of the storm. The *Tribune* quipped, "in other words he struck the 'Banana Belt.'"[19] The second announced, "The Mississippi was open from St. Paul to the Gulf. Good enough for the eastern extreme of the 'banana' belt."[20] On the editorial page of the *Tribune* in January of 1883 there was a clarification and correction of a recent temperature which had reached only nineteen degrees below zero rather than the reported forty-seven degrees below. The writer asked, "Where in the whole United States can a better record be found? The fact is the winters on the Missouri slope are delightful, but of course they would not be so reported by the eastern papers that see their best citizens moving northwest."[21]

Bismarck was "no longer the cowboy's paradise." It was as orderly a place (as could be found) where the Sabbath was "well observed, and where there were now only thirteen liquor licenses in the county and gambling houses were prohibited. Hurdy-gurdy and dance houses are things of the past, never to be known again in our fair city. Peace and prosperity have dawned...."[22]

Porter's farming prospered during 1882 as reflected by his annual report. On sections 8 and 28, township 139, range 80, he grew wheat on forty acres yielding an average of twenty-five bushels per acre and sixty acres of oats yielding an average of sixty-five bushels. Porter added, "Also raised 400 bushels of splendid potatoes on two acres of land. A portion of the land has been under cultivation since 1873 without manure or anything to enrich the soil."[23]

Porter's yields were more than two times the average. In the ten-year period from 1896 through 1905, the United States Department of Agriculture gave as average yield for North Dakota wheat of 12.17 bushels per acre, oats 20.07 bushels per acre, and potatoes 94.8 bushels per acre.[24]

Due to an epidemic of diphtheria in Bismarck during the winter of 1882–83, Lottie and Helen took their two-year-old children to Oberlin hoping to escape the dangerous disease. George wrote on February 11, "Diphtheria has subsided here — no new cases for some time. I cannot tell whether it was necessary to bring the babies away or not. I am sure that it was our best judgment and I think it will come out right in some way."[25]

Four days later Fairchild wrote Helen that the mail might be delayed since the trains were backed up and it was storming "furiously." He advised her, "Don't let the folks bother you about Bismarck. Hope it will be a 'second Winnipeg.' Everything is booming again this spring. Every train brings people here and all say multitudes are coming."[26] At this time his goal was to stay ahead of Raymond's bank.

On Sunday evening, March 4, 1883, Fairchild called on Porter at his home. Fairchild found Porter dutifully writing Lottie. Porter invited Fairchild for tea at the Sheridan House while they waited for the mail train to come in. He wrote Helen, "People ask me when you are coming back. Others want to rent the house."[27] Fairchild told Helen he was reading Adam Smith's *Wealth of Nations*.

Things were not going well between Porter and his wife possibly explaining some of her long visits away from Bismarck. Fairchild wrote Helen in Oberlin, "You can tell Lottie, to comfort her (if you choose) that her husband will *love* her *nights* when she gets back to him and if she could only restrain her temper and not say bad things to him and be perfectly sweet, imitating her actions when she was a bride, as far as practicable, she can make him love her ever so much more — try and think of things to please him, if she knows of anything he likes, do it for him and all that sort of thing — If I had it to do, I should give him a good talk — tell him how my wife is to me and all that — of course she [Lottie] could not carry it out but still I do really think she will learn it in her lifetime and if she could learn soon, it would add to her happiness."[28]

Porter was beginning to make his fortune in real estate. He was encouraging George to go in with him and buy a half a block in the new Fisher Addition and develop sixteen 150 × 400 feet lots with a loan to George of seven hundred dollars at six percent for three years. Harry Douglass would build houses according to Porter. If George wished to bail out at any time, Porter would tear up the note and resume ownership of the land and any improvements that might have been done. George wrote Helen, "The offer is so good, so liberal and does not bind us up very close and I think we had better take him up."[29] Unfortunately, for some reason, George did not buy the half-block. Perhaps it was excessive caution. Porter bought the entire block as will be noted below.

Fairchild was in St. Paul April 29, 1883, on a mission to get the capital in Bismarck. He wrote Helen, still in Oberlin, from the Windsor Hotel that "McKenzie who is one of the commissioners thinks Bismarck can get it if the proper effort is made." Those interested formed a group in Bismarck to push for it. The Northern Pacific Railroad was giving liberal aid to the project. Fairchild claimed, "If we should succeed Bismarck will be a city very soon."[30]

Three days later he wrote from Merchants Hotel in St. Paul that "everything is working well on the capital matter over in Dakota. We had a lot of papers to fix up today. Tomorrow I shall go back home. I think Mellon is the secret service man. He came out from Yankton this noon and went back with papers this afternoon. Don't lisp a word of this to anyone — I don't want even Lottie to know."[31] On May 11 he was back in St. Paul writing, "Someone has to stay here all the time to keep-up communication between McKenzie and the rest of the commission and the NPRR authorities here."[32] Ultimately they succeeded in getting the territorial capital for Bismarck, a major boost for the area.

The great real estate boom of 1882-83 in Bismarck was underway in anticipation of becoming the capital of the territory. With his business acumen, Porter was participating actively. Porter and Asa Fisher owned 160 acres of land known as Fisher's Addition (160 acres in the northwest quarter of section 34).[33] By May 1883 they had sold between nine and ten thousand dollars worth of lots. The property was considered to be very desirable for residential purposes with the land sloping toward "the built up part of the city." It was noted, "Dr. Porter has selected a block for his residence and will shortly build. He has had the entire block plowed and has built the finest fence in town around the property." A row of shade trees was being set around each of several blocks of land. The *Tribune* reporter speculated, "It is safe to say that lots now selling for 100 dollars in this vicinity will in two months be selling at 200 to 300 dollars."

At the corner of Main and Fourth Streets the new First National Bank of Bismarck building was under construction and heading toward completion that was planned to be December 1, 1883. The bank was said to a "marvelous" success.[34] Porter was now both a director and vice president of the thriving institution, and Fairchild was president and director. Other directors were Asa Fisher, Dan Eisenberg, and H.F. Douglass. Porter, Douglass, and Fairchild also organized the Merchants Bank in Glendive, Montana, in 1883 where Porter invested ten thousand dollars in what would become another very profitable venture for him.

Porter returned to Bismarck along with George P. Flannery and business partner H.F. Douglass September 4, 1883, from a hunting trip to the Yellowstone National Park in time for the festivities on September 5, when the cornerstone of the territorial capitol was laid.[35]

Bunting and Chinese lanterns were hung over the streets. Throngs of people crowded the railroad station on the night that Sitting Bull and his party under the care of Standing Rock Indian agent James McLaughlin got off the train from Fort Yates to be part of the celebration.[36] Several "eminent chiefs" came with him including Flying By; Spotted-Horn-Bull; Tall-as-the-Clouds; Crow Eagle; Gray Eagle, brother-in-law to Sitting Bull; Tomahawk; Two Bears, head chief of the Yanktonais; and others. Long Dog, Young Fireheart, and Long Soldier came the next day. All rode in the grand parade.[37] A special train ran from the depot to the capital grounds for the ceremonies.

The *Tribune* commented that Bismarck had been delayed in its development by the lack of clear titles and "none had dared build permanent structures, but the temporary buildings had been enlarged and improved and the necessity of better ones was not felt."[38] With the boom of the early 1880s underway, substantial brick structures had replaced the earlier log cabins, as Bismarck became the capital of Dakota Territory. At this point it was a city of four thousand people, thirty lawyers, five physicians, and two drugstores, and its spirit was filled with great promise and optimism.

Chapter 15

Farewell to Lottie

As Bismarck and its surrounding area attracted more physicians, the first regional medical society of the so-called Missouri Slope was formed in 1884, the Missouri Medical Society. The Missouri Slope consisted of the fifteen Dakota counties, including Burleigh, whose tributaries drained into the Missouri River. Porter was named president; Dr. H.W. Coe of Mandan, vice-president; and Dr. William A. Bentley, secretary.[1]

Dr. Bentley, a native of Lebanon, Connecticut, and eight years older than Porter, served in the Civil War as a private, Company H, 9th Iowa Infantry. He arrived in Bismarck in July 1877 as its third physician after graduating from Rush Medical School, Chicago, in 1869 and after practicing eight years in St. Paul and Rush City, Minnesota.[2] In addition to practicing medicine he became active in Bismarck politics, a field that Porter eschewed. Bentley was twice mayor of Bismarck (1887–90 and 1891–92) and a member of the state legislature.

During 1884 Lottie's health was becoming a cause for the family's concern. George Fairchild wrote his sister June 13:

> Doctor [Porter], Mother, Lottie, and Hallie left here Tuesday and Duluth Thursday A.M. will perhaps be at Oberlin Tuesday or even Wednesday next. I just want to say a word about calling on Lottie — She has seen very few people indeed — is not able to see company much even when she seems bright — When you call on her, let one go in to see her at a time and not stay over 10 or 15 minutes — Mrs. Viets may not think to regulate call aright. Better tell other people the same until she is much better.[3]

From the tone of the letter that suggests limited visits, one might suspect that Lottie was profoundly depressed or might have been suffering from a mental condition since no physical ailment was hinted at. Later, there would be physical problems, rheumatism, mentioned in family letters, but she would live another six years. It is possible that she suffered from rheumatic fever or rheumatic heart disease.

George Fairchild, himself, was not having the best of years. He admitted in a letter to his father that he was burdened by "work, anxiety, and trouble."[4] While he had hoped that the new bank building would have been completed the previous December, it would be June 1884 before it would be "in running order." While Lottie was ill, the Fairchilds were keeping three-year-old Hallie. George Fairchild wrote his father, "Lottie recovers her strength very slowly indeed, but we think she will get up on her feet again ... Lottie is gaining slowly. It will be some time for her to recover even comfortable health."

In August 1884 in spite of Fairchild's hope that there would be no more attempts by other factions to wrest control of the National Bank from him, his worst fears were realized. To George's great distress, the directors elected Asa Fisher as president and demoted him to cashier again. Where Porter was in the matter is unclear. He had been a partner with Fisher in selling residential lots in Bismarck within the previous two years. In any case, Fairchild felt miserable about the action. He wrote his brother Jamie, "It is only the most extraordinary Emergency imaginable involving what I call a *crime* on the part of Mr. F. [Fisher] that led to it. Do not speak to any of the family except the Viets for the present. I am worn out with care, anxiety, and mortification. *The bank was in danger*— is now all right. I made the sacrifice voluntarily to save the bank and my friends' interests."[5] The nature of the problem is unknown. Porter, always a man of probity, must not have considered Fisher's action a crime.

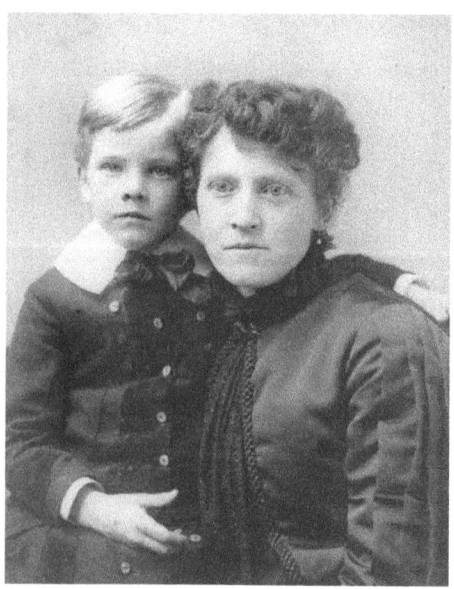

Lottie Porter and son, Hal. Photograph by D.F. Barry. (Courtesy Wyman Family)

Fairchild and Fisher maintained a civil relationship at the bank, but it was always uncomfortable in spite of Fisher being "pleasant" to him.[6] Fairchild and his father took a tour of Yellowstone Park just to get away. They found it rejuvenating. The following year Fairchild's health began to break under the strain of professional disappointment and debt. He wrote his father, "I shall not be able to do much, if any more, active labor or business; that I shall be as Lottie is, comfortable."[7]

In the spring of 1885 Porter was traveling in the south. Fairchild wrote him about the bank situation telling him that he had made up his mind to tolerate his relationship with Fisher for another ten months but if there was no improvement, he would "do almost anything to get out — It is a daily grind unpleasant and miserable and 'tis not worth while to live in this way many years ... I prefer to stay in the business if I can find someone to put in money enough to buy Fisher out — If this can be done, the business will grow and be worth something sometime. If it can't be done, then try to sell out is next."[8]

Porter was not forthcoming with more money for stock and this led to strained relationships. Fairchild's personal finances were a disaster. He owned the George H. Fairchild Insurance Agency which the *Tribune* referred to as one "fast gaining a reputation for stability and prompt settlement of losses and already ranks among the most solid agencies in the northwest."[9] At this time Fairchild was struggling under debts of $16,340 and owed another one thousand dollars to Porter (probably for bank stock). Interest payments amounted to $1,394 a year. With a total income of $2,600 he lacked enough to live on.

His health broke. The *Tribune* reported August 7, 1885:

> President Fairchild of Oberlin College, one of the most prominent of American educators, arrived in the city yesterday to visit his son, George H. Fairchild of the First National Bank, who has been seriously ill for some time.[10]

Meanwhile, Bismarck had a new hospital run by the Benedictine Sisters, who bought out the Lamborn Hotel at the northeast corner of Main Avenue and Sixth Street. It opened as the Lamborn Hospital in May 1885 but was later renamed St. Alexius Hospital in 1905 when it was incorporated. Porter was among the eleven physicians on the staff.[11]

A county board of health was organized for Burleigh in August of 1885. The county attorney, John A. Stoyell, was president by virtue of his position. Dr. Bentley was vice president and Porter was secretary and superintendent.[12] New regulations were mandated by the legislature of the Dakota Territory requiring that a physician "must be a graduate [of a recognized medical school] or a regular practitioner of ten years standing in order to practice medicine." This was an attempt to improve the quality of practitioners in the territory.

Porter left Bismarck on June 22, 1886, to join the party from Fort Yates, Dakota Territory, and headed to Little Bighorn to celebrate the tenth anniversary of the battle.[13] Others who returned were Frederick Benteen; Thomas M. McDougall, commander of B Company; Edward Godfrey, commander of K Company; Winfield Scott Edgerly, second lieutenant in D Company; George B. Penwell, trumpeter in K Company; Chief Gall; and Curley. Bismarck photographer David F. Barry accompanied Porter.[14]

The highlight of the reunion was Chief Gall's description of the battle from the Sioux chief's perspective. The press reported that early in the day he went over the entire battlefield and through an interpreter described "in an intelligent and straightforward manner the exact places in which Custer's command was destroyed."[15] The article was reprinted in *The Custer Myth*, the original being in a contemporary Chicago newspaper.[16]

Gall was contemptuous of the Crow scout, Curley, who had been with Custer's command and scornfully turned his back to him and said, "He ran away too soon in the fight." Gall was then forty-six years old, powerfully built, and "his dignified countenance spoke truthfulness" although at first he "appeared reticent and inclined to act sullen but when he stood on the spot which marked the last sight of Custer on earth, his dark eyes lightened with fire; he became earnestly communicative and he told all he knew without restraint."[17]

Chief Gall answered many questions that remained at that time and was able to add more information. He explained that "a large band of Cheyennes had taken part in the Custer battle."[18] And he told the group that Custer and all his men had been killed in thirty minutes; that the Indians shot arrows after their cartridges were expended and used clubs; that the soldiers did not have enough ammunition because the horses ran away, carrying their reserves, causing the soldiers to use their pistols as a last resort; that the soldiers fought standing up while the Indians fired from behind their horses; and that Sitting Bull was in his tepee "making medicine" during the entire battle and did not fight at all.[19]

Porter and the photographer, Barry, returned June 27, 1886, to Bismarck and according to the *Tribune* gave "a most interesting report of the journey and visit."[20] They were impressed by how "much feeling and pride that Gall showed as he stepped upon the famous battlefield" ten years after the savage killing of squaws and children, soldiers and Indian warriors. According to a reporter:

Curley — Crow scout who was with Custer's column at Little Bighorn but who deserted, survived, and was snubbed by Gall at the tenth reunion of the battle, 1876. Photograph by D.F. Barry. (National Archives [165-AI-4])

The last relic of the battle to be found on the field is now at the *Tribune* office, having been presented by Dr. Porter, and is the foot of a soldier's boot, the leg having been cut off and taken by the Indians at the close of the fight, as was done with all the boots of the soldiers. This the Indians always do as leather is of great value to them; they have not learned the mode of manufacture. There is a bullet hole in the toe of this interesting relic, and the effects of the blood on the coloring of the leather is visible. Photographer Barry has a splendid collection of views of the field which he took during the visit, and which he soon will have completed.[21]

Shortly after returning to Bismarck Porter and his wife sustained a lighting strike to their house, which entered their bedroom during the night frightening them and doing "considerable" damage. Both of them saw a fireball as large as a head and Porter reported that he thought he was dead. "He could not move and it seemed that his head had been severed from his body and that he was doubled up in the throes of death."[22] As he recovered he shook his wife, who had "suffered similar sensations." He rushed upstairs to check on their five-year-old son,

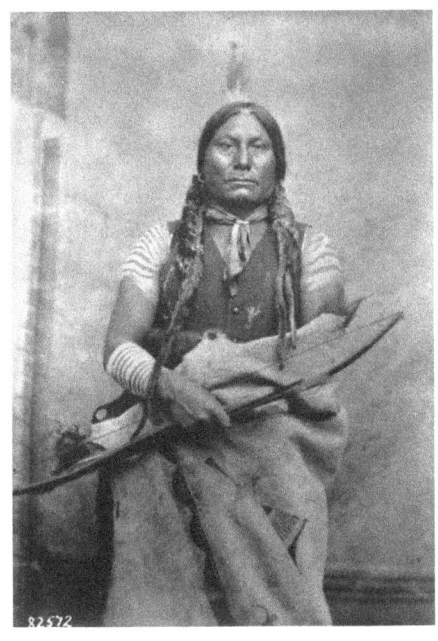

Gall, Hunkpapa Sioux chief who with Crazy Horse led opposition to Custer at Little Bighorn (National Archives [82572]).

Hallie, and found him sleeping without interruption. The walls of the Porters' bedroom were blackened, the gold leaf was knocked from the molding, and shingles were ripped off the roof of the cupola. Lottie Porter, who had been ill since 1884, became worse after the shock and was said to have never fully recovered.

Nevertheless, the Porters were able to attend what was billed as "the great society event of the season," the wedding reception of Asa Fisher's daughter at the parents' home in Bismarck on October 27, 1886. Along with Governor and Mrs. Pierce, Judge and Mrs. Francis and the cream of Bismarck society, the Porters were observed at the reception with Lottie wearing black velvet, jet trimmings, and point lace.[23]

In January 1888 Porter wrote anonymously an article entitled "A Catechism" that was published, with some editing, by William P. Moffet in his weekly muckraking newspaper in Bismarck, *The Settler*.[24] The article asks some sensitive questions about political matters in Burleigh County, specifically about the Alexander McKenzie machine:

> What sheriff of Burleigh County has made brags that he is the only sheriff in Dakota who has made money off the county? Who has robbed this county of

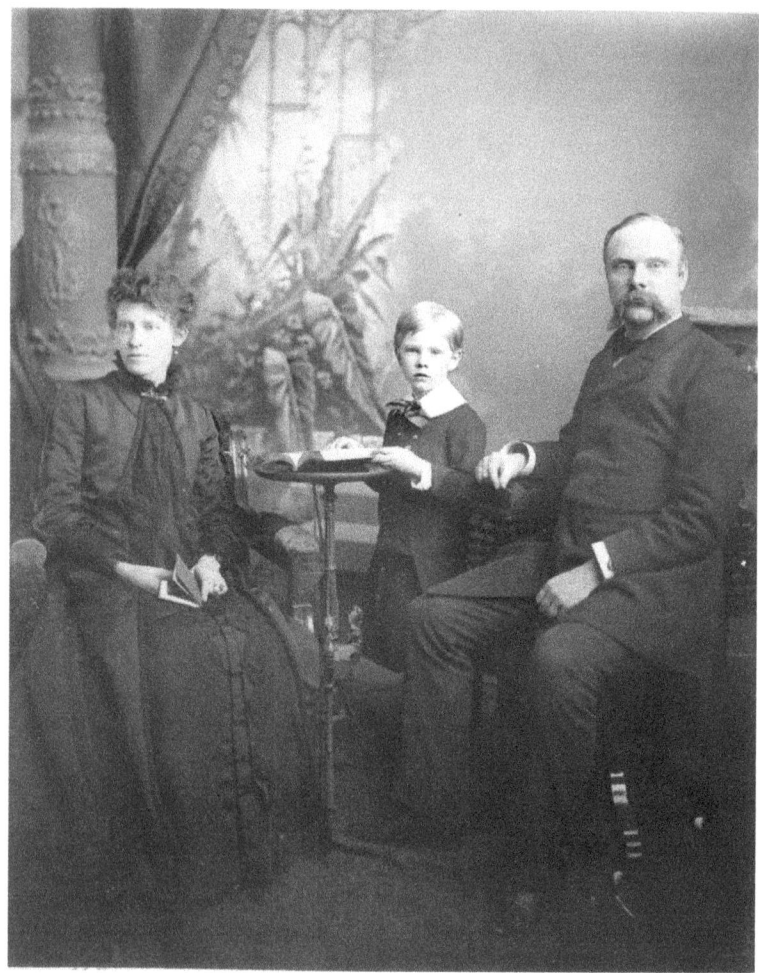

Porter family in Bismarck, left to right, Charlotte (Lottie), Hal, Henry R. Porter, 1886. Photograph by B.F. Barry. (State Historical Society of North Dakota 0264–28)

wood and coal and prison labor for lo these many years...?Why do [*sic*] the ring kick so vigorously when their stealings are cut off? How many empty houses has Griffin now?

The article goes on to implicate several other members of the machine in crooked dealings, led by the most powerful man in the Dakota Territory, Alexander McKenzie.[25] Saloonkeeper and deputy sheriff L.N. Griffin attacked the editor and beat him over the head with his revolver causing a large scalp wound that Porter closed with several sutures. Moffet was incapacitated for some time afterwards and claimed in a civil suit later that he was unable to perform physical labor around the office as before.[26] Porter was unable to testify, since he was in Jamestown on the day of the trial. In spite of several witnesses who had seen and heard from Moffet immediately after the attack, his civil suit against Griffin for fifteen thousand dollars was denied.[27] No one knew that Porter had written the article. A clipping of "A Catechism" is fixed in Porter's scrapbook with the initials H.R.P. placed by Porter at the end of the clipping and a first hand account is available in Moffet's seven page sketch of Porter in the State Historical Society of North Dakota Library in Bismarck.[28]

But Griffin's time in Bismarck was limited. Much to the surprise of everyone, North Dakota and South Dakota voted for statewide prohibition of alcohol on October 1, 1889.[29] This effectively shut down saloons and put Griffin and other keepers out of business. It was with concern that the *Tribune* editorialized: "Prohibition will be disastrous to the financial and business interests of the state, at least temporarily, there can be no doubt. It means in addition to virtual confiscation of thousands of dollars worth of property the loss of a large portion of the revenue necessary to the carrying on of the state, county, and municipal government."[30] Yet the town survived and even prospered. Twenty years later the *Tribune*, in a column reviewing earlier days, reported that L.N. Griffin had been driven out of town by prohibition in 1890. "He went to Centralia, Washington, but soon got out of the liquor business and has since become one of the leading citizens of Whatcom [County, Washington] and is well-to-do."[31]

At the end of 1887 with the bank and insurance business doing well, Fairchild was still under personal economic pressure. He wrote to his father, "Dr. Porter will not take the presidency of the bank [Asa Fisher was still president and Porter vice-president] and there is nothing to do but go on as we are."[32] Further, Fairchild learned to his disappointment that Porter had been "trying to sell an interest in the bank to some friends."

Poor health continued to plague Fairchild. In March 1888 he was feeling better and thought he was even looking better, but he was taking digitalis[33] twice a day.[34] He had developed heart trouble, possibly rheumatic fever as the result of a severe throat infection that he had had while in Oberlin in 1874. Financial troubles mounted. His sister, Mary, sent him some money from time to time, and Porter passed on his *Century* magazine and *Harper's Weekly* to the Fairchilds after he had read them to spare George the expense.[35] The Porters invited them to Sunday dinner occasionally. Everyone in the family realized the pressure that he was under and tried to help.

During 1888 Porter, in addition to his private practice, was again employed by the Burleigh County Commissioners as county physician with responsibility to attend the sick in the county poor home, the county jail, and those we would now call welfare patients. His salary was five hundred dollars per year.[36]

Tragedy struck on August 6, 1888. Lottie died in Bismarck at the age of 35 of "congestion of the lungs" after years of ill health.[37] Details of her death are quite limited. This could possibly have been due to congestive heart failure or to pneumonia, but a more precise diagnosis is not available. We do know that she had a chronic illness of some kind characterized by rheumatic problems. Sometime before her death, Lottie wrote a note to her husband and asked that he take care of Hallie as he would have taken care of her and enclosed clippings of her hair.[38] Her funeral was held at 4 P.M. the following day at the family residence with burial at Oberlin, Ohio, in the Westwood Cemetery. Her parents, Henry Viets and Samantha Joslin Viets, were still living. When they died in 1894 and 1898, respectively, they were buried near Lottie's grave.

Porter was left with Hallie, seven years old, to care for. The marriage, though short, was never described as a happy one. Not one letter exists to our knowledge between Porter and Lottie as documentation. Neither Porter descendants, through his sister Sarah Davis, nor descendants of Katherine Fairchild, who gave some of the Fairchild letters to the State Historical Society of North Dakota and who received the personal effects of Hal (Henry Viets Porter) by his will, have any letters between Henry Rinaldo and Lottie Porter. Unless they may be found some day, one might suspect that the letters were destroyed and most likely by their son, Hal. Regrettably theirs is no love story.

On New Year's Day 1889 Hallie spent the entire day until 9:30 P.M. with his cousin Katherine. Helen considered this very wearing, according to George, because it was hard to keep the house straight and because they were constantly teasing each other as children will do. During the day Porter and Fairchild, together, made social calls on the ladies of the city, as was the custom in Bismarck to welcome in the New Year.[39]

While Porter had been successful, his brother-in-law George Fairchild had not been. He was swamped with debt and could hardly support his family. This led to some resentment. He wrote to his sister, Mary, who had sent him some gifts and money, "thank you for the gifts ... Hallie has very nice things and he looks so knobley [sic] and

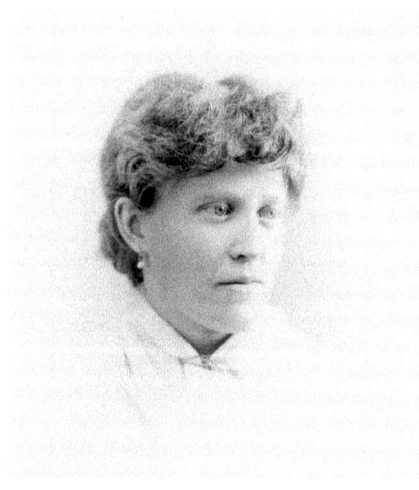

Charlotte Porter. Photograph by H.M. Platt. (Courtesy Wyman Family)

sleek that I had begun to think Katherine looked rather plebeian beside him.... Now Hallie says Katherine's coat (made from Lottie's old cape) is prettier than his and has of all things that which he covets most a good peace [*sic*] for a *bustle*. He has always been fond of girl dresses and is happiest when dressed up with skirts and *bustle*."[40]

Fairchild had obtained papers to go into receivership in March 1889. His sister again offered him money, but this was only in small amounts. He was attempting to get a job with the Department of the Interior and was asking for letters of recommendation.[41] In a letter to his older sister, Lucy Fairchild Kenaston (1842–1912), Fairchild wrote in June, "Dr. Porter and Hallie have gone down to Detroit Lake, Minn. for a few days outing with some friends. Katherine will be eight years old soon and she has not been to school yet. I think she can keep ahead of Hallie easily tho he does go.... Hallie has a pony now and Katherine rides fearlessly."[42]

Porter was active in the Association of Acting Assistant Surgeons, U.S. Army, which met for the first time June 24, 1889, at the Casino, Newport, Rhode Island. These were the surgeons who had served in the Civil War and the Indian Wars on contracts, not as commissioned officers. At this meeting letters of appreciation were read from "Mrs. General Custer" and General W.T. Sherman. Porter agreed to serve on the council of the new organization.[43]

By August 1889 the capital site issue was settled in Bismarck's favor for the upper part of the territory with Pierre for the lower part. It would be November 2 when statehood would be achieved, and this was roundly applauded in Dakota.

On Sunday afternoon, September 8, Fairchild wrote his mother, "I have come down to my office to write you. Hallie and Katherine keep things pretty well stirred up at the house and then my own pen and ink suit me better."[44]

On November 2, 1889, statehood came to North and South Dakota; no longer was it a territory. Porter's life had changed with the loss of his wife. He had been highly successful as a physician and as a businessman and had become wealthy. But he no longer needed or apparently cared to practice medicine. He took more and more time away from work with travels. Consequently, he resigned as county physician in 1890.

Chapter 16

Banking Business

Poor George Fairchild continued to struggle, both financially and physically. To add to his woes, Hallie had become more of a problem. On January 7, 1890, Fairchild wrote to his sister, Mary, complaining, "Hallie spent the afternoon ... which is always hard."[1] Things were not looking much better for him in Bismarck either. Later, he wrote to his father in Oberlin regarding prospects: "Nothing shows in the future of Bismarck. It looks all dark and dull yet — people leaving all the time — can't make a living here. The stock business is growing in the country and promises well, but it will be several years before it will make a show."[2] This contrasted with his earlier sanguine prospects for the future of Bismarck.

In April the *Tribune* reported what it called a good joke on Dr. Porter reprinted from the *Jamestown* (North Dakota) *Alert*:

> Dr. Porter of Bismarck is in the city today to attend the organization of the new board of trustees for the [state] insane hospital of which he is a member. The doctor took the train at Bismarck last night, retired in a Pullman lower and instructed the porter to call him for Jamestown. He was awakened as the train pulled into Eldridge and when the train stopped, the doctor hustled off and the always obliging porter followed and handed him his valise, not even failing to express due appreciation as he pocketed the usual tip. The little hamlet was enshrouded in darkness and the doctor did not discover that he was in the wrong pew until the train was steaming along toward Jamestown at a thirty mile an hour rate. Eldridge is not the most inviting place at 4 A.M., but the doctor after a silent execration of the "accommodation" porter, summoned all the philosophy in his disposition to his aid and composedly waited for the first freight, which he caught and rode into the metropolis in the caboose. This is as the doctor tells it, but the story is abroad in the land that he came in on foot.[3]

He attended the meeting of the asylum board in Jamestown two months later without difficulty.[4] In the same news item it was announced that he was leaving for the Pacific coast for a few days before returning to Livingston, Montana, where he would join Judge John Bowen for a two-week bear hunt in the Rocky Mountains. While he was gone Hallie, age 9, would stay with his aunt, Mrs. Clarke, in Ashland, Wisconsin.

16. Banking Business

Porter was in Tacoma and Spokane Falls where he wrote a letter to M.H. Jewell, editor of the *Tribune*, on June 25 when he added:

"P.S. Who should I meet this morning at breakfast but Joe Hanauer [Bismarck dry goods salesman]. He said, "You are just in time, Doc. I am to be married this afternoon at 2 o'clock." They stood under a solid arch of roses reaching from the floor to the ceiling. The ceremony was witnessed by 250 elite of the city. The bride is young and beautiful and she did look "just too lovely." She wore a long white train, white silk and a lovely white silk bridal vail [sic] — should say six feet or more. She sparked with diamonds. So did Joe. They were as fine a bridal couple as you would wish to see. May they live long and prosper. This letter is like a lady's, viz., the p.s. is the most important part.[5] [Porter had written a spoof on a wedding report in the social pages]

Porter returned to Bismarck from the bear hunt in the Rockies with Judge John Bowen on July 19, 1890.[6]

Porter's care of some mental patients reached the public attention in the press. Two examples follow:

William Howard, a convict at the penitentiary, was found insane yesterday by Dr. Porter of his city and Dr. Read of Mandan, and will be taken to the asylum at Jamestown. Howard is off on a religious mental side track, and his mental balance wheel has been gone for some time. This will be the second time Howard has been at the asylum.[7]

And the following:

Sept. 17th [year?] Dr. Porter, of Bismarck, put up at the Hyatt House on his way to Lake Geneva [Wisconsin], with Frank Buffum, a young man who is demented, and whom he was taking here to be cured. He locked him in a room upstairs while he went out to get a shave; when he returned Frank had got out the window, jumped off the stoop, and disappeared. Since then no trace can be found of him. A reward of $25 is offered. Frank is medium height, slender, dark hair and eyes, no beard, had on a coat vest and soft hat of dark brown, and dark pants. He is shy, sickly, and inclined to hide his face. His mother is here awaiting in great suspense some tidings of her lost son. Later — he was found at McHenry Monday in a box and taken to Lake Geneva. He scratched on a piece of leather and fastened it on the outside of the box these words: "bury me in this box." He still lives.[8]

In February 1891 Fairchild wrote Mary that he was able to go to his office every day but that his strength was slow to return. His heart always went "bad" when he was sick, and it took it weeks to get it "quiet and orderly again." Hallie was ill with measles and couldn't visit his cousin Katherine, but he was improving "nicely" and had a new housekeeper that he [Hallie] liked very much. Fairchild's income for 1890 was $1500 — not enough.[9] In June his cough was worse and he could "just get about." He "had to sit up some to get rest."[10]

In September 1891 Porter traveled to Arkansas, Texas, and Mexico. While he was away, Hallie stayed with the Fairchilds. M.H. Jewell, editor of the *Tribune,* published what he called "a readable letter from Dr. Porter who is recreating at Hot Springs."[11] This is the first of Porter's traveling letters that the editor would share. Over the next thirteen years they became quite popular with *Tribune* readers. Jewell calls this "an extract," but it seems complete and it exhibits Porter's skills at travel writing and shows his ability to tell a good story as do those that follow.

Hot Springs, Ark., Oct., 3rd, 1891.

I must stay here and take the baths a week or ten days anyway. That is the "proper caper" here. This is a beautiful place and called the "Fountain of Youth." Here is where you find the Elixir of Life—fifteen cents a drink or two for twenty-five. Can get anything you want, if you have the ducats. Anything from a free lecture of Y.M.C.A. to a jack pot, and by the way this is where they "play 'em high"—bet whole stacks and then sleep in the streets. It would make your heart sad to see some of the people and watch those arriving on every train. The poor pale mother with her little sickly child and perhaps the last dollar of her hard earned savings to try and recover the health of the little one. On our train was an ostensibly wealthy couple, with their little ten year old boy, all crippled up with rheumatism and scrofula—bright little fellow, with sparkling bright eyes—his hands and legs were bent and twisted, and limping around on crutches. You see people from all parts of the world—the rich coupon cutter from New York to the poor man, sent down here by the county commissioners, at the expense of the overburdened taxpayer.

With a population of about the same as Fargo, Hot Springs has 500 hotels and boarding houses. One small hotel has 600 rooms. How is that for a little one? Hot! Well I should smile—arrived brown, with dust in ears, eyes, nose and mouth, I went direct to a hot bath—115 degrees—to get cooled off. This is called the Baden Baden of America and it is said that "creation has given the Hot Springs no rival. Its springs are the modern pools of Bethseda [*sic*], whose waters are ever stirred by the blessed wings of the "Healing Angel."

Say, did you ever see the Arkansas hog, or razor-back. Mark Twain has an exact picture of the animal in his book. These hogs run faster than the trains and their long snoots and legs are put up for rooting and running. Their hams are just the size of a North Dakota jack rabbit's. The Arkansas beef is good—to chaw on—good as gum, and more lasting. Wish Joe Dietrich had some to give his kickers.[12] Neither do the natives hold their beef very high. En route here we met a steer on the track. I noticed the train shot ahead and beef went up at the rate of forty miles an hour.

Inquiring of the conductor why he did not slow up and give the steer a show he said its cheaper to run fast and knock them out of the way than to stop. If they had to pay at all it was only $5. The fire bell is just ringing and everybody is running.

Yours Truly,
H.R. Porter.[13]

16. Banking Business

By the 23rd of October he was back in El Paso en route to Bismarck.[14] He returned to Bismarck October 29 with rings for Katherine and Hallie from Mexico City as well as Mexican coins, a beautiful dress for Helen, and a coffee wood cane for George. Upon his return, Porter not infrequently entertained the Fairchilds for dinner.

In December 1891 he was involved with the start-up of a new bank in Mandan.[15] His travels did not interfere with his business dealings. Porter and Harry F. Douglass, who were major investors in the new bank in Mandan, had earlier bought some valuable property in Washington, DC, from a black Pullman porter who was also an investor in the bank.[16] Washington property, likely the same, was the subject of a press clipping that Porter put in his scrapbook.

Dr. Porter in Luck

Dr. Porter, of this city, while in Washington a few years ago, was induced by a friend to purchase a tract of broken land on Rock Creek, northwest of the city. It was hinted that it might be a good spec in it, as there was some prospects [sic] of the government seeking a location in that direction for the zoological park. Porter put in a few thousand and the following Associated Press dispatch means that his possessions are worth at least double what they were a week ago.

Washington, May 29 [1889]

The site of the new zoological park for which Congress appropriated $200,000 at the last session, has been selected by the commission to whom the matter was referred. It lies along the banks of Rock Creek, northwest of the city between Woodley Lane and Klingle Road, and comprises about 150 acres, delightfully situated and admirably adapted for the purpose. It is about two miles from the White House. The animals now in Smithsonian Park will probably be removed to the new location late in the fall.[17]

On May 20, 1892, Porter began a month's trip around the eastern United States, leaving Hallie for over five weeks with the Fairchilds while going to New York City as one destination.[18] When he returned on June 25 he brought Katherine a pair of patent leather slippers, black silk bows, a handkerchief, a box of candy, and necktie for George.[19]

Porter had sold out his bank stock leaving poor George Fairchild even more stranded and vulnerable. Asa Fisher began buying up stock, and it was only a matter of time before Fairchild would be ousted as cashier. By selling out at the right time, it made Porter almost immune to the severe economic downturn, or Panic of 1893, that followed.

Telling of his hurt, Fairchild wrote his sister:

I am glad Dr. Porter is out of the bank business—he has hated the whole business for years and has shown it in every way—tho he always tried to be pleasant yet in every way his connection made my situation hard—I am relieved with his relief and while he is interested to have me hold it he would not want to put a dollar in nor would I ask him to—The severance of former relations is agreeable.[20]

This is likely not an accurate assessment of Porter's feelings about the banking business; he was still a major owner in two other banks. Although he had sold his shares in Bismarck's First National Bank, he still had major holdings in banks in Mandan and Glendive. It is probable that Porter left the First National Bank to disentangle himself from a family connection that was proving burdensome.

Porter wrote a colorful letter to his niece in Washington, DC, during the summer of 1892 advising her to tell her father to avoid getting over-heated by working in the garden or pumping water. These activities could be very dangerous and lead to what he called "insolation," or heat stroke, a condition that might prove to be fatal. He told of a number of patients that had died before reaching him, but there were deaths in those who got to him. "Tell him to let the weeds grow and the milk sour, but not to expose himself to this dangerous malady," he wrote.[21]

Throughout his career Porter was a "horse and buggy doctor." He loved fine horses and his were mentioned with some regularity in the *Tribune*. It was said of his beautiful black pacer that it could keep up with anything in town and make a buggy hum. He also had a thoroughbred mare that he enjoyed riding.[22]

Eleven-year-old Katherine Fairchild, normally of a sunny disposition and up to this point apparently unaware of her father's precarious financial condition, entered into her diary on December 18, 1892, the following: "It is now nearly Christmas and I am getting ready for it. My preparations are nearly finished for we are not going to make Christmas the usual holiday as Papa has a business trouble and we have to be careful of expenses."[23] This is a sad commentary by an unusually perceptive and intelligent eleven-year-old girl.

Chapter 17

Travels Abroad

George Fairchild's health continued to deteriorate. In March he blamed his cough on the wind out of the east and complained, "I get best rest at night with wet packs on my chest."[1] And "I sleep short naps sitting up in bed these nights and lie down occasionally to rest my back."[2] He could see the end of an era stating in a note to his sister, "The Doctor closes out and leaves for good in June, and if we go that will be all the old promoters [of the bank]. Fisher stands pretty much alone. None of his associates amount to much."[3]

Twenty years after arriving in Bismarck, Porter was planning a year-long trip, the summer tour in Europe and the winter in Palestine, Egypt, Syria, Asia Minor, Turkey, and Greece. He was taking up stakes and would probably return to Washington, DC, where his parents, sisters, and other family members lived.

In April 1893, anticipating leaving, he resigned as the local surgeon for the Northern Pacific Railway having served for twenty years. He was given, as a memento, a conductor's lantern, now in the collection of the North Dakota Historical Society. On April 13 he sold his Victorian style residence at 824 Fourth Street to Judge Walter Winchester.[4] When Theodore Roosevelt was campaigning for the vice-presidency of the United States, he had dinner on September 15, 1900, with the leaders of the North Dakota Republican Party at Judge Walter Winchester's home, 824 Fourth Street.[5] Porter was not on the guest list for dinner at the home he built.

Porter and Hallie moved into a hotel on April 27, 1893. Katherine Fairchild wrote in her diary, "Last night was the last day Hallie and his papa stayed in the house — it was dreadfully torn up, it was the last time [I] saw [a] frontier household in their house.[6] Finally, he resigned as Burleigh County physician to be replaced by Dr. F.D. Kendrick.[7]

On May 2 and May 9 Hallie appeared in a musical at the Methodist and Episcopal churches, respectively, in Bismarck at The Ladies Concerts. He played a piano solo, "La Gitano" by Franz Behr, and it was said to have drawn "a full share of appreciation and an encore."[8] On May 13 Katherine and Hallie attended dancing school and soon after Porter sent Hallie to stay with rel-

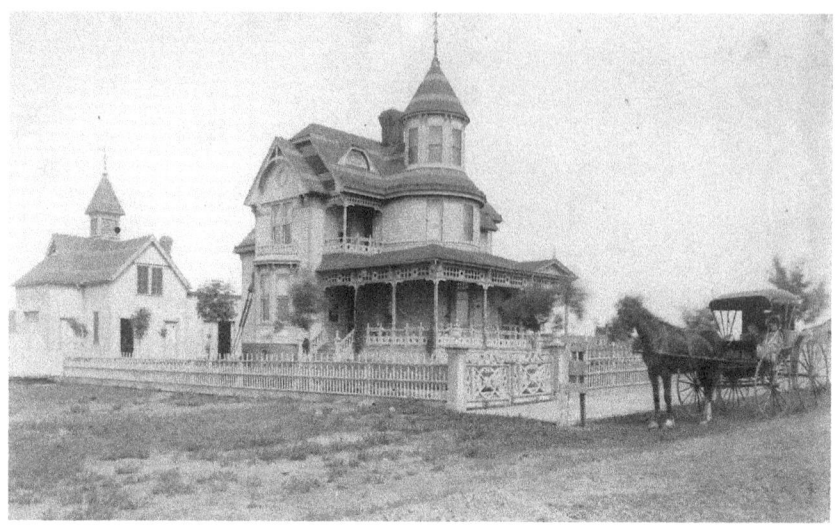

Above: *Dr. H.R. Porter home, Bismarck, North Dakota, late 19th Century (State Historical Society of North Dakota 0264–36).* Below:*Henry (Hal) Viets Porter, son of Dr. Henry R. Porter and Charlotte Viets Porter (courtesy Wyman Family).*

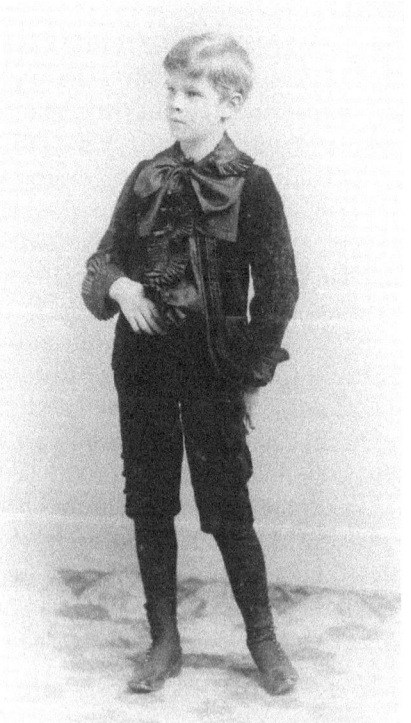

atives in Wisconsin. Hallie, now twelve years old, was to be shifted from place to place, staying with relatives and friends, and attending private schools for the rest of Porter's life. One suspects that his sense of abandonment sadly contributed to his life-long dislike for his father.

On May 5 the New York Stock Exchange crashed ushering in the Panic of 1893. Porter, who had already liquidated his Bismarck bank stock and had sold his home in Bismarck, was untouched. By his timing and good luck he escaped as a wealthy man while others suffered.

Porter and his friend and business associate Harry F. Douglass left Bismarck on the 6 P.M. train for Minneapolis on May 26, 1893, for what Porter thought would be the last time. There was great excitement in

17. Travels Abroad

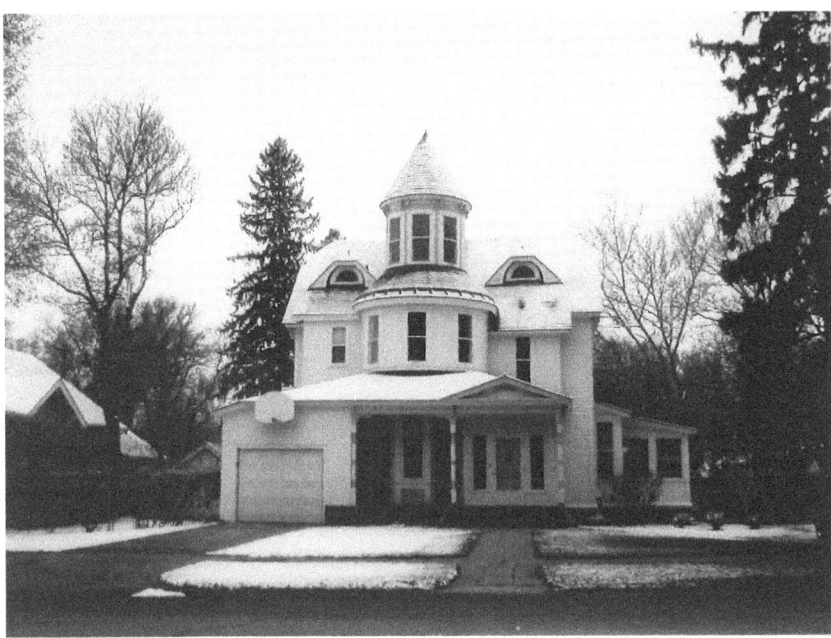

Dr. H.R. Porter's former home, Bismarck, North Dakota, 2003 (photograph owned by author).

the country about the World's Columbian Exhibition in Chicago that President Grover Cleveland had opened on May 1, 1893. People came from all over the country and the world to see the new wonders at what was popularly called the Chicago World's Fair of 1893. Excursion trains brought millions to see the Great White City, as it was called, and the attractions on the midway. This was an event that Porter would not have missed. He brought Hallie along with him in early June to see for the first time such things as the new Ferris wheel. Editor Clement A. Lounsberry went to the fair about the same time and reported after having tea with the Japanese, he enjoyed a Turkish lunch featuring the celebrated *ka ba* "with the accent on bah." While walking on the streets of Cairo, he saw "the voluptuous forms of dark beauties of the Nile" and, therefore, could not fault Mark Antony for lingering in Egypt.[9]

Of special interest to Porter at the fair might have been Sitting Bull's cabin on display and the appearance of Rain-in-the-Face in feathers and war paint and, of course, Buffalo Bill Cody's Wild West Show. He had faced both Sitting Bull and Rain-in-the-Face seventeen years earlier at Little Bighorn. Sitting Bull had been killed in 1890 by Indian police and Rain-in-the-Face was now in show business. After attending the fair Porter left for Washington and New York and sent Hallie back to Ashland, Wisconsin, with the James W. Clarkes.

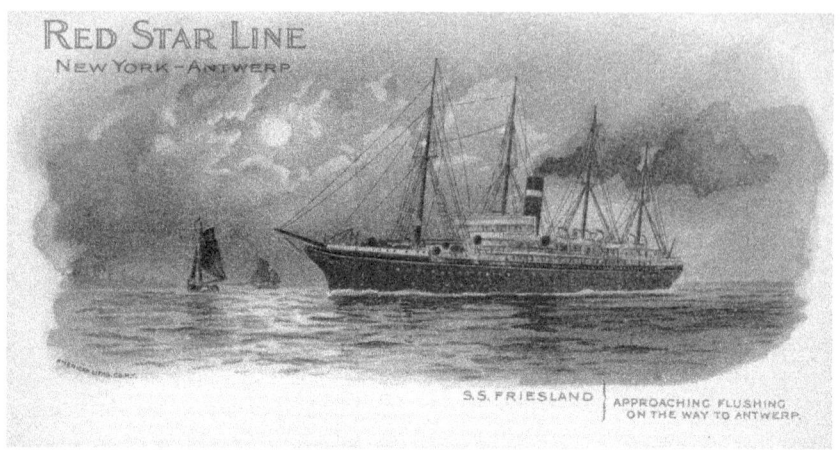

SS Friesland, *Red Star Line. Dr. Porter sailed from New York to Antwerp in 1893 on this ship (photograph owned by author).*

Porter obtained a certificate as "Citizen of the United States" from the Department of State in Washington that would allow him to pass freely between countries and to assist him with "all lawful aid and protection" in case of need.[10] He was now forty-five years old, stood five feet, seven and a half inches tall, and had the following features: round forehead, blue eyes, straight nose, mustache, pointed chin, light hair, fair complexion, and an oval face. Weight was not specified but photographs from this time showed him to be portly.

Porter sailed from New York on Wednesday, June 28, 1893, with the DePotter Special Tour of Europe on the S.S. *Friesland*, Red Star Line, and arrived in Antwerp on July 8. On his passenger list, Porter placed checks by names, presumably of people he met. Most checks are by the names of women. One name not checked was that of Dr. George Dock, one of the most prominent men in American medicine. At the time Dock was chairman and professor of medicine at the University of Michigan, the school that Porter had left after one year.

The S.S. *Friesland* was 437 feet long with a 51.2 foot beam, one funnel, four masts, steel construction and a single screw which produced a speed of fifteen knots. Built in 1889 by J&G Thompson of Glasgow, the ship carried 226 first class, 102 second class, and 600 third class passengers.

Porter stopped in Paris on July 27, 1893, where he saw the most luxurious city in the world with its plush hotels, spectacular cafes, tree-lined avenues, famous gardens and statuaries, and steam-powered gondolas plying the waters of the Seine. He left Paris on the first leg of his yearlong travel with plans next to climb Mont Blanc, the highest mountain in Europe at

15,780 feet, riding a donkey, according to a post card that he sent back to the *Tribune*.[11] He very likely could not have expected to reach the peak by this method.

From Dresden, Saxony, he wrote in a letter to the editor of the *Tribune* around the first of October:

> Have been on the go nearly all the time and have seen quite thoroughly all the large cities in Holland, Belgium, France, Germany, Northern Italy, Switzerland, etc. The Swiss Alps and lakes are fine and well worth a trip to see.
>
> I'm getting on first-rate. My French was a little off in Paris where I went into a sort of general store to purchase a hot water bag. When I told the sweet creature behind the counter what I wanted she said, "*oui, oui*" and I said, "yes, yes." She led me to the next room and commenced to show me a very nice line of ladies' fur-lined cloaks. Well that did knock the pins from under me. After a while, however, and by showing her a piece of rubber and gesticulating and placing my hands over the spot where this hot water bag was to be applied, I succeed in seeing her pull out from under the counter a dozen of them. Berlin is a much finer city than I supposed. Fine streets and buildings, beautiful parks and fountains and everything so clean and neat. Went through the emperors' palace which contains 700 rooms. Had to put slippers on not to soil or scratch the finely polished floors. The Zoo here is the finest in the world and contains every known animal, bird and reptile, fine specimens of buffalo and an American mule even, and probably the only one in Germany.
>
> Dresden is a pretty place, full of parks and fountains also. I meet plenty of Americans here, in fact, the town is full of them. They come here to study German and to educate their children. This place has one of the finest galleries in Europe, only that of the Louvre in Paris and the one in Florence being better. In this gallery is the Sistine Madonna which is considered the finest picture in existence today and it is certainly a marvel of beauty and an inspiring work and Raphael's masterpiece. The gallery is full of works of Raphael, Correggio, Andrea del Sarto, Titian, Tintoretto, Veechio, Veronese, Rembrandt, etc. This country gets away with us on art but that is about all. In our hotels, our railroads, and our steamboats, we can distance them every time. The women here do not have a very soft snap, surely, see them plowing in the fields, sweeping the streets, taking care of the public parks, blacking boots, shoveling coal, and even hitched up with a dog and hauling a load which would make a Dakota mule lie down and bray. These people over here are not too much in the joking way—too matter of fact and practical. Have tried to get off some of our American jokes on them, but 'tis too hard to explain the thing after, and I've given up in despair.
>
> I leave here in a few days for Vienna, thence to Venice, Nice, Monte Carlo, Genoa, Florence, and Rome, where I expect to be a month from this date or about November 1st. I shall remain in Rome and vicinity until January 1894 when I start for Egypt and Holy Land to spend the winter, returning via Greece and Turkey, stopping at these places some little time. I will not return to Paris for the reason that I have been there twice already and have been obliged to go over the ground here twice in order to carry out my plans and see all I had mapped out.[12]

From historical Vienna, a city of magnificent buildings, gardens, and parks, he sent this letter:

Oct. 9

Am having a very nice time in Vienna which is a very fine city and comes very near being up to Paris. Left Dresden on the 5th inst., arriving here the same day. Passed through a beautiful country — very highly cultivated — and followed the valleys and this winding course of the river Elbe for nearly one half the distance. Saw more women working in the fields than men. They were plowing, digging potatoes, and doing every kind of work. Never saw a cow hitched up to a plow or burrow and made to do a horse's work before. A cow and a woman do not have a fair shake in the country. I wish you could see some of the pictures and other works of art here. Great, I tell you.

I visited the emperor's stables today, where there are 400 and fifty horses and five hundred carriages — all for the royal family. Royalty comes high, but they must have it. This kinging [sic] is pretty good business after all. You don't have to set up the wires for re-election every four years, and then 'tis a close corporation; you keep the thing right in the family all the time.

Must tell you a little joke on myself. While in Saxony I went up the River Elbe on a steamer one day to visit the royal vineyard and the king's chateau. After having seen everything else, my attention was drawn to a nice place — the "King's Restaurant" — where I strolled in — and the same looked fine to a hungry Bismarcker. Well, with the aid of a conversation dictionary, I ordered a good dinner. As I did not want to drink any cholera water, I ordered a bottle of "Herdseick Monopal" and of course everything went very lovely for a while. After the repast was over I motioned to the waiter to bring me the bill, and "Ye Gods!" What did I see? "One bottle of *Herdseick* 1,000 and a mark that looked like a $ sign." You can just image that I thought the "King's Restaurant" prices were way up and the Dutch [Deutsch] were trying to ruin me. I soon found, however, that the 1,000 was not dollars but pfennigs, and a thousand pfennigs is only about $2.50. My dinner went on digesting again immediately.

Wines are so much cheaper here than in America. Poor wines are cheap and dreadful to drink. The best qualities are about the same as our prices. If you want a good cigar, you must get a "Henry Clay" from New York. The best and finest shoe store in all Paris has a nice little gold painted sign in the window which says, "These shoes imported from New York." Hotel rates are $3 to $4 a day, by the time you pay for candles or electric lights — when they have them — and fee everybody who is hanging around the door when you leave, expecting it. One man will bring down your umbrella, another your grip, and a third your trunk, and the boots — he is always there — and the charming chambermaid with her clean, white cap on will inquire very sweetly if you haven't left something in your room. Then last but not least is the porter, all dressed up in fine, dark blue broad cloth trimmed with gold braid and gilt buttons and looks like a major general. Why, at first I thought it would be an insult to offer him money, but I soon found that he was insulted if you did not. Everyone expects a fee in this country who does the least thing for you and some do not — the cabman, the waiter, elevator boy, etc., etc. If you stay one night at a hotel and have supper and breakfast and your bill is $1.75, why you will have to pay out about one dollar in fees. Of course, this is not compulsory, but fees are expected and some of the servants get no other pay. Americans have the name of being better than any other on the feeing business. The native fee about five cents a day, or even less. Some of the hotels make an extra charge for ice and writing paper. They all charge extra for tea or coffee for every meal except breakfast. A breakfast in Europe is a mighty slim affair anyway. Just bread and butter and coffee — simply that and nothing more.

The distances here are not like the United States. You can not travel six days and nights continuously and still be in the same country. In going from Paris to Berlin, a ride of twenty two hours, I started in France, passed through Belgium and Holland and landed in Germany, which makes one republic, two kingdoms, and one empire in less than one day's ride, and my baggage examined three times.[13]

He passed through Venice, but readers of the *Tribune* next heard from Porter in Monte Carlo. The editor commented that although he wrote "a gossipy letter, he doesn't say anything about 'breaking the bank.'"

Monte Carlo, Oct. 23 [1893]

As Mr. Pye used to say, "By the Gods" you ought to be here.[14] This beats anything I've seen yet. I thought Nice was the nicest place but this discounts it.

Monte Carlo is in the Kingdom of Monaco which is the oldest and smallest in the world.

The present Prince is a descendant of Grimaldi of the 10th century [sic, thirteenth century] who drove the Saracens from his dominion. You can shoot an arrow today across his lands.

He has a navy of one ship and an army consisting of seventy five men, one newspaper, and a patron saint.

The Casino is also the finest in the world and owned by a French company which pays the Prince an enormous sum for yearly rental. Some told me it was one and others said five millions, so you can take your choice.

Monte Carlo is situated right on the shore of the Mediterranean and at the foot of the hills or mountains. The grounds are laid out in the most beautiful style, all kinds of flowers, orange, lemon, fig, olive trees, and palms and other tropical and semi-tropical flowers, trees, and plants. Most elegant salt and fresh water, both where the temperature is the same summer and winter. This is certainly a perfect paradise so far as nature and ingenuity of man can make it.

I visited the casino where the roulette and *trente et quarante* was going on and it was a sight to behold. There were six tables going, with sixty at a table and not a word spoken. All could not be seated and gents must leave their hats in the check room. The ladies can wear their hats. I never saw the money fly as it did on those tables, which were literally covered with gold pieces. One dollar, or a French franc, was the smallest bet allowed, but I did not see any limit the other way. At one table they were playing nothing but gold coin, and some of them piled a foot high. It was fun to watch them play; gents not more than 19 years old; old ladies dressed in mourning even, and everyone so nicely dressed in silks and diamonds. I noticed particularly one fine looking old man whose head was white as snow and who had only thirteen hairs on top of his head. I'm sure he was 75 or 80 years old, but the thirteen hairs were lucky numbers; he kept winning right along. The ladies sit and win or lose as the case may be, and never move a muscle, although you can detect by close watching an occasional twitching of the corners of the mouth when there are large losses also, a gleam of delight in their eyes when they pull in pile after pile of the golden coins. Tell Dennis Hannafin [a well-known Bismarck politician and gambler] that this is the place where he ought to be.[15] He is a no limit man. They could suit him here.

The weather is hot but should think the climate would be perfect a little later on. Oranges are now green but just commencing to ripen. Ladies are wearing white dresses. From my window I have a splendid view of Monaco, Monte Carlo and out on the Mediterranean as far as the eye can reach; can also see far over into Italy. I want to see a little more of this gaming business but shall start tomorrow or next day to Florence stopping a few days again at Genoa, I believe ... I send you my admission card to the Casino so you can see what it is like.

Wish I could send you some views of this place, but there is duty on the mounted ones and it would spoil the unmounted ones to fold them.

The road from Genoa here was just simply a succession of orange, lemon, fig, and olive groves and close to the sea all the time. I shall go to the Casino in the evening as I've seen it in the day time only as yet. Regard to all friends.[16]

Chapter 18

Italian Journey

While Porter was cavorting across Europe hard times had returned to Bismarck with the Panic of 1893. The Northern Pacific Railroad had fallen into receivership again. With Bismarck's economy so enmeshed with the health of the railroad, its outlook was decidedly dim. It would be another three years after the mortgage on the property was foreclosed and the railroad reorganized before any hope for better times could return.[1]

A battle for control of the First National Bank of Bismarck had occurred at the end of 1892 and culminated in the loss of control by the Fairchild, Porter, Whitaker and Eisenberg faction to the Fisher faction, which had control of 526 votes against a possible 496 votes controlled by the Fairchild faction at the January 10, 1893, meeting. Wildly inflated prices were offered for the few stocks necessary for control of the bank.

Fairchild's offer of five thousand dollars for J.R. Gage's ten shares was trumped by Fisher's offer of five thousand dollars plus the job as cashier for one hundred dollars a month. Porter had held an option on the Strauss stock until January 6, 1893, but then did not exercise it. When Gage's written contract with Fisher was not honored, Gage sued Fisher. In district court, when Fisher was asked why he put Gage on the board of directors, he replied that "he did not want a fight on his hands," and added that "Messrs. Fairchild, Porter, Whitaker, and Eisenberg were exceedingly vicious, and doing all they could to injure the bank when they found that he [Fisher] had control. They went all over town telling all about the depositors, and he did not want to have Gage with his enemies. It was to avoid this, and for this reason alone, that he put Mr. Gage on the directorate."[2]

Judge Winchester rendered a verdict in Fisher's favor with Gage ordered to repay Fisher three thousand dollars and to give him a note for two thousand dollars, and Fisher ordered to return to Gage the ten shares of stock.[3] It appears that Porter was unwilling to pay excessive prices for shares in the battle for control. This led to further ill will in the Fairchild family toward him. The battle between Fairchild and some of Porter's former business partners, including Fisher, may have soured Porter on Bismarck and possibly have been a factor in his plans to leave.

Meanwhile, Fairchild was ruined and left Bismarck on July 24, 1893, a broken man. His twelve-year-old daughter Katherine confided in her diary:

> "Oberlin, Ohio, Saturday, October 13, How circumstances change! The little house is no longer inhabited by us in the bracing air of Dakota. Hallie and I no longer quarrel over croquet or skating for we are no longer there. Hallie is in Ashland — his papa is across the Atlantic. Papa and Mamma and I are in this college town at Grandpa's. I left this journal to use a small red diary but I have come back to these white pages with joy and yet sorrow — joy that my education is begun — joy as that which Grandpa sheds abroad — sorrow that Hallie is not here, that Aunt Grace is dead — that we no longer have a little house of our own — sorrow that I am a year older and my childhood days are passing so swiftly and yet glad I am getting old enough to do some good in the world."[4]

Two weeks later she wrote, "I keep wondering what my circumstances will be — fatherless for dear Papa is so sick — we don't know if he will ever get out of bed again."

Porter was in Venice on November 11 and wrote, "Wanting to see Venice again, here I am. The crown prince is here and the firing of cannon has been going on all day."[5]

Soon after, Porter described the sights of Rome for *Tribune* readers:

> I'm enjoying Rome very much and was agreeably surprised to find such a clean and beautiful city. The recent heavy rains have caused the rise of the Tiber which has done some damage and the people here seem to think 'tis a wonderful stream and large, and while it is the largest river in the Italian peninsula it is nothing in comparison with our own Missouri.
>
> Yesterday I went out about six miles on the Roman Campagna to see a fox hunt. They routed a fox soon after the start, but the dogs did not get him until after a run of about ten miles. Was good sport to see the fox run and jump for his life with the hounds close on to him pell-mell. The horses would take the fences, stone walls and ditches splendidly. The first man who reached the fox after the dogs caught him took the head to have it mounted. The second gets the tail, and the next few each have a foot. Saw large flocks of sheep on the Campagna, and the men attending them had coats and pants made of sheep skins with the wool on, and the wool side out.
>
> Thought I had seen fine churches in Paris and the Cathedral at Milan and Cologne, but they are simply not in it when compared [*sic*] with St. Peter's and St. Paul's here. Words fail to give any idea of their grandeur and magnificence. St. Peter's is the largest and probably the most beautiful church in the world. The bronze statue of St. Peter in this church has the right foot partly worn off by devotees who go there daily by hundreds for this purpose.
>
> A constant stream of people were kissing the foot today. The canopy and high altar stands over the tomb of St. Peter. The confessional is surrounded by eighty-nine ever-burning lamps. The church is full of the most beautiful statuary and

mosaics and it is light and bright and airy and hasn't the dull, dark appearance of most Cathedrals. The air is fresh and good and does not have the "odor of sanctity" which most of the churches have. While I am in love with St. Peter's church I must not fail to say that St. Paul's church is considered by some to be equal and even superior to the former. St. Paul's is outside the city walls, and with her solid columns of oriental alabaster resting on pedestals of solid malachite presented by the emperor of Russian, why it is very difficult to decide between the two. I attended mass at the church of St. Cecelia where a cardinal was officiating.

There is a church here, the Scala Santa, which has a flight of twenty-eight marble steps from the palace of Pilate at Jerusalem which Christ once used. They were brought to Rome in the year 326, and may only be ascended on the knees.

I saw lots of people going up that way but did not try it. The visit to the Catacombs was very interesting where there are twelve miles of passage way hewn out of solid rock. These passages are filled with the dead, one above the other, eight or ten high in places. Each body had a separate hole dug out of the rock where the body was put and it was then closed with a close-fitting stone and cemented so that it was air-tight. A jolly old monk took us through and pointed out the more prominent tombs. The Corso presents a lively scene every evening when the fashionable world comes out and crowds it with elegant carriages and foot passengers. The fountains of Rome are one of its most beautiful attractions. They are everywhere and, what is better, they are always playing. No dry ones like so many of ours in America.

Wish you could see the Sistine Chapel in the Vatican. Paintings by Michael Angelo, and the Vatican Palace is the largest in the world, and the residence of the Pope. The palace contains eleven thousand halls, chapels, saloons, and private apartments—eleven thousand, mind you and not eleven hundred.

In the Vatican gallery are the celebrated pictures, "Transfiguration" and "Coronation of the Virgin" by Raphael. I visited a monastery called Tres Fontana (three fountains) where the monks are all rich, but they are not allowed to speak, and work in the gardens with bare heads and feet. In the grounds is the very spot where the Apostle Paul was beheaded. Saw the block or shaft to which he was bound when he was beheaded. I send you a few leaves from the place.

H.R. Porter[6]

In his next letter in December 1893 he wrote:

Have been in Rome about four weeks and like it first rate, and more I see of it the better I like it, and I must tell about some of the interesting places. Palatine Hill was the original site and center of the mistress of the world. Hortensius, Catiline, Cicero, and other big guns had their private dwellings here. On this hill is where Romulus built his city 735 B.C. Some of the walls are still standing and in fact the whole ruins, called the "Palace of the Caesars" are in good state of preservation, especially the beautiful mosaic floors, and even some of the wall painting, and they have been buried for hundreds of years. Workmen are still excavating. Some of the walls were cased with transparent oriental marble so highly polished as to reflect like mirrors. 'Twas here that Cicero delivered the first oration against

Catiline and the Emperor Caligula was murdered by Cassius A.D. 39. [*sic,* Cassius Chaerea and two other stabbed Caligula in A.D. 41] The cave or grotto was pointed out to us where the she-wolf was found nursing the twins. Immediately below is the valley made famous by the rape of the Sabine women.

From Pincian Hill or "Monte Pincio" we get one of the finest views of modern Rome. The hill is laid out for walks, driveways, parks, flower gardens, fountains, small lakes, and live swans, beautiful tropical trees and plants, etc. The band plays here several times a week and it is where the beauty and fashion of Rome congregate every Sunday, to listen to the music and show off their fine carriages and superbly dressed ladies. On this hill where once were the famous gardens of Lucullus in which Messalina, the wife of Claudius afterwards celebrated her orgies. Wish you could see the Colosseum, which grand old structure has stood from about the time of Christ, and which looks good for thousand of years to come. The interior has seats for 87,000 spectators. The seats where the Vestal Virgins sat are still there, and when they said thumbs up, the prostrate gladiator's life was spared, and thumbs down meant instant death. They have queer ways of doing things here, for instance, in going to the opera they charge 40 cents for admission then $1 or $2 for a seat. In making purchases they ask you [for] 40 to 50 percent more than they will take. It took me a long time to get onto this game, and when I did was ashamed to offer so much less, but soon found out that I was being swindled at every turn. Now, after inquiring the price I cut the price right in two the first pop. Often times they say, "take it," and always come down from 20 to 40 percent. The weather is warm and pleasant. Children barefooted. Orange and olive crops are just being harvested. Some of the olive trees here are 2000 years old. Have had beggars on the run and follow our carriage for two miles. We tried to tire them out but they tired us out, and we threw them a handful of coin to get rid of them. I understand that in some parts the policemen go in pairs for self-protection, as they are afraid to be out after dark alone. These Italians are very apt with a knife, their favorite weapon, it makes no noise and is very sure. You may be certain that I'm not wandering around much dark nights.

The hotel where I'm staying is kept by an American lady who has been here twenty-eight years. Nearly all her boarders are Americans from Maine to California and all splendid people with whom 'tis a pleasure to meet and associate with.

Was driving on the Pincian Hill Sunday where I met the queen, raised my hat to her and received a bow and a pleasant smile in return. Have met the king several times, same way. He is a fine looking person, bright piercing eye, white hair, and mustache and easily recognized from the picture on the postage stamps. Can tell the queen by her driver and coachman, who are all dressed in red and scarlet. They put on no airs and are very popular in Rome and Italy.

Last Sunday I saw the Pope perform mass in St. Peter's, which church seats about 25,000 and holds 80,000, or about one half the population of Minneapolis (as per last padded returns). The Pope was carried in on a golden sedan chair by six men. A passageway was made through the church and guarded. Swiss Guards keep the way clear with spear and sword. As he passed in and out the people shouted "*Viva il papa-re*" (Long life to the pope-king). The ceremony was certainly grand, solemn, and sublime. Many men, women, and children were weeping as the old, feeble pope was carried out, waving his trembling hand and blessing the audience. He must be between eighty and eighty-five years old, and cannot stay much longer. [Pope Leo XIII, born 1810, died 1903, pope 1878–1903. He was eighty-two and was called The Great White Shepherd of Christendom.][7]

New Year's Day found Porter in Naples. From the Hotel Pension Britannique he wrote to his niece, his sister and others telling them about the sights that he would describe more in detail in a letter to the *Bismarck Tribune* that follows.[8]

January 3, 1894 — Naples

How are you today? I'm quite well thank you and I am having a devil of a fine time, can assure you. I was stuck on Rome, and I can tell you that if I ever hated to leave a place, those places were Paris and Rome. Believe I'm seeing everything pretty thoroughly. I left Rome a few days ago at 8:30 A.M. and arrived here at 2 P.M. passing through great mountain scenery and beautiful valleys of olives and orange groves. The latter so full of fruit that one could hardly see the leaves on the trees. Someone said, "see Naples and die." [There is an Italian proverb, "See Naples and then die."[9] It is referred to in James Joyce's *Ulysses*, "the bay of Naples (to see which was to die.)"[10]] Another fellow said, "Live and see Naples." I agree with the other fellow. Naples is the largest city in Italy—population about one-half million—and occupies one of the most beautiful situations in the world. Nature has certainly very bountifully lavished her gifts on this favored spot. In the older parts are narrow dingy streets and high and narrow houses with flat roofs and balconies which are not very attractive but interesting. The origin and name of the city [is] Greek, and its history goes back a thousand years before Christ. This is the greatest place for fast driving, cracking of whips, rattle of wheels, braying of donkeys, shouting of hawkers at all hours of the day and night.

The cabmen all drive their horses without any bits. They have a sort of leather and metal band around the nose and lines are fastened on either side. Men go around the streets driving a flock of goats (ten to fifteen), and when any person wants any milk, they come out with a cup pick out or choose the one they want milk from, when the man halts his flock and calls out the name of this one. She comes to him and he milks her right there and then. Not much chance to chalk and water or dilute that milk. The only way I can see to beat that game would be to pump all the goats full of water before starting out.

The "Museum Nazionale" contains collections from the excavated treasures of Pompeii, Herculaneum, Stabine, etc., and is the first in Europe. The "Neapolitan Aquarium" is a sight and a wonder, and the best in the world. Contains the most curious marine animals of every description, cuttlefish, octopus, electric rays, which you are permitted to touch and receive a shock—many kinds of living coral. Beautiful medusae and crested blubbers, pipe fish, cray fish, and many exquisitely colored fish from the Mediterranean.

Pompeii is only about eighteen miles from Naples, and the visit to this once prosperous town with a population of 25,000 is indeed interesting. This ramble through the city of the dead is well-worth a trip to Europe. The streets are straight and narrow, seldom more than twenty-four feet in breadth—and some only fourteen—but nicely paved with blocks of lava. You can see deep ruts in the causeways made by wagons. The houses are built of concrete. Some of the shop tables are covered with marble, and fitted-up with large earthen vessels for the sale of olive oil; the paintings on the wall are in good state of preservation.

In the museum we see preserved casts of human corpses and one body of a dog. Among the figures are a young girl with a ring on her finger, two women, one tall and old, the other young. Also, loaves of bread charred from the heat but otherwise perfect. One loaf had the baker's name plainly stamped on it, viz. "Celer Slave of 2 Granius Verna." Saw also honey, grain, nuts, figs, pears, etc. and surgical instruments same as we have now, viz: bone forceps, bivalve speculum, syringes.

Did you ever see a beggar on horseback? Well, I saw one yesterday on a donkey. He rode up and held out his hat for coin, and I was walking. Wasn't that gall? Talk about western gall, why, we are not in it with the Italians....

We go up Vesuvius tomorrow. Can see the smoke rolling out by daylight and the fire by night. The mountain side is covered with luxuriant vineyards which yield the famous "Lacrimae Christi [wine]." I sail for Egypt Saturday.

H.R. Porter[11]

In Egypt he met another DePotter tour, the Long Oriental Excursion, that left New York January 4, 1894, on the Hamburg-American steamship *Columbia*.

Chapter 19

Up the Nile

Porter's next letter, as usual, related his adventures as he traveled from Italy to Egypt and then up the Nile. It went to the editor of the *Tribune*, M.H. Jewell. At the time Porter was staying at the Grand New Hotel for six days before leaving on a month's cruise up the Nile. Jewell published the letter on February 15 under the heading, "Among the Pyramids, Dr. Porter Rambling About Among the Obelisks and Pyramids of Ancient Egypt."

Cairo, Egypt Jan. 20 [1894]

Instead of sailing from Naples I sailed from Brindisi, which gave me an extra day of rail and one day less of water. Left the latter place on the 7th inst., and we had only got well into the Adriatic before the steamer rocked and plunged and flopped about like a fish out of water. Of course we all took to our heels and the most of us to our beds. The second day, passed into the Mediterranean where it was even worse and that night we were obliged to brace ourselves and hang on in order to keep from tumbling out. The waves dashed over the ship, the water squirted through the keyhole [porthole?] and wet us from head to foot. I found my shoes in the morning floating under the berth, and an inch of water on the water-tight floor. One of my shoes was waterlogged so that she could not sail as fast as the other, consequently did not have so much trouble to catch it. After three days and nights of this sort of traveling, for pleasure, we sighted the coast of Africa and one hour later we landed in Alexandria, a seasick party of nine — now happy Americans. Also many others from different countries. We visited Pompey's Pillar, the bazaars, Mahomeden cemetery, and other places of interest, and then started for Cairo by express train, an only three hour run which was very pleasant and interesting, Arab towns all along the way, built of mud, long lines of camels loaded with cotton and all kinds of truck. Dusky Arabs plowing with buffaloes hitched to wooden plows and also watering the land by dipping the water up in baskets and thus irrigating thousands of acres.

The weather here seems simply perfect. So much finer than Italy. Warm, bright, and pleasant, no rain. Ladies are dressed in white and gents wear straw hats. Must tell you about a nice little shooting match I saw last evening between two editors of rival papers. They met on the street a block from the hotel and pulled their guns. At first I thought some Arab boy had lighted a pack of firecrackers, but in a second saw one of them fall with five bullets in him. He is very good editor now. The other fellow wasn't much of an editor for handsome I can tell you. He was blood from the crown of his head to the soles of his feet. He had a furrow plowed through each cheek, part of his nose shot off, and two of his fingers dangling from his pistol-hand, but game to the last. Eight policemen had their hands full to arrest him, and he would have killed them if he had more guns. Come to Cairo, good opening for your business, just now.

I visited the Citadel and Mosque of Mohamed Ali which are situated on the same high point where you get one of the finest views. At the foot of the Citadel northward lies Cairo with its innumerable domes and minarets, beyond are the green delta. On the right is the tombs of the Memlooks and Obelisks of Heliopolis. On the left is old Cairo, the Nile, Grand Aqueduct, the Pyramids of Ghizeh [Giza] and Sakkurah [Sakkara]. The citadel is garrisoned by English troops, and 'twas here that the Memlooks were invited to a feast and entertainment and then slaughtered. Four hundred and fifty were killed here and 800 in the city. Only one escaped by leaping his horse from a very high terrace. The mosque is very beautiful, the whole of the interior being lined with Oriental alabaster. On the left, a golden grill enclosed the tomb of Mohamed Ali, with lamps kept perpetually burning. The museum at Boulak is a wonder. We saw paintings between six and seven thousand years old, and bright and fresh looking mummies of nearly the same age; one of Ramses II. Cairo has a population of about 400,000, and sitting on the hotel porch, here is what you will see any day — donkeys, donkeys everywhere. They use them here same as people use street cars in Chicago; camels loaded with everything- hay, boards, heavy timbers and a whole family of eight on one camel; snake charmers, dressed in leopard skins with a bag of snakes and a monkey man with him. He will commence to pull out the snakes until a sidewalk is covered with them, and punch and bother them and make them fight him, throw them on the monkeys, and frighten them nearly to death. The monkeys will yell and jump on the men's shoulders in trying to get away. A half-dressed and half-wild Nubian will sing and dance and play on his harp for ten cents; funerals where they carry the body and coffin on their head; an Arab prince on his fiery steed and the rich heavy swell in his fine carriage, and two Arab outrunners who run ahead, straight as an arrow, crying out in Arabic, "look out, look out, get out of the way." They run that way for miles, look fine and are dressed in wide, white pants — wide as a grain sack — which comes down to the knees, then bare legs and feet, red Turkish cap, richly embroidered Persian jacket, silk sash, etc. The English swell is here in all his glory. Men sprinkle the streets from goat skins filled with water from the Nile, and carried on their backs. Could fill a dozen pages with the apparent fakes we see every day. In one of the bedrooms of the khedives' palaces we saw six curtains which cost $2,500 each, or the snug little sum of $15,000. Visited the university where there are now 8,000 and sometimes 12,000 dirty Arabs who sit in groups and circles of about thirty, with the teacher in the center, expounding knowledge and the law. Mohammed knew what he was doing when he made his people pray five times a day, and wash before every prayer. If there is anything on earth needs washing five times a day, 'tis an Arab. We leave on the 25th inst. for a month on the Nile, and to the first cataract. Will have about twenty-four in our party — all Americans. We go in two steam-towed *dahabeahs*, with a crew of sixty, including sailors, servants, dragomen, etc. We fly the American flag, and as one boat is new, have named her *Columbia* and have a long steamer flag flying from her mast, with that name on it. Saw the dervishes the other day, and they are a howling success. The Sioux ghost dance or sun dance is not in it with them. We visit the great pyramids and sphinx on Monday.

H.R. Porter[1]

While Porter was in Egypt, George H. Fairchild, age 49, died in Oberlin, Ohio, on February 9, 1894, of heart trouble. Fairchild had left Bismarck and had gone East when his health began to fail the previous July. This coincided with his banking and personal financial problems. He left a wife, Helen Viets Fairchild, and a young twelve-year-old daughter, Katherine, who wrote in her diary, "I did not have to wait till I was twenty to be fatherless for dear Papa left us at 3 o'clock on the morning of the ninth just two days after I last wrote. Oh, how I will miss him. If I could only have had him till I was a little older, but it would have been no easier — only Mamma and I are left now — The undertaker came and fixed him nice and we had him in his room till Sunday — he looked so natural."[2] His was a sad story of struggle and failure of one not suited by temperament for the rough and tumble of frontier banking. There is no record of Porter's reaction to the death, no letter or public comment.

Porter's party left Cairo on January 25 on two *dahabeahs* towed by a steam tug, which was underpowered. Consequently the tour director, Dr. DePotter, returned to Cairo to charter a steamer that could do the job. It had accommodations for twenty-six. Since there were only twenty-four in the party, there was plenty of room, so they transferred "bag and baggage" to the steamer.

The group seemed to have a wonderful time with music from a piano and dancing until late every evening. They reached Kom Ombo near Assuan on February 13 at the first cataract. This was the end of their journey up the Nile and the place where they turned around.[3]

Two days after writing to his family, Porter wrote to M.H. Jewell another of the "for publication" letters, which had attracted a sizeable following. The editor wrote, "The *Tribune*'s letters from Dr. Porter are read with interest all over the state."[4]

Assouan, Upper Egypt, Feb 14 [1894]

Your letter of January 1st reached me a few days ago on the Nile steamer, where it had been forwarded from Rome to Naples, then to Cairo and Luxor, etc. The extra postage on it was only 40 cents, but your letters are very welcome, and cheap at any price. There is one good thing about the postal arrangement here; they do keep a letter hot on your trail, and it will catch you nearly every time, but papers, they just chuck them into the fuel pile and never bother anymore about them.

The trip on the Nile is delightful. We stop at all the places of interest and take donkey rides to those that are any distance from the river.... We visited the city of Memphis, and very little remains to remind us of the most ancient city in the world. Here is the colossal statue of Rameses II, the brick pyramids of Sakhara, tombs and gigantic Sarcophagi of Sacred Bulls, the Mausoleum of Thi, etc. At Beni-Hassen the donkeys are the worst in Egypt and the donkey boys the finest. They would light, and five or six of them grab for our saddles, so then we have to use their donkeys. We furnish our own saddles. Beni-Hassen is a very bad town and was once completely destroyed by Ibraham Pasha on account of the insubordination of the people.

On our way to the tombs we were guarded by soldiers to protect us from being robbed. While we were tied up at his place, quite a storm came up in the night which caused a good deal of excitement. Our boats and tugs broke loose, crashing into each other and floating downstream. All was yelling and confusion, the sailors calling on Mahomet and every other prophet to save us from destruction. We finally landed on a sandbar and were safe. In the morning, after getting off, while the storm was still raging, we were obliged to land or rather cast anchor on a fine onion patch. The owner came down, wild with excitement, and ordered us off. Our crew said no and peeled for a fight, when this Arab grabbed up a handful of sand, threw it up in the air, and gave a yell that would cause a Sioux chief to blush with envy. With this yell the Arabs seemed to spring up from the ground and in less than no time a hundred of them were on the spot, all armed with sticks and ready to cut our ropes and pull up our anchor. They were too many for us, and we had to pull in our horns and pay the damage for the onions, and thus ended the row and the fun....

We are always on deck from morning until eve. Have four meals a day, viz: breakfast, 8 A.M.; lunch, 12 m.; tea, 4 P.M.; dinner, 6:30 P.M.; then dance every night until 11 or 12 o'clock. During the day some are reading, writing, card-playing, sewing, loafing, drinking, smoking, playing a piano or guitar, one or two couples in a quite shady nook making love. I believe this country is conducive to love and laziness. I'm quite sure the latter and do not require much argument to convince me of the former. No wonder Anthony and Cleopatra killed themselves when they found their little game was up. This Nile trip is really the perfection of travel. From Cairo to Assouan is about 600 miles—the valley of Egypt is 600 miles long and 10 to 30 miles wide. You can see from one side to the other nearly the whole distance. One side is the Libyan and on the other the Arabian mountains. Arab towns, large sugar factories, employing 2,000 hands, and beautiful palm groves all along the river. Should think it would be the hunter's paradise for we are all the time seeing large flocks of ducks, geese, cranes, pelicans, and other game birds. The weather is very warm and the air soft and balmy. [There are] plenty of men and boys, perfectly naked. The women are more modest with the exception of a pair of earrings or a string of beads around their necks. This seems a little queer at first, but 'tis a very light and airy costume—very little trouble to dress and withal has many good points, especially for this country and lazy climate. One drawback to traveling in this country is the everlasting begging or *backsheesh*. It seems a small matter to give 5, 10, or 25 cents but when you consider that sometimes 100 hands are held out to you at once, why, it will not take much figuring to use up $100.

19. Up the Nile

We have one in our party who weighs more than the donkey she rides, and 'tis one of the sights of Egypt to see 300 pounds of female loveliness on a 250 pound donkey. All you can see of the donkey is his ears. We have another very nice personage in our party, but he will insist and persist in picking his teeth, also his ears with his spectacle bones at the table.

I send you program of the camel, buffalo, and other races we saw at Luxor. They were very funny. The camel is not so bad as he is painted, but 'tis a long time between drinks with him. Yesterday I rode one eight miles over the Nubian desert to the Island of Philae. All the others took [the] *dahabeah* and laughed at me, saying, "you will wish you hadn't," but I was the first one in and the old camel and myself laid down under a tree in the shade and ate dates until the party arrived. Our dragoman told me not to ride the camel. Said it made some people have hemorrhage of the lungs. This one was an exceptionally good and easy one or I'm a natural camel rider (probably the latter) for the motion was pleasant, very pleasant when walking and when going, no harder than a trotting horse. On our way we saw the huge obelisks partially quarried from the native rocks. At the island of Philae we visited the Temple of Isis, one of the most elegant structures amidst the most beautiful scenery on the Nile. The whole island is covered with ruins and here is the splendid temple known as "Pharaoh's Bed" where we had a fine lunch in the temple. Returning we took a boat and shot the first cataract stopping on the way to see the half-wild Nubians jump about twenty feet into the boiling rapids and swim out. Others shoot them on a log after taking off all their clothing. All this for one piaster or five cents. It seems strange how much people will do here for a few cents. The other day when I was visiting the tombs of the kings at Thebes, one of the pretty little water girls came along side of the donkey and said, "Me your girl today." I said no. She put her hand on her heart and said, "You no like me; I feel very sad because you no like me; I like you; you very nice man. You pretty man. I think you American man. Me like Americans." Well what would you do in a case like this? Of course I let her be my water girl after all that. She was tall and straight as an arrow, dark-skinned, snow white pearly teeth, black eyes, bare feet and legs and so little clothing that it is not worth mentioning. Well this dusky maiden followed me and kept close to my donkey either walking or trotting, with her water jar on her head always ready to give me a drink or pour water on my hands or wet my head, all this for twelve miles in the hot sand and burning sun for 10 cents. Some only give 5 cents. I gave her 25 cents, and blushed for giving so little. At Thebes we saw the statue of Rameses the Great which is the largest in the world. The weight is 1,000 tons a foot, eleven feet long and one of the toes larger than a man's body. How in the world they ever transported this massive statue of stone is a wonder. Assouan has a population of about 10,000 about 600 miles from Cairo and steam boat terminus from lower Nile. It is a beautiful place in a fertile strip of fine date palms. Considerable trade is carried on in products from Soudan and Abyssinia, brought on camels and shipped north to Aksiut and Cairo. The chief articles are ostrich feathers, ivory, indian rubber, senna, tamarinds, wax skins, horns, dates, etc. Can get ostrich feathers from 40 cents up. Egypt is full of temples and tombs and the mountains are literally honeycombed with the latter. Human skulls and bones are scattered around everywhere, and if they were in Dakota, they would be gathered up and shipped and ground into fertilizer the same as our Dakota buffalo ones are. The enterprising Egyptians, however, do rob the tombs of the mummies and they have them for sale on every hand.

You can purchase hand, foot, head, or any part you want. I have two mummy hands and bones of various parts of the anatomy which I have picked up and purchased. [Porter seems to have been attracted to collecting human body parts, scalps in the west, bones at the catacombs, and mummy hands in Egypt.]

I have seen a dog and a man hitched up together in Belgium, a woman and a cow in Germany, but the queerest of all was seen the other day—a camel and a small cow hitched up and plowing. They plow and dip the water from the Nile for irrigation and tread out the grain with the patient ox—separate the wheat from the chaff by throwing it in the air, exactly the same as it was done six or seven thousand years ago. This is progress. The tombs and temples, however, they were far ahead of us. At Thebes and Luxor especially at Karnak, we see the most interesting part of ancient Thebes. Under the Pharaohs, the temples here were considered the most striking creation of the age famous for architectural achievements. Much has been destroyed, yet after centuries there is no building that equals in size and grandeur the temple of Amon at Karnak.

H.R. Porter[5]

The tour returned to the Grand New Hotel in Cairo on February 23 for a few days before leaving for the Holy Land.

Porter's letters to the *Tribune* lifted the spirits of Bismarck citizens who were suffering through the Panic of 1893 and gave them needed diversion from their woes. The price of wheat had plunged when money could not be borrowed from back East to ship it to the markets. Money was scarce and unemployment was rising. But the witty and informative accounts from a well-known friend brought them some relief.

Chapter 20

Travels to the Holy Land and Around the Mediterranean

Porter's next account for Dakotans came from the Holy Land, which was then under Turkish control. Tour guides had no problem relating contemporary geographical features to biblical history. Porter jotted notes and biblical references on one of his prescription pads and dated it March 2, 1894, Joppa, on which he cites Jonah 1:3. "But Jonah rose up to flee to Tarshish from the presence of the Lord, and went down to Joppa; and he found a ship going to Tarshis." There were other references to Acts 9, 2 Samuel, 2 Chronicles, Genesis, Ezekiel, 1 Kings, and 2 Kings.

He arrived in Jaffa, Palestine, on March 2 and traveled by rail through the plains of Sharon, by way of Ramleh, through the Valley of Ajalon [where Joshua commanded the sun to stand still], to Jerusalem. He started the next letter after staying in Jerusalem at Hotel Howard from March 2 to March 6, when he left for Jericho, and completed it after he arrived in Damascus at the Hotel Demetri on March 19. He seems to have been a most gullible tourist when in the Holy Land. His biblical information does not bear close inspection.

Jerusalem, March 9 [1894]

We left Alexandria a few days ago and after twenty-four hours ride on a steamer where nearly every person was sick, we landed at Jaffa, or rather anchored out about one-half mile from the shore which is as near as ships or steamers can come on account of the dangerous, rocky coast.[1] All passengers and freights must be landed in small row boats which is slow, difficult, and dangerous.

Right here at Jaffa is the place where Jonah was taken out of the wet by the whale. We visited the house of Simon the Tanner [where Peter lodged, Acts 9:43], and also saw the rock to which [the mythical] Andromeda was chained in order that she might be devoured by a huge sea monster, but was released by Perseus. We left Jaffa in the morning and passed through the valley of Sharon and over the mountains of Judea. What was my surprise when I went forward to see the engine which drew us up the grade and to notice that it was a Baldwin,

Philadelphia, United States of America.² The engine was all right but the coaches were just horrible — and first-class too. It rained very hard on the way to Jerusalem and the rain came through the roof of the cars so that we actually had to put up our umbrellas in order to keep dry. On our arrival here every hotel was full, and we were obliged to put up at a hospice, or Austrian convent where we were well taken care of. Visited the Church of the Sepulcher, saw the place where Abraham was on the point of sacrificing Isaac. Here is the Stone of Anointment on which the body of Jesus laid when it was anointed by Nicodemus and the Holy Sepulcher; the stone said to be the one the angel rolled away from the mouth of the grave. This place is constantly guarded by soldiers and fifteen lamps kept burning all the time. Here are the sticks in which the feet of Christ were put during his preparation for crucifixion, and the chapel of St. Helena where the cross was found. At Mount Zion we saw the home of Cariaphas [Caiaphas, the high priest]; the prison of our Lord; the spot where the cock crew, etc. Jerusalem is full of interesting places, and we visited all of them with a guide to explain and to brush up our memory. I will mention some of the most interesting: The Mosque of Omar standing on the site of King Solomon's temple, which is on Mount Moriah; the stable of King Solomon. Here is the Holy Rock, 57 feet long and 43 feet wide on which Abraham worshiped and offered sacrifices and burnt offerings. Elijah [sic] and David, Jesus and Mohamet have all prayed here; St. Anne's Church, where Mary, the mother of Christ was born; the Judgment hall, where Christ was condemned, and the room where he was scourged; the street through which he was made to carry the cross.

We made a visit to Bethlehem in carriages. On the way I saw the tomb of Rachel; David's well; the place where the three wise men saw the stars; church of the Nativity; and the exact spot where Christ was born. Returning to Jerusalem, I saw the tomb of the Virgin, nearby is the rock where Peter, James, and John slept and the place Judas betrayed Christ with a kiss; visited the gardens of Gethsemane, and rode horseback through the valley of Jehosaphat and Hinnom, passing the village of Shiloah.

On the 6th we all left Jerusalem on horses for Jericho, leaving at 8 A.M. and arriving at 5 P.M. We enjoyed the ride as the roads were fine and the mountain scenery very picturesque. The way is very winding and the mountains of Judea all rocks and very little vegetation and no signs of life with the exception of a flock of goats here and there guarded by a dusky native clad in sheep skins and sitting on a rock playing a sort of flute. The mountains and rocks are so steep and only a blade of grass occasionally, it seems impossible that the goats can pick a living. I should think they would require a dentist to keep their teeth in order and a set of climbers on their feet. We also meet long caravans of camels, of poor little donkeys about the size of a large dog, with men, women, and children on their backs. We passed Bethany on the way which is a dirty place of about forty hovels. At noon we lunched at the house of the Good Samaritan and saw where the great Elijah was fed by the ravens, also where Christ was tempted. After a good night's rest in camp, we mounted and started for the Dead Sea where we waited an hour, took a bath and then to the River Jordan where we had bathed again to get rid of salt for the Dead Sea which is very irritating to the skin. We rested and lunched on the banks of the Jordan at "Pilgrims Bathing

Place" where Jesus was baptized by John. Gilgal is near here and we had it pointed out to us.

I started this letter in Jerusalem but did not finish it as we were hurried away on our journey to Damascus where we are now (March 20). Talk about Jordan being a hard road to travel —'tis not so— Jordan is easy, very easy, but when you travel from Jerusalem to Damascus, two or three hundred miles on horseback, and a bucking, kicking stallion at that, and over the roughest roads in the world, when going up the mountains you must hang on to your horse's neck to keep from sliding over his tail and going down, you must grab his tail to keep from riding on his neck and ears. Why, you may call that a hard road, and that is just what it is. All this for $10 a day, rain, dust, blistered nose, face and ears and other parts of the anatomy also blistered. Some of our party had never been astride a horse before, and the third day out from Jerusalem they could not walk and it was painful to ride. All the riding horses here are stallions, and such a kicking, biting, fighting lot I never saw. One lady was kicked from her horse. Several more thrown and it is a wonder they were not killed. My horse was a fine one, but a bucker and kicker, he nearly landed me several times but never got me off, although I rode all over, that is from his ears to his tail. However, I like the ugly brute, for he never fell or got tired and carried me through safely, and I was the first one to reach Damascus, nearly two hours ahead of the party. I must say that I really enjoyed the trip, and our camping outfit and arrangements the best I ever saw. Five Turkish tents, good beds and we were allowed plenty of baggage, all packed on horses and mules. When we would reach camp every evening our tents would be up, beds ready, Turkish rugs on the floor, and an elegant lunch or dinner ready. We made the trip in ten days, and the trip, though hard and rough, was full of interest. Will simply mention some of the places where we visited. Bethany, place where David fled to get away from Saul [sic]; Tomb of Samuel; Old Shiloh, where the Ark of the Covenant stood 300 years; Jacob's well and tomb; Synagogue of the Samaritans at Nabulus, where we saw the pentateuch, which is 3,525 years old. Nabulus is the meanest place we have yet seen; children followed us and hooted, made faces, and threw mud, and spit at us, and tried to snatch our riding whips. Samaria, we saw where John the Baptist was buried, passed Remeth (of Joshua XIX-21) March 13th after a hard pull up the mountain, passing ancient Jezred [Jezreel]. Close by is the scene of the great battle by Saul against the Philistines. Saul, himself, fell here and Elisha restored child to life. In Nazareth we saw Gabriel's Column [?], which marks the spot where the Virgin received the angel's message, and also the kitchen of the virgin, the workshop of Joseph, etc. The 14th we reached the Sea of Galilee where we camped on the shore and I had several good swims. The sea is only fourteen miles by six, and would only make a fifth or sixth class lake in the United States. Was shown the place where Simon was born and also the birthplace of the Prophet Jonah and the Mount of Beatitudes or scene of the Sermon on the Mount, where our Lord fed so many hungry people on so little material [sic]. At Canna, the original water jars were shown in which Christ turned water into wine. We sailed down the Sea of Galilee to Capernaum, and after viewing the ruins of that ancient city, found our horses waiting for us, where we mounted and started again for Damascus. But my letter is getting too long. Arrived here yesterday,

March 19th, and remained long enough to see the city and will start in a few days in carriages to Baolbec [sic] [Baalbec or Ba'labakk] and Beyrouth [Beirut] thence by steamer to Constantinople and Greece. Hope to be home in May.

Yours truly,

H.R. Porter[3]

In Beirut, an Ottoman provincial capital with a large port and a major economic center, he stayed at the New Hotel d'Orient and sailed from there on March 26 for Asia Minor, Turkey, and Greece on an Austrian Lloyd steamer with calls at Alexandretta (Iskenderun), Mersina (Mersin), Rhodes, Samos and Scio, and Smyrna. He arrived in Constantinople on April 1 where he stayed at the Grand Hotel de Londres.

Porter showed no sign of questioning the authenticity of many of the sites that he visited, but tourists are ever at the mercy of their guides for information.

Constantinople, Turkey, April 6 [1894]

Reached this city last Sunday and found a newsletter from Editor Jewell waiting, for which I was thankful. On March 22nd we left the oldest city in the world, Damascus, in fine carriages, three horses to each carriage, and after a 70 mile ride over a beautiful and very smooth winding mountain road, we found ourselves in Baalbek where we saw the most wonderful ruins in existence. Here is the great temple, huge columns of the peristyle, the sole remains of the once world renowned temple. Some are sixty feet in height. Here is the Temple of the Sun. The portal of the temple is the gem of the structure, well preserved, and the finest stone carving in the interior of anything we have yet seen. Some of the huge stones are a marvel, and how they were ever transported and raised in position is a wonder and shows that those old fellows knew as much, if not more, than we smart ones of the present day. One stone, by actual measurement, I found to be 64 feet long, 13 feet high, and about the same thickness which is the largest stone ever used in a building. Visited the quarry where these stones came from and found one even larger moved about twenty yards. Evidently they could get it no further and there it remains even unto this day and probably will for all time to come.

Another ride of seventy miles over and around the Lebanon mountains and we were in Beyrouth [Beirut] where we rested a few days and then boarded an Austrian Lloyd steamer for Smyrna and Constantinople. Our trip to this place was all that could be desired for a rough, uncomfortable, mean, dirty passage of five days. It was too stormy to stay on deck; too crowded with four in a cabin to breathe. First class passengers were obliged to take second class accommodations and sleep on the floor, but pay first class rates all the same. The wind and the waves were so strong and high one day that the steamer could make no headway and had to turn tail and find shelter near an island, and cast anchor for twenty-four hours. We called at Rhodes, Samos, Scio, and remained a day at Smyrna. Our last day, however, was fine and leaving the Grecian archipelago behind us, we steamed through the Dardanelles and the Sea of Marmora to Constantinople

20. Travels to the Holy Land and Around the Mediterranean

with hardly a ripple on the water. The view and changes were grand as we neared Constantinople, the chief city of the Ottoman Empire and the home of a million souls; the sight was simply too magnificent for my feeble power of description. I thought Naples beat the world, but Constantinople goes ahead of Naples. Yesterday I visited the Sublime Porte, the Seraglio, the Mosque of the Sultan, etc.

In the afternoon we chartered a steamer and sailed up the Bosporus into the Golden Horn and the "sweet water of Europe." Today we were present at the Selamlik which is the ceremony that takes place whenever the Sultan goes to the Mosque to perform his devotions. We had a fine window in a building opposite the mosque, reserved for persons of distinction and to foreigners of which we were one, and where we could get a splendid view of the Sultan and the troops as they passed by. The Sultan was dressed in a stambouline, wearing a fez without ornaments or other distinctive sign. Two or three carriages followed carrying some ladies of the harem. After the prayer His Majesty approaches a window and the troops filed by which takes nearly two hours, and a splendid lot of soldiers they were too. The cavalry are especially fine, the finest horses I ever saw. Some of the infantry marched like a horse with a stringhalt [lameness in a horse due to muscular spasms], but they kept good time and are fine looking men. The Turks, contrary to my expectations, are a fine noble race. They have large eyes, aquiline noses, white complexion, sometimes flaxen hair. The prominence of their cheek bones and their square jaws show well their Asiatic origin. The Turk is obliging, generous, and renowned for his hospitality. The present Sultan, Abdul-Hamid Khan II [Sultan 1876–1909 and known for his fierce repression of the "Young Turks"], is the most remarkable sovereign in his dynasty. He is said to be good, mild, generous, and enlightened; he joins to brilliant intellectual abilities, lofty views and a quick understanding, etc. However, I was not much impressed with his looks. He had a large, aquiline nose and the skin seemed to be drawn tight over his face, and he seemed to me like a too much married Turk. I understand, however, that he is not very much in that line for a Turk—for a Sultan, I mean. No one knows how many wives he has, but from the best authority, I learn that the lowest estimate is 200, and he has been married once since my arrival, so that would make 201 at the present moment, and probably more tomorrow. The present Sultan, when one of his wives gets a little cranky or unmanageable, does not sew her up in a sack with a big piece of lead and throw her in the Bosporus. He has a better way now, and one that does not shock the people so much. He has built a very nice private insane hospital on the banks of the Bosporus, which will hold more women than the North Dakota Insane Asylum. When he has had enough of the ladies, or they get a little too much for His Royal Nibs, why he gives the grand wink to the High Mogul and Chief Eunuch of the Harem and from that moment she is insane and goes to the ground palace for treatment on the beautiful banks of the Bosporus and is never seen again.

Tomorrow we take a trip to the Black Sea and Monday leave for Athens. Some cholera here and I am afraid we will be quarantined on our arrival in Greece. I think I'll make a trip through Spain before my return, but hope to be home in May.

Regards to all,

H.R. Porter[4]

His next letter was from Athens. He missed a major earthquake by a few days as his letter was described in the heading of the *Tribune* as written before the "late earthquake" there.

Athens, Greece, April 25 [1894]

Have been in Athens four days, and will remain here a day or two longer and then take steamer for Brindisi. Our trip from Constantinople was simply delightful. We were on the large French steamer, *Senegal*.[5] The weather was perfect and the water smooth and we were among the islands of the Grecian archipelago or near the coast of Greece all the time so that the trip was as pleasant as it could possibly be. Every spot of ground was of historic interest and beautiful withal.

We were fortunate to get away from Constantinople just as we did for the reason that a quarantine has just been established since we left and lots of American travelers are kicking themselves for going to and remaining too long in Constantinople.

We avoided all but twenty-four hours quarantine by taking steamer from Constantinople to Smyrna, then changing to the French line, and going back to Thessalonica, then to the seaport town of Athens, Piraeus, which is six miles away and where we were held up twenty-four hours.

All the hotels and steamers are crowded and so many of them are American; Americans everywhere. Our party is gradually breaking up and I will soon be left alone and traveling on my own hook. I do not like to see them go having enjoyed their company since January 1st. We have formed friendship and ties which are hard to part. Three of our party left us at Constantinople, four more left this morning for Paris and another goes tomorrow.

Athens is a beautiful, clean, white city, located in a valley with a population of 80,000 or 90,000. The whole population of Greece is less than that of the cities of New York and Brooklyn, but she has an army of fighters considerably larger than the United States, viz., over 30,000 strong. They do not appear, however, to be made of the same stuff as the Athenians who drew up in line to fight King Darius of Persia with more than 200,000 men; but contrary to all expectations the Athenians totally defeated the Persian army, although fifteen times larger than their own.

The museum here contains treasures which are the finest in the world although such vast quantities have been sent to other countries. Dr. [Heinrich] Schliemann's (now dead) [1822–1890] house is one of the finest in Athens, white marble and richly adorned with paintings and sculptures. You will remember he is the person who had been devoting years of his life in locating, studying and digging up treasures which have so long been buried and lost. Other parties are still carrying on the work, and we saw them still excavating where new discoveries are being made every day. The visit to the Acropolis is well worth a trip to Athens. Built on a solid rock, it is several hundred feet in height, and although a ruin, enough still stands to give a good idea of its former greatness and exquisite grandeur. Some of the most delicate carving over and around the doors looks just like lace work. The whole temple was made of Eleusinian and Pentelic marble. In the Parthenon stood the gold and

20. Travels to the Holy Land and Around the Mediterranean

ivory statue of Athena Parthenos, forty-seven feet in height, the most admired work of Phidias. The nude portions were of ivory and the rest of the stature and the removable mantle were of solid gold. We visited the temple of Victory and Minerva's, the theater of Bacchus, Mars Hill, etc. The Temple of Jupiter, Olympus or Zeus, the Pnyx, which is the place where the Athenians held their political meetings and the exact spot where the citizens listened to the stirring eloquence of a Pericles and a Demosthenes. The King's palace is only one block from our hotel, a few blocks further is a large rock called Mount Sycabettus, 948 feet high, on the top of which is a very small church. The proper thing to do is to climb this mountain, and, of course, I tackled it, a good climb I can tell you, up a rough, steep winding road. At the top I found a neat little church, a dirty old Monk and a sick cat, and one stunted olive tree. The Monk was pouring olive oil into the cat, but he let her go when he saw me and was very polite—handed me a chair—held out his greasy paw and we shook. He talked Greece and I talked United States for about half an hour, neither of us understanding a word the other said. We had a very animated conversation and finally he pulled out a bottle of benedictine and we both smiled and I handed him a franc and started down the hill again.

H.R. Porter[6]

He left Athens by train to Corinth on April 16 and to Patras where he embarked on the 17th for Corfu and Brindisi, arriving in Italy on the 19th. On the evening of the 20th a major earthquake struck northern Greece causing many deaths and much destruction, hence the headline for Porter's letter in the Bismarck Daily *Tribune*, "NO EARTHQUAKE YET, Doctor Porter in Greece, and Writes, But Before the Late Earthquake."[7]

Porter crossed Italy by train to Naples on his return and while there, at Hotel Royal des Etrangers, cabled Burleigh County treasurer J.P. Dunn to forward his tax bill to him at the Corner of Third and Spruce Streets in Washington, DC, where he planned to make his home about May 25.[8]

From Naples he traveled to Rome and Genoa and sailed to Tarragona, Spain, where he reported to his readers in Bismarck the following:

Madrid, Spain, April 30 [1894]

Arrived in this city after a twenty-four hour ride from Taragona [*sic*]. I was glad enough to get here I can tell you. Have been three days getting here, and find it will take two or three days more to get to the south of Spain, one thing is certain, they do not know or care much about railroading. The trains are slow. Only the express trains run sleepers; consequently you cannot hurry in Spain. This makes travel very disagreeable and tedious. I find you cannot hurry a Spaniard any more than you can an Italian, which is not at all. He will smoke and talk and look pleasant and happy, while you are worrying and rushing around for your ticket and baggage, and he will let the train slip out from under your nose just as if it did not matter at all, and then you have another day's hotel bill to pay. The hotels, how they do go for the American dollars, and the exchange, how slick they manage that! You take a twenty franc piece and change it back and forth a few times and you will wonder where your money has gone. You won't have a cent left. Someone asked where all the brigands of Spain were, and the answer was, "Why, they are all keeping hotels," which is quite true. If they can't rob you in the slickest, smoothest style of the art, and smile and pretend to be doing you the greatest favor, why, I'm no judge of the grand and sublime. Four dollars a day for a little rat hole of a dirty, dark room, and though bull beef and black coffee is all right for the hotel man, but you don't care for that kind of diet and price for a very long season. The hotels, however, are all full and I had a hard time to get a room even on those terms. Madrid is a beautiful city, situated in the midst of a vast sandy plateau. The streets are wide and clean, fine buildings, public gardens, fountains, and statuary, all making one of the most attractive cities. The picture gallery here is a gem and contains many Murillos and quite a number of Velasquez, Raphael, Titian, Tintoretto and many other celebrated painters.

This afternoon I witnessed a bull fight at the Plaza de Tores which is a vast amphitheatre calculated to hold 20,000 people. Every seat was taken. The first bull that was let into the ring came with head and tail high in the air, a noble beast certainly. He looked at the vast audience as he came proudly in, and then at the gaily clad bullfighters (Banderilleros) and quicker than a flash he plunged for one and then another only, of course, to miss them and to hit the red cloth held before them. The bull looked surprised and became furious, pawed the ground and lashed his tail and started for a man on horseback. The man did not falter but rode toward the bull and charged him with a spear.

The bull was equal to the occasion and rushed on horse and rider with the speed of lightning and the force of a battering ram. Down went horse and man. The bull turned immediately in pursuit of more game, which he found in another horse and rider and another and another until in thirty-five minutes he had actually killed seven horses. The first poor animal was torn open so that portions of the intestines came out and dragged on the ground. Still the rider urged him on and rode around the ring until he fell down dead. And this they call sport. It is one of the most cruel, barbarous, and disgusting sights I have ever witnessed and I never want to see another one. In the mean time the bull was charging around from one man to another with his tongue out, his sides panting, blood shot eyes, and his sides covered with blood and dripping on the ground from sharp, arrow-shaped instruments, which were thrust into his flesh, and barbed, so as to tear and cut his flesh, and that maddened him more. Well, this sort of thing lasted until the last suffering bull could not stand it much longer from loss of strength and blood. A trumpet was sounded which was the signal for the finishing stroke and one of the fighters, the matador, rushed up on the bull and thrust a long sword into his shoulder up to the hilt. The blood rushed from his nose and mouth. He stood still a few seconds, quivered, and fell down dead upon the body of one of the seven horses which he had killed only a few minutes before. Ropes were fastened around the neck of the poor bull and the seven dead horses and they were dragged out during the uproar of 30,000 voices with the exception of one poor, lone Dakotan from Bismarck, by gaily decked mules and the thing was over in less time than it took me to tell it. This, however, was only one-sixth of the fight as they had five more bulls left to go through the same performance. One was enough for me, and I left, sorrowful and disgusted. The men in Madrid are a fine looking lot. The women are simply beautiful. Large, well formed, fair complexion, red cheeks, dark hair and eyes, white pearly teeth, smiling and pleasant. What more do you want to complete the picture?[9]

Chapter 21

Washington and Bismarck

Porter returned to Washington, DC, in late May 1894 in good "health and happy spirits."[1] His plans were to remain there at least for the short term and practice medicine but retain his business interests in Bismarck as well as continue to maintain a home there. Editor Jewell reported visiting him in Washington soon after his return. Porter told him that he had "been on the frontier a long time and want[ed] a little diversion." Jewell concluded that he would practice medicine there only to dissipate idleness.[2]

While Porter had been on his tour his son, Hallie, now thirteen, had at first lived with relatives in Ashland, Wisconsin (his mother's half-sister), but when Porter returned, he was in Minneapolis with Porter's friend and former business partner H.F. Douglass.

Porter had no intention of practicing medicine in Washington but only wanted to be with his family. His mother, father, and unmarried sister, Frances, were living there after his father's retirement from practice in New York Mills, New York, and were at 1922 Third Street N.W. His sister, Sarah, was there with her family and husband, an employee of the Bureau of Printing and Engraving.

On July 2nd, a month after his return to Washington, he and Hallie paid a four week visit to Oberlin much to the delight of young Katherine Faircloth. She and Hallie played tennis on July 4th and Porter set off fireworks in celebration. Katherine entered in her diary on the 12th, "Uncle Harry and Hallie came to see us two weeks ago and we have had lots of fun together." Porter and Helen Fairchild attended the first church in Oberlin together on the 15th leading to speculation that he was courting the former sister-in-law since Porter's church attendance up to that point had been sketchy. Porter and Hallie returned to Washington on the first of August. Hallie, now thirteen, was unhappy in Washington, so Porter sent him back to Oberlin to go to school in September for the 1894–95 session.

Porter returned to Oberlin for an extended stay in mid–April 1895. He gave Katherine a "pretty little pocketbook" and five dollars to start her fund for a bicycle. Porter took the children on carriage rides to Elyria and entertained them in other ways such as boat rides, sailing, and swimming. He invited the family to dinner at the hotel and in turn had dinner at the home of Helen and Katherine. Porter escorted Helen and Katherine to the Baccalaureate Sermon for the College on June 16th, and on August 2 he attended church with Helen, Katherine and Hal. Porter left Oberlin August 22 headed to Detroit.[3]

Meanwhile, back in Bismarck, former judge of probate, state senator, and honorary colonel Clarence Belden Little liquidated Capital National Bank in Bismarck, of which he was president, and bought a controlling interest in Porter's former bank, the First National Bank of Bismarck in 1895. Little, a native of New Hampshire, graduate of Dartmouth College, and former law student at Harvard, had gone west to Bismarck in 1883, much as Porter had done ten years earlier and had been extraordinarily successful. Little's home, or mansion, at 504 North Washington Street, built between 1902 and 1906, is now home of the State Bar Association of North Dakota and a showplace in Bismarck.[4]

In September 1895 Porter returned to Bismarck to make it once more his home.[5] He had become a westerner and could no longer be comfortable living in Washington. "Washington was a beautiful city, no city that he had ever visited was more so," Porter had said, but his frontier spirit could never be tamed. His friends were overjoyed with his return. He was one of Bismarck's most popular and beloved figures and was known by all.

Not wishing to have a house, Porter obtained elegantly appointed rooms downtown for himself and Hallie, which he maintained throughout the remainder of his life in Bismarck.

The *Washburn* [North Dakota] *Leader*, edited by Joseph Henry Taylor, a pioneer journalist and author of *Sketches of Frontier and Indian Life on the Upper Missouri and Great Plains* as well as an expert on hunting and wildlife, reported sometime after his return to Bismarck the following:

> Dr. Porter and son of Bismarck came down to the county capital Saturday, from a few days outing among the stock ranges and the beaver dams of Douglas River. The doctor is an old timer to this section as time goes. In the debut he first saw service as a "saw bones" with Crook in 1872; was transferred to Camp Hancock in 1873, and came down from Little Big Horn, the sole surviving surgeon of 1876 — took a leap in the dark in Bismarck suburban property and came out of the capital boom of 1882 riding a Trojan horse filled with the wads of the sluggards who invested on the top of a carefully cultivated "rise." Since then the doctor visited the Mecca of all scholars, scientists, and dreamers who can afford it — old Rome, the Holy Land, the Pyramids of Guiza's plain, the catacombs of the Nile and Memphis' splendid ruin. Familiar with the wild Sioux and their haughty pose with its scenic effect on everyday life in frontier days, the doctor was surprised to see in the Arab horsemen who drew reins in the shadow of the Sphinx or along the green shores of the broad Nile River, almost a counterpart of our own Sioux of the Dakotas....[6]

Aside for Porter's visits around the world this article indicated that his travels may have been funded by the fortune he made in real estate in the 1882–83 boom, which led up to Bismarck becoming the territorial capital in 1883, thanks to the efforts of Alexander McKenzie, also known as the Big Boomer, Northern Pacific Railroad interests, and local support that included people like George Fairchild.

His two years away marked another major watershed in his life. He had not re-married after his wife's death in 1888. His son was not close to him and would never be. Porter returned to Bismarck without any interest to be at the center stage of either the medical profession or the business world. He was wealthy, secure, and, in effect, semi-retired, yet only 48 years old. He continued to send Hallie back to Oberlin to the preparatory department of the college up until the fall of 1901. While there Hal lived in a boarding house and was a frequent visitor and close companion of his childhood playmate and first cousin, Katherine. She would help him with getting his room organized and help him with his homework, since he was considerably less academically talented than Katherine. Katherine led an active social life as a college student at Oberlin, while Hallie's seemed more limited. Hallie and Porter often spent Christmas vacations together with family in Washington, DC, and sometimes Oberlin, and would vacation in the summer at Lake Chautauqua, New York.

One of his former patients in 1939 remembered this era, almost fifty years later. He had been delivered by Porter and recalled that the doctor had driven the first rubber-tired buggy in Bismarck. "I remember climbing the stairs in the Dakota Block, turning to the left and seeing the words, 'H.R. Porter, M.D.' ... Dr. Porter practiced medicine when he felt like it and for those who were his personal friends. He had a mirror fixed to the wall outside his window so that he might see who climbed the stairs. Some people go in and more did not. He was the most successful surgeon in the Northwest because he discovered a great principle nearly 70 years ahead of his time."[7] That principle must have been to select your patients wisely.

Porter attended a social event on January 28, 1896, at the Sheridan Hotel, a Leap Year's Party, as one of the eligible bachelors of Bismarck. It was a dance given by the young ladies of Bismarck in honor of the men.[8] But no romance developed in his case.

A tragedy occurred in March when a prisoner undergoing rectal surgery by Dr. Francis R. Smyth of Bismarck died under chloroform anesthesia prior to the operation. At the coroner's inquest held the following day at the office of the state's attorney, Porter, formerly the prison surgeon, testified that the administration of the anesthetic had been proper and that the death, in his opinion, had been unavoidable.[9] At that time chloroform was widely used as an anesthetic for operations and childbirth, but it was replaced by safer agents later. The risk of overdosing was well recognized and caution urged in its usage.[10]

The worst snowstorm on record hit Bismarck on Thanksgiving Day 1896 with drifts of snow up to fifteen feet deep. All traffic including the railroad was halted with the eastbound train stuck in a snowdrift. Since it was a holiday, only a few people were downtown; some checked in hotels and a few struggled home. Others were taken in at houses on their way after near exhaustion. The *Tribune* reported that "Dr. Porter got bewildered at about nightfall, in hunting for the Dakota Block, and finally encountered a light, which led him to a house, whose tenant led him to his destination only a short distance away."[11]

Like all physicians, Porter had to deal with questions about health issues from family members. When his niece, Helen (Nell) Davis, wrote from Washington asking about her neuralgia, he replied, "In the first place, I'm not sure 'tis neuralgia. If it is pure and simple, there is nothing better for it than 'Dr. Gross Neuralgia Pills,' same as your Father used. They should not be used continually if you are not cured by them for fear of the morphine habit."

She had been to New York recently and had told Porter about it. "You are ahead of me on Bernhardt. I have never seen her but always wanted to. Looks like you. Why, I thought she was tall, angular-bony and ugly. You are not. You are plump-smooth, slack- pretty. If you saw the pictures at the Hoffman House, you must have been loafing around the throne — the bar. I mean for that is where the pictures are. [Hoffman House, Broadway at West 25th Street, New York City, was an elegant hotel that had W.A. Bouguereau's famous eight by ten foot painting, *Nymphs and Satyr*, hanging in the bar, which shocked the Victorian sensibilities of some of its patrons.] You can get a very nice Manhattan cocktail there for 25 cents. The pictures look much finer through the bottom of a cocktail glass. I stop at the Hoffman but 'tis not the best hotel by any means. Did you go through any of the finest hotels?"[12]

This letter shows, among other things, Porter's familiarity with the bar at Hoffman House in New York and its famous painting by Bouguereau. He frequently visited New York City and often departed from there on foreign tours. Now that he was no longer involved in real estate deals, bank start-ups, and railroad organizations, he could indulge his thrill of adventure in travel.

Porter brought suit against Collier Publishing Company in October 1897 after he had traded a parcel of land for five hundred dollars worth of books and had failed to receive the books.[13] He was known to have a large personal library and was considered one of the most educated and literate citizens of Bismarck.[14] He almost certainly received satisfaction from the Collier Company, since nothing more came of it. Five hundred dollars worth of books in 1897 would have been a library in itself.

Porter, a man of wit and good humor, loved nothing better than to tell a joke or find the funny side of a situation. He collected jokes and pasted them in his scrapbook along with his own newspaper clippings of some of the many letters that he had written. One such clipping from his scrapbook is a letter to a medical journal that was published.

To the Editor of the *Medical Record*,
Sir: In answer to the query, "Should Ministers Pay Doctors?" I say, "Ay, verily." For twenty-five years your humble servant has been pouring physic down and pumping other medicines up into the ministers, their wives, and other members of their family, free of charge and sometimes without even a thank you. Why should we do it? Are not the ministers well paid, as well fed and clothed — house rent very little, and often free? When they travel, 'tis either D.H. [D.G.? *Deus gratius*, thanks to God] or half-fare.

Don't we pay when they marry us? Don't we tip them when they baptize our children? Don't we give them a few ducats when we die?

They do not have the expense of keeping a horse or two, nor of the wear and tear of carriages, cutters, harness, etc. No getting up "o' nights" for a drive of forty miles in the country with the wind howling at a speed of forty miles an hour and the mercury forty below zero—furnish the medicine free—all for the love of your fellow—man. Not a cent in sight, but we must go—*bon gre,' mal gre'* [like it or not]—or we are heartless, cold-blooded, cruel.

Ministers sometimes show their gratitude, as when I attended one through a severe sickness, and during his convalescence he advised one of my good pay patients to try a rival M.D.; said he would "get him on his legs quicker." This minister, however, was an exceptionally mean one. As a rule, they are jolly good fellows; but I say, let them pay and then they will better appreciate us.

H.R. Porter, M.D.

Bismarck, N.D., November 17, 1897[15]

As war clouds gathered in Washington in early 1898, Porter sought one more great adventure. Porter, now age fifty, tried to do something that Theodore Roosevelt, age forty, was able to do, volunteer to serve in the military in the Spanish American War. He advised his congressman, M.N. Johnson, that he would give fifty thousand dollars to the government if he could be allowed to join the army as a surgeon or serve in the ranks. This is equivalent to more than one million dollars in present day value. His request to the president was referred to the secretary of war, and the request was ultimately refused.[16] Press reports of his offer headlined it as "He Comes of Fighting Stock, North Dakota Physician Ready to Take to the Field Again."[17] The *Tribune* in its account called him one who had "achieved note through his connection with the Custer massacre," and retold the whole familiar story of the battle.[18]

When Senator James K. Jones of Arkansas proposed in 1898 to purchase an oil painting of Sitting Bull at government expense of one hundred and fifty dollars, Representative Johnson of North Dakota protested vehemently, saying that although Sitting Bull had been one of his constituents, it was his opinion that someone more worthy of memorializing should be chosen, since Sitting Bull was a medicine man and not a warrior and had spent his time during the battle of Little Big Horn with the squaws "cooking mysterious herbs, dancing, and chanting incantations to the devil." (Utley calls this view one "abetted by Indians currying favor with the Great White father" and one totally unjustified in light of Sitting Bull's known bravery and leadership of his people in the battle.[19]) Johnson said that Gall, Grass, Running Antelope, and Rain-in-the-Face did the fighting so why not have one of Gall painted "if we are to glorify any of the executioners of our poor, brave fellows who were caught in that cruel trap." But if the honor were to go to a medicine man, "let us buy a picture of gallant Dr. Porter, who successfully planned and superintended the transportation of the wounded of Reno's command on improvised stretchers to the steamboat twenty-five miles from the battlefield, and then a thousand miles by water to Bismarck, N.D., the nearest place he could get shelter and medicines. The doctor is one of my constituents, and the handsomest man in Bismarck today." The *Tribune* duly noted that Congressman Johnson was pulling Porter's leg.[20]

A tragic fire swept through downtown Bismarck on the night of August 8, 1898. It started in the Northern Pacific warehouse where "all manner of inflammables" were stored. No lives were lost, but economic losses were great as the wooden structures quickly caught fire. The *Bismarck Tribune* office and plant burned to the ground with complete loss of its files. The *Bismarck Settler* allowed the *Tribune* to publish from its presses. Katherine Fairchild in Oberlin heard about it from a friend and recorded how she "hurried around and found that it was so. Papa's old bank [First National] and three, no four blocks right in the heart of the city are in ashes. Uncle Harry, I think, did not lose anything — neither did we, but I guess it has ruined the town. We have not heard from Uncle Harry [Porter] since."[21] Porter was listed in the newspaper as having five hundred dollars in property loss, if this was indeed the doctor.[22] The Sheridan House Hotel was said "to have [had] a narrow escape, but was saved." The destroyed area extended northward from the Northern Pacific tracks to Thayer Street and east and west from Third to Fourth Street.[23]

In Porter's scrapbook there is his invitation to a hanging. Frank Vyzralek, North Dakota's first state archivist, has in recent years reviewed this case and the seven other death penalties exacted in North Dakota from 1883 in northern territorial days to 1915 when the state legislature eliminated this punishment except in the case of an inmate who while serving a life sentence kills a prison guard.[24] Vyzralek stated that, "by custom, condemned criminals of that day were apparently accorded the right to invite certain of their friends or acquaintances to view the execution. Such invitations to the hanging of both Cole and Hans Thorpe, are known to exist; Cole's message is accompanied by a jail photograph." Porter's invitation was dated March 19, 1899, with a photograph of the prisoner dressed in a suit, white shirt, and striped tie with the inscription. "Complements of James W. Cole. Requests the pleasure of your company at his execution on Friday, March 24, 1899. (signed) H.P. Bogue, Sheriff." Under the photograph there is the note, "Jim, the ole? Indian friend of H.R. Porter. To be hung March 24, 1899." Cole, a well-known African-American resident of Bismarck, had shot and killed a fourteen-year-old black schoolgirl when she did not respond to his advances. He turned himself in, pleaded guilty, and did nothing to delay his execution to which he was sentenced by Judge Walter Winchester. He was hanged shortly after daybreak on March 24 on an enclosed scaffold built next to the county courthouse to which access was achieved through an office window. It was reported upon in detail in the *Tribune* of the same day.[25] Porter was not there.

Dr. Henry Norton Porter, father of Henry R., died September 12, 1899, in Washington, DC, at age eighty-two. Since retirement from practice in New York Mills, New York, he and his wife had lived at 1912 Third Street, De Droit Park in Washington. Helen Polson Porter, his wife and Henry R.'s mother, died eight months later. They were buried in Rock Creek Cemetery, Section K, Washington, DC.

Porter left Bismarck, probably Sunday night, September 24, 1899, for New York City to attend the Victory Celebration of the Spanish-American War and the Admiral Dewey Jubilee on Saturday, September 30.[26] He may well have taken advantage of a special offered by the Nickel Plate Road, Chicago to New York, and advertised in the *Tribune*.[27] Three trains daily with "vestibuled" sleeping cars were leaving Chicago September 26, 27, and 28 and returning before October 4 with round-trip fare of twenty-four dollars. While thwarted in serving in the army, he could not be denied the celebration of victory.

Porter was a Freemason. In October 1899 he, along with his friend M.H. Jewell, were initiated "into some of the hidden mysteries of the order" in Mandan.[28] A later biographical sketch described him as being "a Mason of high degree."[29] He had been a member of a lodge of some type as a young man in New York Mills. A number of Masonic ceremonial items of clothing that belonged to Porter are among the holdings in the Archives of the North Dakota Historical Society.[30]

Porter advertised in the newspaper November 27, 1900, under "Lost" three checks of one hundred and sixty-five dollars, two hundred and forty, and one hundred dollars, all endorsed and drawn on the First National Bank of Bismarck, North Dakota. The *Tribune* proudly reported a few days later that Porter had walked to the bank the day before and had placed a fourth check in the watch pocket of his trousers and to his surprise found there the three previously lost checks and the paper concluded that "it all proves the value of advertising beyond a question."[31]

In November 1900 Porter made improvements in the Dakota Block. He had new stone walks laid in front, reinforcement made to the stairs, and repairs to the woodwork. He was proud of this landmark building of Bismarck from which he practiced medicine in his upstairs office.[32]

Meanwhile, new doctors were arriving in Bismarck trained in antiseptic and aseptic techniques and were replacing the older doctors of Porter's generation whose educations were fast becoming obsolete. Of necessity, Porter's practice had been a very general one. The nearest surgical specialists were in St. Paul, Minnesota. His practice encompassed medicine, obstetrics, trauma, pediatrics, psychiatry, and minor surgery. From his office equipment now in the State Historical Society of North Dakota, it can be seen that he had a rudimentary laboratory for testing urine, instruments for diagnosis, gynecological instruments, syringes for injections, scalpels and sutures for trauma, and a selection of drugs generally available at the end of the nineteenth century.

The story is told that when young Dr. Eric P. Quain came to Bismarck in June 1899 just out of his internship at City County Hospital in St. Paul and was called upon to treat an injured baseball player bleeding from the nose, he arrived at the emergency department at Old St. Alexius to find the sister mopping the man's face with un-sterilized cotton. He asked for sterilized gauze and was told that he would have to bring his own; they had none. He asked to have some surgical instruments sterilized to which the sister replied "with some annoyance" that if he would wrap them up in a towel she would take them to the kitchen and have them boiled.[33] But to Porter the newer medical techniques and procedures were of no concern. He was pleased to turn the practice over to younger surgeons. For several years his limited and selective practice had permitted him to pursue his own interests leaving him plenty of time for hunting and traveling. These were the things he really cared about now. He was still a respected figure in Bismarck. In December 1900 Governor Frederick B. Fancher of North Dakota made Porter an honorary colonel on his staff, an honorific not associated with the state militia.[34]

Chapter 22

Final Years

Forever restless, Porter sailed from New York in January 1901 on another adventure aboard a 450-foot yacht with two stacks and two masts and a displacement of 4,419 tons for forty days to South America and the West Indies that included Puerto Rico, Jamaica, and Cuba. He wrote to the *Tribune* from the Hamburg-American Line vessel.

> On Board *Prinzessin Victoria Luise*
> Feb. 1.

Yesterday we landed at Port-au-Prince and spent the day sightseeing. You would laugh to see the way things are done in Port-au-Prince and the manner of conducting the city government. To say they are 200 years behind the times would be drawing it mild. Water pipes lie on top of the ground. Soldiers look like mere boys, and act like them, too. The policemen look and act the same, all are barefooted; the latter get fifty cents a week for pay and board themselves. They do their own cooking in the streets or on the edge of the sidewalk with an old tomato can for a pot to boil or stew their frugal meal.

This is the capital of the Haytian [sic] Negro republic, a city of fifty to seventy-five thousand colored people. The Haytians say (and also act) on the theory of Hayti [sic] for the Haytians.

A white man cannot own any land here. The president is a full-blooded Negro and they don't want, nor will they allow any poor white trash around. Such a poor looking, tumble down dirty city and the people are so poorly clad and ragged, and some of the children are perfectly nude. With all this they seem jolly, smiling and a happy, contented lot. Their wants are few and it requires very little exertion to live. Hardly any fuel or clothing [are needed] and light food and fruit suffices but Oh ye Gods! What a climate. __ in the shade now and this is their winter. Fruit did you say? Well, you ought to see the cocoanuts, pineapples, oranges, limes, mangoes, bananas, etc., growing here just now, and the prices—well, they will make you smile. Oranges 15 for 10 cents, limes, 25 for 10 cents; cocoanuts, 12 for 8 cents; bananas, one whole bunch for 10 cents. A bunch may have 75 up to 200 in it. How does that strike you on fruit? Tomorrow we expect to reach San Domingo, then to San Juan and St. Thomas; thence to Martinique and Trinidad and South America. The *Princess Victoria Louise* is a brand-new steamship and this is her first trip. She is a floating palace: laundry, barber shop, bathroom, smoking room, library, gymnasium, and four meals a day and lunch

22. Final Years

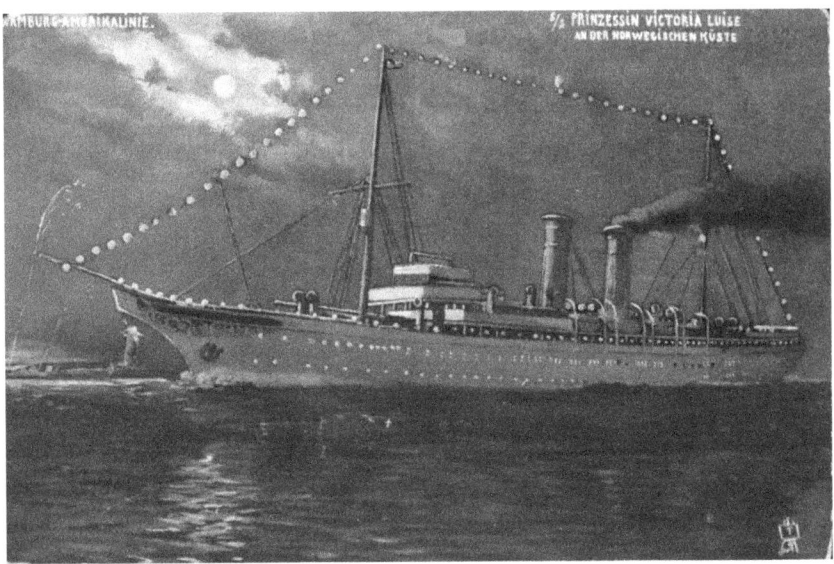

Princezessin Victoria Luise, *Hamburg-American Line. Dr. Porter sailed from New York to South America in 1901 on this ship (photograph owned by author).*

and lemonade brought to you on deck every hour. We have a very pleasant lot of passengers—100 of them and a crew of 195 all told.

Well, "s'long." I'm writing this on board steamer and she is rocking too much for steady writing.

H.R. Porter[1]

Three weeks later he wrote to his niece in Washington, DC, from Havana that the *Princess Victoria Luise* was "anchored within 500 feet of the *Maine* which is partly above the water and can be plainly seen." He had enjoyed the cruise and the people aboard and called it "the trip of my life." He told of one woman who gave her life history "while sitting in a cozy corner on deck" while there was "a warm and balmy breeze cooling one hot and fevered brow, a tropical moonlight and the Southern Cross just above the horizon, and both of us a little moonstruck." He complained, "I haint heard a word from Hal. I wonder why he don't write?"

By mid–March Porter was back in Bismarck telling all his friends about the trip and describing it as "full of pleasurable surprises [with] a jolly company on the yacht [making] it all the more enjoyable."[2] The newspaper recorded, "Dr. H.R. Porter returned from his tour of the West Indies—glad to get back to the balmy air of North Dakota."[3]

He returned to his real estate and business ventures. An entire block across from the governor's mansion in Bismarck that he owned that was

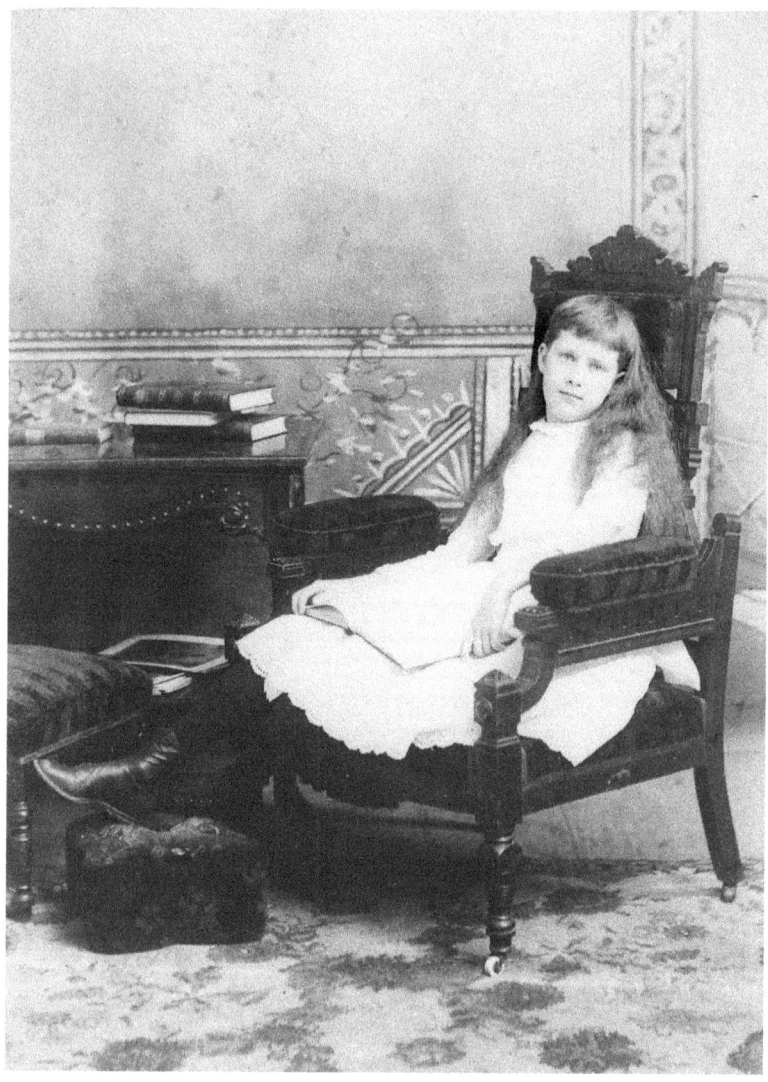

Katherine Fairchild, daughter of George H. and Helen V. Fairchild. Photograph by W.H. DeGraff. (Courtesy Wyman Family)

"level as a floor," and he had seeded it in grass to turn it into a "beauty spot."[4]

During the summer of 1901, Katherine and Helen Fairchild returned to Bismarck for a visit by a voyage from Cleveland through the Great Lakes to Duluth and then by train to Bismarck arriving on July 25. Hal met them at the train and chauffeured them around town in his father's Stanhope carriage with rubber tires and pulled by two fast horses. Katherine described Porter's "rooms": "I never saw anything so beautiful. He has a $100 Graphophone and he played it nearly an hour for us and we looked at all his curios."[5] During their visit Porter showered mother and daughter with flowers. Katherine admitted, "I would like to like him very much, only I am afraid of him." His rough-hewn manner and imposing figure caused her to feel intimidated.

In September 1901 Porter sent his son, Hal, now twenty years old, to St. John's Military Academy, "a school for gentlemen's sons" in Delafield, Wisconsin. A family story has it that Hal had been expelled from Oberlin preparatory department for smoking.[6] Hal's relationship with his father continued to deteriorate. Perhaps Porter hoped that the discipline of military school might be good for him. The uniforms and drill were based on the West Point model. It was a small school. In 1890 there were only eighty-three students. They attended chapel daily, participated in drills and athletics, and went to classes that ranged from the seventh to the twelfth grades. The school's motto was "Work Hard, Play Hard, and Pray Hard."[7] Although Hal hated being at the school, he completed a full year there.[8] The rigors of military school ended Hal's formal education. In August 1902 he boarded a train for Glendive, Montana, to work in a bank co-owned by his father.[9]

Porter advertised for bids in February 1902 to construct a frame ironclad bank and store building in Wilton, twenty-three miles north of Bismarck.[10] It indicated his continued interest and passion for the banking business and accumulation of wealth. He visited the area and spent some time enjoying himself at Neal's ranch nearby.[11]

Porter's final world trip began when he was fifty-five years old at a time when he was described as "in the prime of life and vigor."[12] He was unaccompanied, as was his custom, as he crossed the Pacific. He seems never to have invited his son, Hal, to travel with him. He had asked John J. Jackman, friend and pioneer farmer and businessman of Bismarck, to go along on this trip in case of an accident or trouble, but he had declined as did his old hunting friend, Judge Bowen.[13] Could he have suspected impending health problems? We don't know.

Nevertheless, Porter traveled in grand style befitting one of the best dressed men in Dakota. He carried a frock coat, a black waistcoat, a blue serge waistcoat, a gray silk coat, an overcoat, a dress coat, white shirts, colored shirts, a silk shirt, six collars, cuff links, silk handkerchiefs, neckties, and shirt studs mounted in gold, diamond, and ruby. To protect his feet from the cold and dampness of the decks, he brought along a traveling rug.[14]

From Manila, where he stayed at the Oriente Hotel, he sent a postcard saying, "This is the best place to leave I've struck. Return to China in five days."[15] He forwarded to editor Jewell a copy of the Hong Kong *Telegraph* dated January 28, 1903, and from Calcutta he sent the last of his letters, which was published in the *Tribune* posthumously.

Calcutta, India Feb. 18, 1903

Dear Jewell: — We arrived here today from Ceylon after six days on the P&O steamer *Somali*. The Bay of Bengal was smooth — the weather beautiful and the journey delightful.

The thermometer stands at 85 degrees. Hotels are all full and I'm sleeping in a tent on the roof of best hotel in the city. Population one million. On our left is the coast of India and on the right Burma and Siam. After a week in Manila I returned to Hong Kong just in time to see the Chinese celebrate their New Year's which lasts two days, Jan. 29 and 30. They certainly know how to celebrate and have a good time. The coolies even would not work for double pay, but on the contrary came out in their silk gowns and vests and pants, and they did look clean and fine in their gaudy attire. Some wore green pants, yellow vest and long flowing pink gown, white stockings, black skull cap, all silk and their long braided pigtail down below their knees. The Chinaman in China is very different from the ones we see in America. Here they are tall, large, clean, fine looking men. A Chinaman will not wear a badge of servitude during the New Year's festival. Thought I had seen firecrackers shoot off and fireworks, but we Americans are not in it with John. On the night of Jan. 28 at midnight, I awoke to hear the beating of tom-toms, and the loudest and continuous firing of crackers ever made. After dressing I went out in the streets and spent the balance of the night watching the performance. In China they never fire less than a pack and from that up to hundreds of packs, yes, thousands at one time. Saw hundreds of strings touched off that were twenty to thirty feet long and braided close into a central fuse so that the round braid would be as large as a person's thigh, or ten or twelve inches in diameter. All kinds and sizes of crackers and plenty of giant ones which made the roar of a cannon. They would go up to the third story and let this string of crackers down by a rope run over a pulley to within four feet of the ground and then light the central fuse and slowly lower it as the crackers went off and fell on the ground. At the end or top was a grand explosion and fireworks of every color and description. It seemed as if the infernal regions were let loose. After one of these long strings [was] done another was started and this was kept up for three days and nights. Seemed as if they would tear the city all to pieces. The paper and burnt firecrackers were six inches deep in places and men were constantly employed to take it away. All the stores were closed and everything given up to feasting and drinking. We were twelve days steaming from Hong Kong to Ceylon, remaining at Singapore and Penang long enough to see the cities and visit the wonderful Botanical Gardens, said to be the finest in the world. In Colombo I was fortunate enough to see the wonderful Tallpot palm in bloom; it only blossoms at the age of about fifty years and only once and then dies. 'Tis in bloom, however, for about one year. At some of these places it rains 36 inches in thirty-six hours. I went seventy-five miles out in the jungle from Colombo in Ceylon and saw monkeys, wild elephants, and horrible-looking monsters like snakes with feet. At one place where I remained one day in China they were having the bubonic plague very bad; the people were panic-stricken and concealed the dead bodies and at midnight they would carry them out in front of another house and dump them in the middle of the street. The authorities were puzzled to know how to stop or to find the proper houses where the dead came from. One bright light whom we would call the chief of police issued an order and posted it over town that "any house where a dead body was found in the street in front of said house, said residence would be held strictly responsible and have to bury and pay all expenses connected therewith."

The next morning he had thirteen dead ones in front of his house and in his yard. Evidently the Chinaman has a sense of humor in his make-up. We meet Americans from New York, Chicago, Pittsburg[h], D.C., San Francisco, every place on land and sea and railways. Leave here in a few days for Darjeeling and the Himalayas, then across India by rail, twenty days' trip to Bombay. In Ceylon I rode through Sir [Thomas] Lipton's tea plantation. Saw the natives picking tea and the tea houses where 'tis dried and fitted for packing and consumption. During a certain part of the process 'tis handled by the bare feet of the natives. The tea is picked every eight or ten days and then only certain leaves. The P&O steamers are patronized by everyone, but the majority are English. They are very stylish and always wear full dress for dinner. The result is a very swell affair every day at 7 P.M. dinner. If you don't appear in full dress, they will very politely ask you to put it on. One poor American traveler who had never been abroad before and who was sitting next to me did not have a dress suit, was in a bad plight. He consulted me and at the first port we had him into a full dress suit in just twenty-four hours after landing. He is the biggest toad in the puddle now and wants to wear it all the time.

The P&O Steamship company do everything for the comfort and pleasure of their passengers in the way of games—ping pong, quoits, shuffle board, tennis, cards, checkers, chess, music, etc., etc.

Yours truly,

H.R. Porter[16]

On the six day cruise from Ceylon to Calcutta Porter, who was always an affable traveler, met new friends who would ultimately tell the story of his final illness. From Calcutta the group traveled north 412 miles to the foothills of the Himalayas at Darjeeling, a city 7,000 feet above sea level. There the group left at 4 A.M. for a partial ascent of Mt. Everest, and on this trip Porter became sick. He was thought to have over-exerted himself, but in retrospect the altitude provoked symptoms of a heretofore unrecognized heart condition. He was able to return with the group to Calcutta, but the next day he worsened on the train while en route to Agra by way of Benares. He felt that he could not get warm and suggested that he was suffering from cardiogenic shock. At the Metropole Hotel in Agra he was put to bed and attended by a Dr. Lucas and a nurse, Mrs. McGann. Dr. Lucas brought in another doctor in consultation as Porter continued to worsen. One of the members of the tour group, A.T. Rutter of Ronderboach, South Africa, actually slept in the room to look after him. He asked Porter for his son's address as he was failing, and Porter told him, "I am not going to die yet." Then Porter asked, "What time is it?" Rutter replied, "3 A.M." These were Porter's last words early in the morning of March 3, 1903.

On the following day services were conducted by an English clergyman with burial in the British Cantonment Cemetery. The hotel manager made the arrangements.

Thus, Porter never got to see the Taj Mahal that he had come so far to see nor did he make it around the world as planned. The Rutter family left Agra the following day to resume their trip to London where Porter had intended to go, but never reached.[17]

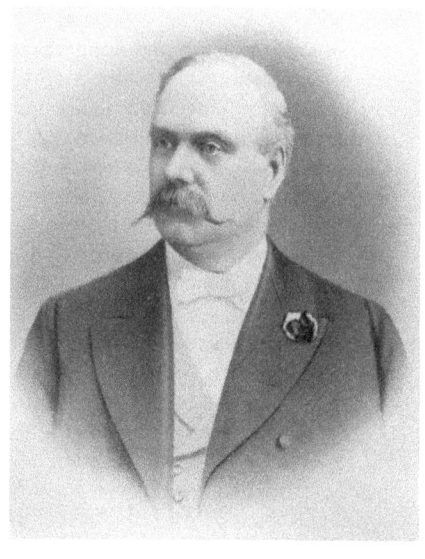

Dr. Henry R. Porter (State Historical Society of North Dakota A-4390).

His friends in Bismarck were shocked at the news. Hal was called back from Glendive. Hal requested to have Porter's body shipped to Oberlin, Ohio, for burial, but it never happened. His name is on the family marker in Section Q of the Westwood Cemetery, Oberlin, but his remains are in India. The marker in Oberlin states:

Henry R. Porter
Died March 4 [sic], 1903
Agra, India

On another side of the rectangular stone is the following:

My wife
Charlotte Viets Porter
Died August 6, 1888
Age 35 yrs, one month, 6 days.

In ceremonies at Porter's grave in Agra on April 16, 1989, a marker placed there by the Little Big Horn Associates was dedicated by Les Wollemborn, New Delhi consul general of the United State; Admiral and Mrs. Huntington Hardisty, Commander in Chief Pacific Forces; and Vice Counsel Douglas Kelley.[18]

The plaque states:

Dr. Henry Rinaldo Porter
13 February 1848 — 4 March 1903 [sic]
Acting Assistant Surgeon U.S. Army

22. Final Years   177

On 25–26 June, 1876, Custer's 7th U.S. Cavalry suffered a defeat in battle with Sioux Indians at the Battle of Little Big Horn, Montana, USA. It is now famous in American Folklore.

As the only Surviving Medical Officer, Dr. Porter's surgical skill and cool personal bravery were responsible for preserving the lives of some 60 wounded men. He won the praise and respect of all surviving officers and men.

Placed by Little Big Horn Associates

Although both markers in Oberlin and Agra date Porter's death as March 4, he actually died March 3 and was buried on March 4 in Agra. The *Bismarck Daily Tribune*, in reporting his death, copies the cablegrams to Hal as follows:

> Agra, British India, March 3, '03
> H.V. Porter, Bismarck, N.D.
> Your father died this morning heart affection
> Instruct about burial.
>
> Hotel Metropole[19]

Further confirmation was a cablegram to H.F. Douglass that indicated Porter died on the 3rd and was buried on the 4th.[20] Notably accurate on his plaque in Agra was Porter's date of birth, February 13, a date that has been incorrectly stated in Hammer's books and articles as well as in *Men with Custer* in 2000 as February 3.

His personal effects were lost for a time in India but were forwarded to Judge Bowen in Bismarck by William Thomas Fee, United States consul in Bombay, in January 1904 after they were discovered being held by the Railroad Company there for storage charges. Fee negotiated their release and forwarded them by way of United States Express Company, 49 Broadway, New York City. In addition to his clothes, there were personal items such as his open-face gold watch with gold and platinum chain and charm, a pair of gold pince-nez glasses and cord, and souvenirs that he had bought on the trip.[21]

Some of the things said by people who knew Porter best are found in his obituary and editorial the same day in the *Bismarck Daily Tribune*.[22] His personal bravery was unquestioned. He was kindly and sympathetic, universally popular, and a genial fellow. He was said to have been somewhat reserved, but to those who knew him well, he was a wonderful friend. An eager student and traveler, he was "of a literary nature" and left "by all odds the finest selected private library in the city, if not the whole state." His success in business was recognized by all, yet at other times his methods might be perceived as ruthless to the point of provoking ill will even within his family circle. He was both a rugged westerner and a cosmopolitan sophisticate.

Porter had made a will on July 15, 1902, in which he left all income from his property to be paid to his son, Hal, twice a year as long as he lived. After his death all property would go to his children, and if he had no children, Porter bequeathed everything to his two sisters, Sarah and Frances, both in Washington, DC, or to their heirs.[23] He left Hal all his personal effects, household goods, jewelry, books, silver, engravings, horses, carriages, etc. He named Henry F. Douglass, his business partner then living in Minneapolis, and Francis H. Register, attorney from Bismarck, as trustees.

In 1906 Register and Douglass filed an appeal with the district court in Burleigh County against Hal V. Porter, Sarah E. Davis, Frances E. Porter, Dr. H. Porter Davis, David M. Davis, and Helen W. Davis.[24] Judge M.J. McKenzie had ordered that Porter's will of 1902 be made invalid and indicated that he had died intestate since Henry R. Porter "was not of sound mind and did not have sufficient mental capacity to make a will." The will had been ruled invalid based on the fact that it had attempted "to create and does create a perpetuity in the title to the lands, tenements, and personal property," which was in violation of the law of North Dakota. Thus, Porter's will, which had in effect left only the proceeds of property to his son for his lifetime, was declared null and void and allowed Hal, as sole survivor, to gain the entire estate. Porter, no doubt, feared, when he made the will, that Hal could not be trusted with the large sum of money that would accrue if his property and partnerships were liquidated and suspected that Hal would leave no heirs.

The *Tribune* reported that Hal was spending the winter of 1907–1908 abroad, and a personal letter from Paris indicated that he was having a good time.[25] On the same trip Hal wrote his cousin Helen W. Davis in Washington, DC, from the Grand Hotel de Russie et D'Angleterre, Marseille on February 12, 1908, "that he had decided to go on from Cairo to Constantinople and Greece with the party. We have decided to omit the Holy Land camping tour and trip to Jerusalem so we can arrive in Rome by Easter." His address would be the Hotel Pera Palace, Constantinople.[26]

In 1910 Judge M.J. McKenzie authorized the sale of Dr. H.R. Porter's one-third interest in the Merchants Bank of Glendive, Montana, which he had acquired in 1883. His initial ten thousand dollars investment had been rewarded with "splendid" dividends and was sold for seventeen thousand dollars. The sale was permitted by the judge because the partnership expired January 1, 1910.[27]

The matter of the Porter estate dragged on for years. In June 1916 Hal was in Bismarck "closing up some matters relating to his father's estate. He disposed yesterday [June 7, 1916] of many Indian pictures and his father's medical library, one of the finest in North Dakota in its day. Relics of pioneer life and of the Indian Campaigns have already been taken by Mr. Porter to his Minneapolis home."[28] A wealth of Dr. H.R. Porter's surgical, medical, and personal items are now mostly held in the museum of the North Dakota

Historical Society (see Appendix A). Most spectacularly, there is a U.S. Army wooden field surgical kit probably used by Porter at the Battle of Little Bighorn.

For a time Hal lived in New York City at 315 East 68th Street. He would often spend his winters on the Riviera and presumably never held gainful employment while living off the proceeds of his inheritance. He had as a companion a second-rate Broadway actor by the name of Ralph Glover.

Hal spent his final years in a white frame duplex next to his first cousin and childhood playmate, Katherine Fairchild (Frost) Leslie, at Beebee Lane, Storrs, Connecticut, one and a half miles south of the University of Connecticut. He read avidly but did no writing. Relatives remember him as a crotchety old man given to profane and ritualized outbursts in his old age. By all accounts he was never heard to speak a kind word about his father. He asked to be buried in Mansfield, Connecticut, and when he died in 1968 at age eighty-seven, he was interred in the Mansfield Cemetery on Spring Hill Road off Highway 195.[29] His cousin and closest friend, Katherine Fairchild Leslie (August 15, 1881 to December 15, 1959), had died in Storrs, Connecticut, seven and half years earlier and was buried in the Fairchild plot in Westwood Cemetery, Oberlin, Ohio.

Chapter 23

Forgotten Hero

The *Bismarck Tribune* in 1986 called Henry Rinaldo Porter the "Forgotten Hero of Little Big Horn."[1] This is highly appropriate, since the name of this once prominent citizen of the city has all but disappeared. One reminder is Porter Avenue in Bismarck. The street was named for him, but this came from a section of real estate that he co-developed and carried no honor with it.[2] There have been attempts in 1898 and in 1986 (posthumously) to have Porter awarded the Medal of Honor for his bravery; however, the fact that he was a contract surgeon rather than an active duty army surgeon seems to have derailed both attempts.

Twenty-four Medals of Honor were given for bravery at Little Bighorn; all were to enlisted men and all except three were for bringing water up from the river to the wounded or acting as sharpshooters covering the party.[3] The other three were for continuing to fire while wounded, recapturing a pack mule, and bringing up the pack train, respectively. It would seem that Porter's bravery should not continue to go unrecognized irrespective of his lack of a military commission and that he should be remembered as a true hero of Little Bighorn.

A review of Porter's life and what he meant to Bismarck and Dakota is warranted. He was a nonconformist and one who kept his own counsel. Raised by devout parents who promoted evangelical Protestant religion and temperance, he abandoned their teachings some time after his early tour of Scotland and England where he had been a model of temperance, abstaining from alcohol at parties. In London he had visited the great Spurgeon's Tabernacle and heard him preach.[4] Yet in his maturity he neither eschewed alcohol nor was he a regular churchgoer or even a church member. At the time of his death the *Tribune* editorial writer, probably his friend M.H. Jewell, wrote that "he was always confident of a future state in which broken ties would be mended and fond associations renewed."[5]

Perhaps family pressure led him into a career in medicine, the one that his father, grandfather, and great-grandfather had pursued before him. He obviously rebelled after one year of medical school by running away from

23. Forgotten Hero

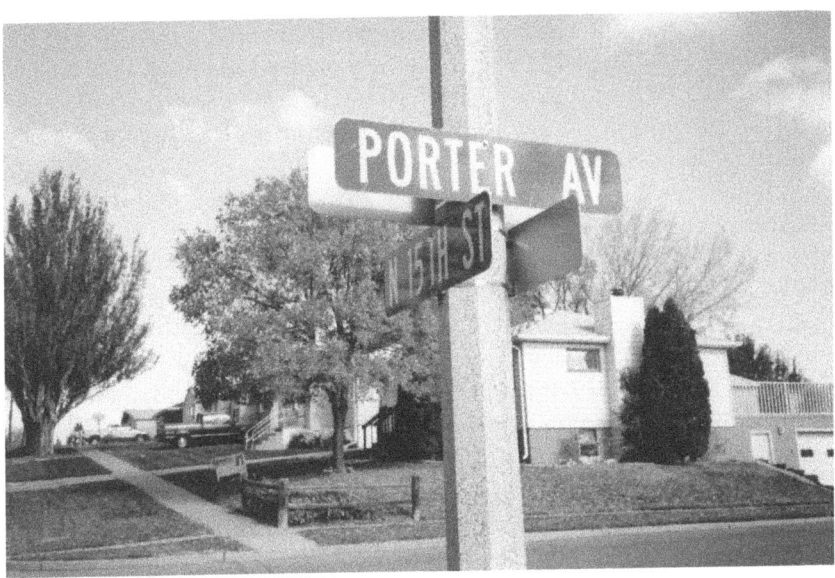

Porter Avenue, Bismarck, North Dakota (photograph owned by author).

medical lectures in New York City to Scotland and England. While there he wrote to his father from London, "It was my intention to go to France or Prussia — if I could not go any other way, to go as a soldier." His love of adventure and a military career at age twenty-two are clear. He added, "I always wanted to cross the ocean and I never would have been satisfied until I had."6 Rather than establishing a practice after graduating from medical school and serving a brief internship, he signed on with the army to work as a contract surgeon in the Arizona Territory. This was his first trip west of the Mississippi. After this he signed an army contract to work in the Dakota Territory. Medicine was never his passion. It was a life that he seemed to enjoy, but he had no problem leaving it for travels and adventure.

When he arrived in Bismarck in November 1873, he was similar to other frontier doctors who tended to be adventurers first and foremost, but he was a cut above. He had graduated from one of the top medical schools in the country. He was a conscientious and caring medical man who was well respected by his peers and his patients and who gave the best care that was possible at the time. At no time was he known to have strayed from the highest ethical standards of the medical profession. It would be up to the next generation doctors to bring in modern scientific advances.

The Battle of Little Bighorn was the defining point in his life. Before that he had been the post surgeon at Camp Hancock, a bachelor in his mid-twenties who had tried to build a practice as the second doctor in the frontier town of Bismarck, and had failed twice in the drugstore business during the Panic of 1873 and its aftermath. He seemed doomed to always play second fiddle to the first doctor there, Dr. B.F. Slaughter. Had Porter achieved early success, it is possible that he could not have been enticed to join Custer's Expedition in 1876.

A question not infrequently asked is, "What did Porter think of Custer?" The answer is not an easy one. Prior to the battle, he seemed to have held him in the highest regard. Custer was Porter's kind of man, a hunter, a fighter, one who loved dogs and horses, and a man with a literary bent who wrote magazine articles about his adventures. Porter was obviously flattered when Custer asked him if he would replace the ailing Dr. George E. Lord on the day of the battle. After Lord demurred in the swap and saved Porter's life in so doing, Porter found himself in the middle of Reno's beleaguered troops on the hilltop. At that point Custer's stock sank pretty low with his fellow soldiers and probably with Porter; however, with his usual reserve in such matters, Porter did not criticize Custer publicly. Benteen was the most vocal critic of Custer's actions and spared no words in saying so.

Porter could not be considered an expert in analyzing the battle. His own account is wrong in details and he always deferred to that of Godfrey's as the most reliable. He was in the battle but saw it from the point of an overburdened military surgeon trying to do his job in the most adverse conditions possible. He never considered himself as a military historian.

When he returned to Bismarck from Little Bighorn, he was at once a war hero, and for as long as he lived he was a local celebrity, a character that everyone knew and admired. His courage and dedication to duty were legendary. As an educated gentleman who was both well-traveled and widely read, he stood at the top of the social ladder with Bismarck's business elite where deals were made on Main Street. His early farming venture on his pre-emption claim north of downtown was one of his first entries into business. With a group he established the First National Bank of Bismarck where he served as director and vice-president and with partners established banks in Mandan and Glendive, Montana. He and Asa Fisher invested in property suitable for home lots and developed it in Bismarck as Fisher's Addition. He was owner of the center section of the Dakota Block, which still stands in downtown Bismarck.

Unfortunately, he lost his wife to an early death in 1888 leaving him with the sole responsibility of raising a seven-year-old son. He left the boy with relatives for long periods at a time while he traveled extensively. His relationship with Hal suffered to the point where Hal was distant and angry. He may well have felt abandoned. Porter's affection for his son was not returned.

How important was he in the development of Bismarck in the nineteenth century? It would be difficult to over-estimate his impact. In addition to his business ventures, he gave Bismarck twenty years of devoted service as physician and surgeon rendering care to all including the destitute, prisoners, insane, railway employees, and the general public.

His strength of character and feelings for humanity were most evident on November 21, 1877, only one year after the Battle of Little Bighorn, when he, Colonel George Sweet, and Dr. William Bentley, as a self-appointed committee of three, invited Chief Joseph, Yellow Bull, Shaved Head, and Yellow Wolf to a banquet at the best hotel in town "as evidence of warm feelings from the people of Bismarck."[7] These captives of the recent Nez Perce War were on the way to Fort Leavenworth, Kansas, under military escort. Porter, one who had barely escaped with his life in Indian warfare, jointly signed an invitation to Chief Joseph that said, "Desiring to show you our kind feelings and the admiration we have for your bravery and humanity, as exhibited in your recent conflict with the forces of the United States, we most cordially invite you to dine with us at the Sheridan House...."[8] This courageous act was, without doubt, the most noble act done by any citizens in the country during the brutal Indian Wars of the nineteenth century. It is one that Bismarck should forever remember with gratitude to Sweet, Bentley, and Porter for their leadership.

His last legacy to the community was a series of travel letters that he wrote from 1893 until 1903 at a time when foreign travel was only a dream for the average citizen. He lived life to the fullest and he shared it with his community.

At one time, in 1893, he sold his home and some of his property with the intention of retiring in Washington, DC. After a year, the West lured him back to the city he loved, to the great joy and satisfaction of his friends in Bismarck. It was from Bismarck that Dr. Henry Rinaldo Porter, survivor of Little Bighorn, left on an around the world trip that ended in Agra, India, in March 1903, with his death. He was fifty-five years old.

The Little Big Horn Associates have placed a plaque on his grave in India that describes his valiant deeds. But in North Dakota, his chosen home, he is yet to receive full recognition as a hero and as one of the pioneers who helped build and develop the city of Bismarck.

Epilogue

"The life he lived was the only one he could ever live; he must go on to the end. The end often comes early to such men, whose spirits are so wrought that they know rest only in action, contentment only in danger, and in confusion find their only peace."

From *Savrola*[1]
By Winston Churchill
Cavalry Subaltern in India,
Sudan and South Africa

Appendix A

Holdings of Dr. H.R. Porter Items, North Dakota Historical Society, Bismarck

Item Name	Description
Surgical Kit	Pocket surgical case
	Instrument, made by Leach and Green
	Instrument, tortoise shell handles
	Instruments, probes, Leach and Green
	Instrument, Belloc's canula
	Instrument, blades
	Instrument
	Instrument
	Instrument
Lantern	Railroad, conductor's — H.R. Porter, MD
Lamp	Lamp, carriage — candle
Candle Stand	Candle holder, hammered iron
Necktie	Ties, collars, & cuffs
Splint	Levi metallic splint, adjustable, child #22
Measure	Medical graduated glass, 4 oz.
Vial	3 tubes aseptic vaccine & bulb, made in Detroit, Michigan
Mask, Anesthesia	Kelene applicator/ethyl chloride, Fitz Brothers, New York.
Kit	Material for uric acid tests, Keaseby Mathers Company, Ambler, Pennsylvania. Litmus paper, test for albumen and sugar, Londonderry Spring Water Co., Nashua, New Hampshire.
Kit, Medicine	Pocket case cocaine treatment, hydrochloride of cocaine, William R. Warren and Co., Philadelphia and New York.
Kit, Medicine	Pocket case, 4 glass vials of pills, opium 15 white pills, mor-

	phine powder, pillcath [?] 3 whole 2 broken, aconite (see below), empty.
Syringe	Pocket case, hypodermic test, sodium tungstate 26 tablets, urinary test tablets, citric acid 26 tablets, potassium ferricyanide 26 tablets, litmus (missing tablets), lead oxide, atropine sulfate, indigo and sodium carbonate, potassium mercuric iodide, picric acid, bismuth subnitrate, test tubes 2, silver test tube holder 1, graduated dropper with white rubber bulb made by Parke Davis and Co.
Kit, Medicine	Pocket case, Codeine 2.5 g, quinine 2.5 g, salol [?] 2.5 g, never used, Antikamnia Chemical Company, St. Louis, Missouri.
Kit, Medicine	Pocket case, vials of tablets, card of Dr. Marion Mead [?], diarrhea—opium 1–4, camphor 1–4, ipecac 1–4, heart stimulant—digitalis minima 2 [also called gratiola officianalis, a plant native to Southern Europe used as antihelmenic, purgative, emetic, and diuretic. Reference: Dunglison's *Medical Dictionary*, 1874], strophan, belladonna, extonoihi [?], tonsillitis—alconite [possibly aconite, from the dried root of *Aconitum napellus*, a cardiac and respiratory sedative, analgesic, diaphoretic, and diuretic], tincture of belladonna 1–10, hydro iodide rub[?] 1–100, ipecac, cathartic active-podophyllin, extrac. colot. co. [?], *nux vomica* [the poisonous seed of *strychnos nux-vomica* that contains several alkaloids, the principal one being strychnine], *oil tiglii* [?], *oil eorcapo* [?], sodium bicarbonate and calomel, ergonate g 1–4.
Suitcase	Leather travel bag, Dr. Porter
Diploma	Oak frame, Georgetown College of Medicine, Dr. Porter
Hod	Coal bucket or hod, brass
Chest, Medicine	U.S. Army Field Surgical Chest No. 2 [see notes Chapter 5]
Vest	Vest
Vest	Vest
Vest	Vest
Vest	Vest
Trunk	Small leather trunk
Hat, Fraternal	Mason's hat with plume
Sash	Mason's heavy shoulder sash
Belt	Leather belt with blue cloth (Mason's)
Glove	Mason's tan cloth gloves
Belt	Mason's rust-colored leather belt
Hat, Fraternal	Mason's hat with brim

Hat, Fraternal	Rain-cover for hat (Mason's)
Print, Photograph	Photo
Frame, Picture	Frame with oval mat and photo removed
Print, Photograph	Photo
Frame, Picture	Frame with oval mat and photo removed
Dish, Chafing	Chafing dish set
Bit	Bridle bit
Bit	Bridle bit
Plate	Baby dish
Kit, Surgical	Field surgical kit (U.S.A. Hospital Dept.) [see notes Chapter 5].
Kit, Surgical	Surgical instrument, pocket kit, dissecting forceps with lock, surgical knives, grooved director 4½ inches, syringe needle, irrigating catheter tip, suture needles— one self-threading. Instruments made by Gemrig
Syringe	Syringe in leather case, 2½ inch barrel, 3-way stop cock, 2 needles, Whitilltata and Co., New York and Philadelphia.
Syringe	Improved antitoxin syringe, metal case, Mulford Co., Philadelphia.
Syringe	Syringe in metal case, small, mark crown over dollar sign, 3 needles.
Sign, Trade	Shingle for medical doctor
Receipt	Checkbook, stubs missing (Dr. Porter's)
Sound	Urethral catheters and Sounds, 5, (male)
Sound	Urethral sound (male)
Tenaculum	Grasping tenaculum
Speculum	Sims vaginal speculum, Shepard & Dudley, New York
Sound	Uterine sound
Speculum	Sims anal speculum
Trocar	Wood handle
Stethoscope	Stethoscope (medical doctor's)
Dipper	Medications dipper, steel
Syringe	Long-nosed syringe
Forceps	Long-nosed forceps
Forceps	Medical forceps
Instrument	Medical instrument
Scissors	Bandage scissors
Scissors	Bandage scissors and tissue clasp, Fensel (German)

Instrument [?]	Double-edged medical instrument, ebony handle, Tiemann
Chair	Desk chair, small, collapsible
Suitcase	Suitcase cover, Dr. Porter
Suitcase	Leather overnight bag, Dr. Porter
Map Case	Leather (owned by Dr. H.R. Porter)
Belt, Money	Travel leather money-belt
Papers	2 boxes cigarettes papers (Austria) Dr. Porter's European Tour?
Cane	Cane, walking, handmade leather washer
Horn, Powder	Powder horn (possibly from the American Revolution era)
Probe	Probe — medical instrument
Rod	Medical instrument, straight steel rod
Clamp	Surgical spring clamps for tubing
Depressor	Steel tongue depressor
Instrument	Celluloid
Stethoscope	Earpiece from examining instrument
Instrument	Unidentified medical instrument
Instrument	Medical instrument rubber handle with bla[de] [?]
Instrument	Unidentified medical instrument
Crank	One-piece steel crank
Stethoscope	Stethoscope bell
Pad	Dr. Porter's prescription pad
Slippers	Pair of leather slippers, dark red
Slippers	Pair of leather slippers, dark red

Appendix B

Porter Lineage

1 Richard PORTER
   b. c. 1611 to 1617 Dorset, Dorchester, England
   - Left Weymouth, England, March 30, 1635
   - Arrived in Wessagusset, later named Weymouth, MA
   - Served in town offices and grew reeds used for thatching houses
   d. c. 1688–1689 Weymouth, MA
   m. Ruth (Porter) c. 1615 in England
         2   John PORTER

2 John PORTER, Sgt
   b. c. 1638
   - Built first sawmill in South Abington, MA, in 1693
   - Held town offices
   d. August 7, 1717
   m. Deliverance BYRAM 1660
      b. 1638 Weymouth, MA
      d. September 30, 1720, Weymouth, MA
         3   Samuel PORTER

3 Samuel PORTER
   b. March 20, 1670, Weymouth, MA
   - Schoolmaster and shoemaker
   - Town officer of Weymouth, MA, in 1705
   - Selectman 1714
   - Tax assessor 1716
   d. August 31, 1725
   m. Mary NASH 1698
      b. March 20, 1675, Weymouth, MA
         4   Jacob PORTER

4 Jacob PORTER
   b. August 10, 1704, Weymouth, MA
   - Selectman, built first mill on Beaver Brook
   d. October, 26, 1778
   m. Esther FORD January 6, 1732
      b. March 8, 1714 (Abington) Plymouth, MA
      d. November 20, 1789

5   Noah PORTER
    b. August 16, 1744 Abington, Plymouth, MA, moved to Cummington, MA
    • Physician
    d. before 1777
    m. Mary NORTON February 2, 1766

6   Norton PORTER
    b. 1771 Abington, Plymouth, MA, moved to Oneida County, NY, 1791
    • Physician
    d. November 18, 1852
    m. Sarah Cobb February 10, 1796, Cummington, MA

7   Henry Norton PORTER
    b. November 5, 1816
        • Physician, Lee Center, NY, 1841 to 1862 then moved to New York Mills, Oneida County, NY
    d. September 12, 1899, Washington, DC
    m. Helen Fulton POLSON 1842
        b. September 20, 1818, Scotland
        d. May 19, 1900, Washington, D.C.
            8   Henry Rinaldo PORTER

8   Henry Rinaldo PORTER
    b. February 13, 1848, Lee Center, Oneida County, NY
    • Physician and surgeon
    d. March 3, 1903, Agra, India
    m. Charlotte VIETS September 4, 1877, Oberlin, OH
        b. July 1, 1853
        d. August 6, 1888
            9   Henry Viets PORTER

9   Henry Viets PORTER
    b. May 23, 1881, Bismarck, D.T.
    d. June 30, 1968, Mansfield, CT
    Never married

Chapter Notes

Chapter 1

1. Alexis de Tocqueville, *Democracy in America*. Trans. and ed. by Harvey C. Mansfield and Delba Winthrop (Chicago: University of Chicago Press, 2002), 634.
2. The following biographical sketches identify Lee Center, NY, as Porter's birthplace: *Compendium of History and Biography of North Dakota* (Chicago: Ogle, 1900), 160; *History of the Great Northwest and its Men of Progress* (Minneapolis: Journal, 1901), 145; *The Medical Fortnightly*, August 1896, 421. The last sketch was affixed in Porter's own scrapbook. In addition, J. Grassick, *North Dakota Medicine: Sketches and Abstracts* (Grand Forks: North Dakota Medical Association, 1926), 234, cites Lee Center. The error of New York Mills may possibly be traced to a 1960 article by Kenneth M. Hammer, "Frontier Doctor," in *The Westerners New York Posse Brand Book* 7, no. 3 (1960): 55. This article also mistakenly reports Porter's date of birth as February 3; the correct date is February 13. Both of the errors are carried forward in "Henry Rinaldo Porter," *Men with Custer*, Ronald H. Nichols, ed. Rev. ed, (Hardin, MT: Custer Battlefield Historical and Museum Association, 2000), 263.
3. *History of Oneida County, NY: Illustrations and Biographical Sketches of Some of its Prominent Men* (Philadelphia: Everts and Farris, 1878), 198–9, 617–8.
4. Henry J. Cookinham, *History of Oneida County, New York From 1700 to the Present Time*. Vol. 1. (Chicago: Clarke, 1912), 392.
5. Weymouth Historical Society. *History of Weymouth Massachusetts*, vol. 1 (Boston: Wright and Potter, 1923), 72–5. Previous citation contributed and transcribed by Sheila Tate, member of the Immigrant Ship Transcribers Guild, June 6, 2000. http://www.immigrantships.net/v3/1600v3/hullcompany16330320.html. (accessed August 18, 2004).
6. Joseph W. Porter, *A Genealogy of the Descendants of Richard Porter Who Settled at Weymouth, Massachusetts 1635* (Bangor: Burr & Robinson, 1898).
7. Thomas Bulfinch, *Bulfinch's Mythology* (New York: Modern Library, [1855, 1858, 1863] 1998), 680–2, 808–14.
8. "A Brave Doctor," *Bismarck Weekly Tribune*, May 24, 1878.
9. Map of Lee Center, NY (1858), Oneida County (NY) Historical Society, Utica, NY.
10. *Catalogue of the Officers and Students of Whitestown Seminary at Whitestown, Oneida County, N.Y. For the Year Ending March 1869* (Utica: Roberts, 1869), 23.
11. "Seminary Had Its Origin in Old Oneida Institute," typescript, June 23, 1931, File of Whitestown Seminary, Oneida County Historical Society, Utica, NY.
12. *Catalogue of the Officers and Students of Whitestown Seminary*, 30–1.
13. Ibid., 23–7. Textbooks for the lower classes included Parker and Watson's *National Fifth Reader*, Webster's or Worcester's *Dictionary*, McNally's *Geography*, Robinson's *Arithmetic*, Kerl's *Grammar*, Davies' *Intellectual Arithmetic*. Textbooks at the higher levels included Warren's *Physical Geography*, Parker's *Natural Philosophy*, Willson's *U.S. History*, Willson's *Ancient and Modern History*, Robinson's *Algebra*, Davies'–Legendre's *Geology*, Gillespie's *Surveying*, Yeoman's *Chemistry*, Dana's *Geology*, Gray's *Botany*, Quackenbos' *Rhetoric*, Upham's *Mental Philosophy*, Paley's *Evidences of Christianity*, Wayland's *Moral Science*, Butler's *Analogy*, Bryant and Stratton's *Bookkeeping*, Cutter's *Physiology*, Burritt's *Astronomy*, Davies' *Trigonometry*, and Mahan's *Civil Engineering*.
14. *Whitestown Seminary Reunion 1881–1931*, typescript. Various Records Collected for the Dunham Public Library by a Member of the Class of 1881, 1931, Call Number 374.9, W582NY, Oneida County Historical Society, Utica, NY.

Chapter 2

1. Ruth Bordin, *The University of Michigan: A Pictorial History* (Ann Arbor: University of Michigan Press, 1967), 34.
2. Hillsdale (MI) *Standard*, January 5, 1869.
3. Bordin, *The University of Michigan: A Pictorial History*, 21.
4. Ibid., 35.
5. Ibid., 39.
6. Howard H. Peckham, *The Making of the University of Michigan* (Ann Arbor: University of Michigan Press, 1967), 37.
7. Ibid., 60.
8. Bangor (ME) Daily *Whig and Courier*, April 29, 1870.
9. St. Joseph (MI) *Herald*, December 10, 1870.
10. Ibid., 61.
11. Porter Family Papers. Most of the original letters have been lost. Almost all references to Porter Family Papers are typescripts of the lost letters. Obtained from Cathy Davis, White Stone, VA.
12. Ibid.
13. Norway-Heritage: Hands Across the Sea, "S/S *Australia*," http://www.norwayheritage.com/p_ship.asp?sh=aust1. Accessed May 11, 2003.
14. "The Anchor Line Steamers," *New York Herald*, September 10, 1870.
15. "Foreign Ports," *New York Herald*, October 15, 1870.
16. "Immigrants to Canada," http://ist.uwaterloo.ca/~marj/genealogy/allan.html. Accessed May 11, 2003.
17. H.R. Porter to Dr. and Mrs. Henry N. Porter, October 3, 1870, Porter Family Papers.
18. H.R. Porter to Mother, October 17, 1870, Porter Family Papers.
19. S/S *Australia* of the Anchor Line arrived in Glasgow on October 1, 1870. See "Foreign Ports," *New York Herald*, October 15, 1870.
20. The S/S *Cambria* of the Anchor Line left New York October 8 and wrecked off the coast of North Ireland en route to Glasgow on October, 19, 1870, causing the deaths of some 170 passengers and crew. See "Lost at Sea, Wreck of the Steamer *Cambria* Off the Irish Coast," *New York Herald*. October 22, 1870.
21. Henry R. Porter to Mr. and Mrs. David M. Davis, October 24, 1870, Porter Family Papers.
22. H.R. Porter to Frances E. Porter, October 31 and November 3, 1870, Porter Family Papers.
23. H.R. Porter to Dr. Henry N. Porter, November 16, 1870, Porter Family Papers.
24. The term "smog" was not invented until 1905 to describe London's natural fog and the smoke from fires burning soft coal that issued from more than a million homes by 1800. These so called "pea-soupers" were responsible for much lung disease and many deaths. See David Urbinato, "London's Historic 'Pea-Soupers,'" U.S. Environmental Protection Agency, History. http://www.epa.gov.history/topics/perspect/london.htm. Accessed March 14, 2004.
25. Claims of the United States against England during and after the American Civil War for damages done by eleven Confederate ships built or outfitted there, including the *Alabama*. An arbitration board awarded the United States $15,500,000 in gold, which was paid in 1873. See Mark M. Boatner III. *The Civil War Dictionary* (New York: David McKay, 1959), 4–5.
26. H.R. Porter to Dr. and Mrs. Henry N. Porter, November 25, 1870, Porter Family Papers.

Chapter 3

1. *Catalogue of the Officers and Students of Georgetown College, District of Columbia for the Academic Year, 1871–72* (Baltimore: Murphy, 1872), 36–41.
2. Ibid., 38.
3. Johnson Eliot, Herbert Boardman, and R.D. DeL. French, *Addresses Delivered at the Twenty-third Annual Commencement of the Medical Department of Georgetown College* (Washington, DC: Tomlinson, 1872), 1–33. University Archives, Lauinger Library, Georgetown University, Washington, DC.
4. Newspaper clipping, marked '72 [1872]. University Archives, Lauinger Library, Georgetown University, Washington, DC.
5. Matthew Cella and Jon Ward, "Columbia Hospital to Close," *Washington Times*, May 8, 2002. http://www.washtimes.com/metro/20020508-24150208.html, Accessed November 20, 2002.
6. H.R. Porter Papers, Surgeon General of the Army, Entry 561, RG94, National Archives.
7. James W. Wengert, "The Contract Surgeon," *Journal of the West* 36, no. 1 (1997): 67–8.
8. H.R. Porter to Dr. H.N. Porter, San Francisco, July 6, 1872, in "A Soldier with Crook: the Letters of Henry R. Porter," Gene M. Gressley, ed., *Montana, the Magazine of Western History* 8, no. 3 (1958): 34.
9. Ibid., 35.
10. Ibid.
11. Laudie J. Chorne, *Following the Custer Trail of 1876*. Rev. ed. (Bismarck, ND: Trails West, 2001), 111.
12. H.R. Porter to Dr. and Mrs. H.N. Porter,

Mullins Station, A.T., September 10, 1872, in "A Soldier with Crook," 36.

13. Ibid.

14. H.R. Porter to Dr. and Mrs. H.N. Porter, Fort Whipple, A.T., September 20, 1872, in "A Soldier with Crook," 36–7.

15. H.R. Porter to Mother, Camp Hualpai, A.T., September 28, 1872, in "A Soldier with Crook," 36–7.

16. John G. Bourke, *On the Border with Crook*, (New York: Time-Life, [1891] 1980), 170.

17. H.R. Porter to Mother, Camp Hualpai, A.T. September 28, 1872, in "A Soldier with Crook," 37–8. See also "Crushing Defeat of the Indians," *New York Herald*, October 7, 1872.

18. H.R. Porter to Mother, Camp Hualpai, A.T. September 28, 1872, in "A Soldier with Crook," 37–8.

19. H.R. Porter to Dr. and Mrs. H.N. Porter, in the field near Camp Hualpai, A.T., November 5, 1872, in "A Soldier with Crook," 40.

20. Ibid.

21. H.R. Porter to Mother, in the field near Camp Hualpai, November 15, 1872, in "A Soldier with Crook," 41.

22. H.R. Porter to Dr. and Mrs. H.N. Porter, in the field near Camp Verde, December 2, 1872, in "A Soldier with Crook," 42, 47.

23. Henry R. Porter to Dr. Henry N. Porter, In the Field near Camp Verde, December 20, 1872, in "A Soldier with Crook,"43.

24. John G. Bourke, *On the Border with Crook*, 212.

25. Ibid., 210.

26. "The Indian War," *New York Herald*, December 15, 1872.

27. "General Crook in Active Pursuit of the Hostile Indians of Arizona," *New York Herald*, December 24, 1872.

28. Ibid.

29. The collection of fifteen letters to his family by Porter from Arizona Territory was given by his son, Henry Viets Porter, to the American Heritage Center, University of Wyoming, Laramie, WY 82071.

30. It has been suggested to me by Dr. Phillip Walker, Charlotte, NC, based on his medical experience practicing in Arizona in the military, that these fevers may well have been due to cocciodomycosis, a fungal disease caused by *Coccidiodes immitis*, a soil saprophyte found commonly in the area, causing a disease endemic to the area.

31. General Orders No. 14, Department of Arizona, Prescott, April 9, 1873. Dr. H.R. Porter's Scrapbook.

32. Dr. H.M. Matthews attested to the marks made as signatures by the chiefs and headmen of the Oglala band on the Fort Laramie Treaty of 1868. See "The Avalon Project at Yale Law School: Fort Laramie Treaty, 1868." *http://yale.edu/lawweb/avalon/ntreaty/nt001*. Accessed March 31, 2004.

33. H.R. Porter Papers, Surgeon General of the Army, Entry 561, RG94, National Archives.

34. Ibid.

35. Ibid.

36. Clipping, undated, Dr. H.R. Porter's Scrapbook.

Chapter 4

1. U.S. War Department, *Camp Hancock and Camp Sykes Post Returns, 1872- 1877*, State Historical Society of North Dakota Library, Bismarck.

2. Linda W. Slaughter, "Fortress to Farm: Or Twenty-three Years on the Frontier," *Bismarck Daily Tribune*, March 31, 1894.

3. "Early Days of Bismarck," *Bismarck Tribune*, June 8, 1883.

4. "Yankton, Burleigh County Organized," *Bismarck Daily Tribune*, July 11, 1873.

5. Robin W. Winks, *Frederick Billings: A Life* (New York: Oxford University Press, 1991), 186–7.

6. Linda W. Slaughter, "Fortress to Farm," *Bismarck Daily Tribune*, March 3, 1894.

7. John K. Brown, *The Baldwin Locomotive Works, 1831–1915* (Baltimore: Johns Hopkins University Press, 1995), 33.

8. "Early Days of Bismarck," *Bismarck Tribune*, June 8, 1883.

9. "Old-Time Notes," *Bismarck Daily Tribune*, September 5, 1883.

10. Frank Vyzralek, information to author via Mark Halvorson, February 25, 2004.

11. "First Train over the Missouri," *Bismarck Tribune*, October 20, 1882.

12. Edward C. Murphy, "The Northern Pacific Railway Bridge at Bismarck," *North Dakota History* 62, no. 2 (1975): 2–19.

13. Sandy Barnard, *I Go with Custer: The Life and Death of Reporter Mark Kellogg* (Bismarck, ND: Tribune, 1996), 78.

14. "Twenty Years Ago," *Bismarck Daily Tribune*, November 4, 1893.

15. *Bismarck Daily Tribune*, May 20, 1874.

16. "Notice of Dissolution" and "Notice of Co-partnership," *Bismarck Daily Tribune*, May 27, 1874. Also, see Nat Brandt, *The Town That Started the Civil War* (Syracuse: Syracuse University Press, 1990), 108–10. George Hornell Fairchild was the second of eight children of James Harris Fairchild (1817–1902) and Mary Kellogg Fairchild (1819–90).

17. Fairchild's mother was a Kellogg and her mother lived in Keokuk. Thus Fairchild was related to the owner.

18. John Jay Knox, *A History of Banking in the United States by John Jay Knox, assisted by a corps of financial writers; the entire work revised and brought up to date by Bradford Rhodes and Elmer Youngman* (New York: Rhodes, 1900), 801.
19. "Personal," *Bismarck Daily Tribune*, May 13, 1874.
20. *Bismarck Daily Tribune*, June 17, 1874.
21. "The Chase for Gold," *Bismarck Daily Tribune*, July 8, 1874.
22. "The Black Hills Country," Traverse City (MI) *Grand Traverse Herald*, September 3, 1874.
23. "The Black Hills," *Bismarck Daily Tribune*, September 2, 1874.
24. George H. Fairchild to Helen Viets Fairchild, Bismarck, June 21, 1874, George H. Fairchild Papers, SHSND A227/1/1.
25. George H. Fairchild to Helen Viets Fairchild, Bismarck, Undated, George H. Fairchild Papers. SHSND A227/1/1.
26. George H. Fairchild to Helen Viets Fairchild, Bismarck, July 5, 1874, George H. Fairchild Papers. SHSND A227/1/1.
27. "Aunt Sally in the Black Hills," *Bismarck Daily Tribune*, September 9, 1874.
28. *Bismarck Tribune*, July 8, 1874.
29. The Reverend I. Oliver Sloan (1820–99) served as a hospital chaplain in the Civil War, was captured by the Confederates, and after the war went to the West as a missionary where he organized the first Presbyterian church in the territory. See "Father Sloan Dead," *Bismarck Daily Tribune*, November 3, 1899.
30. First Presbyterian Church, Bismarck, Manuscript Collection 1873–1900, 1957, SHSND MSS 20490, Bismarck.
31. Clyde L. Young, *85 Years: The First Presbyterian Church 1873–1958* (Bismarck, ND: Tribune, 1958), 9.
32. *Bismarck Daily Tribune*, May 27, 1874.
33. Fannie Dunn Quain Papers, SHSND A23/1/2.
34. "Bismarck, Dakota Territory," *Bismarck Daily Tribune*, December 22, 1875.
35. George H. Fairchild to Helen Viets Fairchild, Bismarck, July 26, 1874, George H. Fairchild Papers, SHSND A227/1/1.
36. George H. Fairchild to Helen Viets Fairchild, Bismarck, August 2, 1874.,George H. Fairchild Papers, SHSND A227/1/1.
37. George H. Fairchild to Helen Viets Fairchild, Bismarck, August 9, 1874, SHSND A227/1/1.
38. George H. Fairchild to Helen Viets Fairchild, Bismarck, August 16, 1874, SHSND A227/1/1.
39. Word had come back from Custer's Black Hills exposition that gold and silver were present in "immense quantities." See "Gold! Confirmed," *Bismarck Daily Tribune*, August 12, 1874.
40. Charles Alexander Reynolds (1842–76), son of Dr. Joseph Boyer Reynolds, college-educated, served as a guide to the 7th Cavalry at Little Bighorn and was killed in the valley fight near Dr. Henry Porter. See Ronald H. Nichols, ed., *Men with Custer*. Rev. ed. (Hardin, MT: Custer Battlefield Historical and Museum Association, 2000), 277.
41. George H. Fairchild to Helen Viets Fairchild, Bismarck, August 23, 1874, George H. Fairchild Papers, SHSND A227/1/1.
42. George H. Fairchild to Helen Viets Fairchild, Bismarck, September 6, 1874, George H. Fairchild Papers, SHSND A227/1/1.
43. *Bismarck Daily Tribune*, May 6, 1874. Also, see Cathy A. Langemo, *Images of America: Bismarck North Dakota* (Chicago: Arcadia, 2002), 70.
44. "Times in Bismarck in 1872," *Bismarck Daily Tribune*, September 5, 1883.
45. *Bismarck Daily Tribune*, May 6, 1874.
46. *Bismarck Daily Tribune*, December 2, 1874.
47. "Nicholson and Porter's," *Bismarck Daily Tribune*, January 13, 1875.
48. "Rapid City," *Bismarck Tri-weekly Tribune*, July 30, 1877.
49. "Dissolution," *Bismarck Daily Tribune*, April 14, 1875.
50. "An Elegant Establishment," *Bismarck Daily Tribune*, May 5, 1875.
51. *Bismarck Daily Tribune*, July 14, 1875.
52. *Bismarck Daily Tribune*, November 8, 1875.
53. *Bismarck Daily Tribune*, June 23, 1875.
54. A trocar to perform such a procedure is among Porter's instruments in the SHSND, Bismarck.
55. "A Successful Operation," *Bismarck Daily Tribune*, December 8, 1875.
56. "Bismarck, Dakota Territory," *Bismarck Daily Tribune*, December 22, 1875.
57. Kenneth Hammer, "Frontier Doctor." *Westerner's New York Brand Book* 7 (1960): 55.
58. The House Military Committee in Washington reported a bill that set the army pay at the annual rate of general, $10,000; lieutenant general, $8,000; major general, $6,000; brigadier general, $5,000; colonel, $3,500; lieutenant colonel, $3,000; major, $2,500; captain (mounted) $2,000; captain (not mounted) $1,800; first lieutenant (mounted) $1,600; first lieutenant (not mounted) $1,500; second lieutenant (mounted) $1,500; second lieutenant (not mounted) $1,400. See "Congressional Summary, March 22." Burlington [IA] *Hawkeye*, March 30, 1876. Pay for enlisted troopers was $13 a

month, quarters, meals, and uniforms. See "The Buffalo Soldiers," http://ushist.com/buffalo-soldiers.htm. Accessed March 31, 2004.

59. James M. DeWolf to wife, Bismarck, May 17, 1876, in "The Diary and Letters of James M. DeWolf," Edward S. Luce, ed., *North Dakota History* 25, nos. 2, 3 (1958): 70.

60. *Bismarck Daily Tribune*, October 28, 1875.

61. James W. DeWolf to wife, Bismarck, April 14, 1876, in "The Diary and Letter of Dr. James M. DeWolf," Edward S. Luce, ed., *North Dakota History* 25, no. 2, 3 (1958): 59.

62. Samantha Viets to George H. and Helen V. Fairchild, Oberlin, OH, May 27, 1876, George H. Fairchild Papers, SHSND A 227/1/1.

Chapter 5

1. James W. Forsyth and F.D. Grant, *Report of An Expedition Up the Yellowstone River, Made in 1875* (Washington, DC: Government Printing Office, 1875).

2. "Personal," *Bismarck Tribune*, June 16, 1875.

3. "Return of Forsyth and Grant," *Bismarck Tribune*, June 16, 1875.

4. "Belknap and Grant," *Indiana (PA) Democrat*, April 6, 1876.

5. *Chicago Tribune* as cited by *Decatur (IL) Republican*, May 18, 1876.

6. Helena (MT) *Independent*, March 24, 1876.

7. Helena (MT)*Independent*, May 7, 1876.

8. "Crook's Army," Helena (MT) *Independent*, June 6, 1876.

9. J.W. Vaughn, *With Crook at the Rosebud* (Mechanicsburg, PA: Stackpole Books, [1956], 1994), 11.

10. "An Indian War Anticipated," *New York Times*, February 21, 1876.

11. "Expedition Against the Indians," *Burlington (IA) Hawk Eye*, March 2, 1876.

12. James M. DeWolf to wife, Dakota Territory, May 25, 1876, in "The Diary and Letters of Dr. James M. DeWolf," Edward S. Luce,, ed., *North Dakota History* 25, nos. 2, 3 (1958): 75.

13. Sandy Barnard, *I Go with Custer: The Life and Death of Reporter Mark Kellogg* (Bismarck, ND: Tribune, 1996), 204.

14. Sibley stoves are small: 28¾ inches tall, 18 inches in diameter at the base, a 5½ × 6 inch door, and a smokestack 3¾ inches in diameter and made of 16 gauge steel. They are portable, and are still commercially available for use in Civil War re-enactments. General Henry Hopkins Sibley (1816–86) was a Confederate officer. See Mark M. Boatner III. *The Civil War Dictionary* (New York: McKay, 1959), 759–60. Sibley also devised the Sibley tent, "a bell shaped tent, often quite large ... allegedly on the pattern of the Sioux tepees and often used in the U.S. Army in the west." See catalogue, http.//www.pantherprimatives.com/pdf/67.pdf. Accessed December 11, 2003.

15. Vaughn, *With Crook at the Rosebud*, 12.

16. Laudie J. Chorne, *Following the Custer Trail of 1876*, rev. ed. (Bismarck, ND: Trails West, 2001), 131–33.

17. Ibid., 136.

18. Ibid., 144.

19. Special Field Orders No. 11, Department of Dakota, June 10, 1876. NARA as cited by Ronald H. Nichols, *In Custer's Shadow: Major Marcus Reno* (Norman: University of Oklahoma Press, (1999) 2000), 151.

20. Chorne, *Following the Custer Trail of 1876*, 149.

21. Nichols, *In Custer's Shadow: Major Marcus Reno*, 153.

22. Vaughn, *With Crook at Rosebud*, 1–245.

23. Edward S. Godfrey, "General Godfrey's Narrative," in W.A. Graham, *The Custer Myth: A Source Book of Custeriana* (Harrisburg, PA: Stackpole Books, 1953), 130.

24. Vaughn, *With Crook at the Rosebud*, 9.

25. John S. Gray, *Centennial Campaign: The Sioux War of 1876* (Norman: University of Oklahoma Press, [1976] 1988), 274.

26. James M. DeWolf to Wife, Rosebud Creek, June 21, 1876, in "The Diary and Letters of Dr. James M. DeWolf," 80–1. (Second Lieutenant Henry Moore Harrington, C Company and Second Lieutenant Benjamin Hubert Hodgson, B Company.)

27. E.S. Godfrey, *Mounts, Uniforms and Equipment*. Cited in Chorne *Following the Custer Trail of 1876*, 188.

28. George E. Lord Papers, Surgeon General of the Army, RG 94, National Archives. For biographical sketches of Drs. Lord and DeWolf see Edward S. Petersen, "Surgeons of the Little Big Horn," *Westerners Brand Book* 31, no. 6 (Los Angeles Westerners: Los Angeles, 1974): 41–3.

29. George E. Lord Papers, Surgeon General of the Army, RG 94, National Archives.

30. See "Descendants of Simon DeWolf," http://guweb2.gonzaga.edu/~dewolf/perry/chapter2.htm, Accessed October 4, 2006. Also, "The DeWolf Family of Bristol, Rhode Island-Part I, http://rhodeisland-philatelic.com/rhodeisland/stampless66.htm. Accessed October 4, 2006. A documentary film of the family history and its involvement in slavery has been made by family member Katrina Browne, *Traces of the Trade: a Story from the Deep North*.

31. Ronald H. Nichols, ed., *Men with Custer*

(Hardin, MT: Custer Battlefield Historical and Museum Association, 2000), 85.
  32. This surgical kit is at the SHSND, Bismarck.
  33. Also, it contains the following:
  Bone rongeur, 10 inch
  Needle holder
  Spring forceps, artery
  Straight and curved needles
  Silver wire, 5 rolls
  Liston knives, 10½ and 7¾ inches
  Catlin knives, 8½ and 4 inches
  Metacarpal saw
  Tennacular
  Scalpels, 6
  Tenotome
  Bone elevator
  Scissors
  Catheters, metal
  Eye spatula
  Bullet probe
  Curettes
  Probe
  Hey saw
  34. Kit is in SHSND, Bismarck.
  35. This chest belonged to Porter and was said to be used at Little Bighorn. It was given to the SHSND by Dr. E.P. Quain, Eugene, OR, in 1949. U.S. Army Field Surgical Chest No. 2, made by F.G. Otto and Son. Inventory when stocked.
Tray:
  Tablets in 120 cc bottles
  Acidum bericum 324 mg
  Antiseptic, 2 bottles
  Carthartica compostre
  Opium, 65 mg
  Potassium bromide, 325 mg
  235 g bottles
  Carbolic acid, 1
  Chlerphormun [Chloroform ?], 2
  Glycerin, 1
  Opium tincture, 1
  Spiritus fermenti [brandy], 2
  Ether, 100 g tins, 5
  Bucket, folding canvas, 1
  Catheters, flexible, 6
  Corks, for ether, 6
  Dressing papers, roll 1
  Felt for splints, 2 pieces
  Muslin, 3 sq meters
  Petrolatum, ½ kg
  Pocket case, aseptic #1
  Razor strop, 1
  Tumbler, 1
Drawer 1:
  Bandages rubber, 1
  Nail brush, 1
  Plain gauze, 2 sq meters
  Gargles, 2
  Iodoform sprinkle, 1
  Catgut ligatures, 2 spools
  Silk worm gut ligatures, sterilized, 1 spool
  Common pins, 1 paper
  Needle, thread, etc. in case, 1
  Pencil, indelible, 3
  Safety pins, assorted, 12
  Ear and nose speculum, 1
  Tape, 1 piece
  Tape measure, 1
  Esmarch's tourniquet, 1
Drawer 2:
  Tooth extracting case, 1
  Absorbent cotton, 2 packages
  Rubber drainage tubes, 3 meters
  Split chain links for pack saddles, 4
  Adhesive plaster, 15 mm spools, 4
  Adhesive plaster, 30 mm spool, 1
Drawer 3:
  Roller bandages, 36
  Suspensory bandages, 2
  Beef extract, 100 g tins
  Shaving brush, 1
  Absorbent cotton, 2 packages
  Graduated measure, 5 cc, 1
  Medicine measuring glass, 1
  Sail needle
  Upholsterer's needle
  Needle holder, 1
  Indelible pencil, 1
  Isinglass plaster, 9 meters
  Razor, 1
  Book, *A System of Operative Surgery* by Henry Hollingsworth Smith (Philadelphia: Lippincott, Grambo, 1852)
  Syringe, 2
  Universal tool
Drawer 4:
  Flannel bandages, 4
  Roller bandages, 12
  Emergency case, 1
Drawer 5:
  Plain gauze 4 meters
  Jute or equivalent, 100 g package, 6
  Castile soap, 2.25 g
Drawer 6:
  Roller bandages, 6
  Hemostatic forceps in case, 12
  Trays for instruments, 2

Chapter 6

  1. Edward S. Godfrey, "General Godfrey's Narrative," in W.A. Graham, *The Custer Myth*, 130.
  2. Ibid.
  3. Frederick W. Benteen, "A Transcript of Benteen's Narrative," in W.A. Graham, *The Custer Myth*, 178.

4. John S. Gray, *Centennial Campaign: The Sioux War of 1876* (Norman: University of Oklahoma Press, [1976] 1988), 151–71.
5. Henry R. Porter, in *Compendium of History and Biography of North Dakota* (Chicago: Ogle, 1900), 163.
6. Joseph H. Taylor, *Sketches of Frontier and Indian Life on the Upper Missouri and Great Plains* (Pottstown, PA: Self-published, 1889), 106. Linen dusters came into use by railroad travelers to protect their clothes from dirt and grime in the latter half of the nineteenth century. They had practically disappeared by the turn of the century only to return with the advent of the open-air automobiles. See "Decline of the Duster," *Bismarck Tribune*, September 7, 1898.
7. "Several Indian Tribes Uneasy," *New York Times*, July 9, 1876.
8. Daniel Kanipe, "The Story of Sergeant Kanipe, One of Custer's Messengers," in W.A. Graham, *The Custer Myth*, 249.
9. Grant Prince Marsh (1834–1916) was the most celebrated Missouri River steamboat captain of his era. His story, including his dramatic dash after the Little Bighorn battle, was described by Joseph Mills Hanson in *The Conquest of the Missouri* (Mechanicsburg, PA: Stackpole, [1909] 2003). Marsh spent seventy years on the great rivers of the country with the greater part on the Great Muddy, or the Missouri River, and its tributaries. He died of pneumonia at St. Alexius Hospital in Bismarck on January 2, 1916, and was buried at St. Mary's Cemetery, Bismarck. He had many adventures and many friends including Mark Twain, "Buffalo Bill" Cody, and Custer. It was recalled in his obituary that the *Far West* was moored at the mouth of the Little Bighorn as the supply boat of the expedition. Marsh had taken her up the Bighorn farther than any other boat and with Porter aboard to take care of the wounded and adjutant Edwin Smith carrying official dispatches and a hundred other messages. He commanded the boat and reached Bismarck in fifty-four hours. See: "Captain Marsh River Pioneer Answers Call," *Bismarck Daily Tribune*, January 4, 1916.
10. Gray, *Centennial Campaign: The Sioux War of 1876*, 279.
11. Frederick Benteen, "A Transcript of Benteen's Narrative," in W.A. Graham, *The Custer Myth*, 181.
12. L.G. Walker, Jr., "Military Medicine at Little Bighorn," *Journal of the American College of Surgeons* 202 no. 1 (2006): 191–6.
13. Gray, *Centennial Campaign: The Sioux War of 1876*, 297.
14. Ibid., 13.
15. William David Nugent, "From Memory's Store," typescript, "copy of, in part and excerpts from the statement of W.G.[sic] Nugents [sic]" May 13, 14, 1933. Re: Battle of the Little Big Horn. Frank Ander's Papers, Box 6, File 43–6-5. Elwin B. Robinson Department of Special Collections, Chester Fritz Library, University of North Dakota, Grand Forks.
16. Fannie Dunn Quain to Mr. Simons, May 15, 1944, SHSND A23/1/1, Bismarck. See Godfrey's article reprinted in W. A. Graham, *The Custer Myth*, 125–149, and in Paul A. Hutton, ed., *The Custer Reader* (Lincoln: University of Nebraska Press, 1992), 257–318.

Chapter 7

1. Wilmot P. Sanford, "The Fort Buford Diary of Private Sanford, 1876–1877," Michael Hill and Ben Innis eds., *North Dakota History* 52, no. 3 (1985): 16–7.
2. Roy P. Johnson, "Jacob Horner of the 7th Cavalry," *North Dakota History* 16, no. 2 (1949): 83.
3. Ibid.
4. Fifteen water carriers were awarded the Medal of Honor. Madden was not. According to Lieutenant Luther Hare in a 1910 interview, "Madden was an intemperate fellow whom no one had much respect for, and when he volunteered to go for water everyone was much surprised." See Walter M. Camp, *Custer in 76: Walter Camp's Notes on the Custer Fight* (Norman: University of Oklahoma Press, (1976) 1990, 67–8. He was given a promotion to sergeant on the field for gallantry by Lieutenant Edward S. Godfrey. See Edward S. Godfrey, "Custer's Last Battle," Paul Andrew Hutton ed., *The Custer Reader*, 309.
5. Typescript of letter from H.R. Porter to Dr. and Mrs. Norton Porter, July 4, 1876, from Porter Family Papers. Also, letter published in Patrick S. McGreevy, "Surgeons at the Little Big Horn," *Surgery, Gynecology, and Obstetrics* 140, (May 1975): 777–8.
6. "Who Broke the News," *Bismarck Tribune*, January 3, 1896.
7. Dr. Isaiah Ashton boarded the *Far West* at the Powder River Depot on July 4 to assist in the care of the wounded for the rest of the trip. See John S. Gray, *Centennial Campaign*, 282.
8. U.S. War Department. *Fort Abraham Lincoln Medical History, 1872–1891.* Roll # 4283, SHSND.
9. Nichols, *Men with Custer*, 19.
10. Ibid., 63.
11. Ibid., 202.
12. Ibid., 33.
13. Steven Solomon, e-mail message to author, September 6, 2003.

14. Photocopy of telegram, Porter Family Papers.
15. George H. Fairchild to Helen Fairchild, Bismarck, July 6, 1876. George H. Fairchild Papers, SHSND Box A227/1/1.
16. W. A. Graham, *The Custer Myth* (Harrisburg, PA: Stackpole Books, 1953), 280–1. G.W. Flannery lived in Bismarck from May 1874 until June 1887 when he moved to St. Paul as president of the Northwestern Trust Company.
17. Ibid.
18. Orlando H. Moore, "The Skirmish at Powder River," August 2, 1876, in Jerome A. Greene, compiler, editor, and annotator, *Battles and Skirmishes of the Great Sioux War 1876–1877, The Military View* (Norman: University of Oklahoma Press, 1993), 92–5.
19. John S. Gray, *Centennial Campaign: The Sioux War of 1876*, 210–1.
20. H.R. Porter Papers, Surgeon General of the Army, Entry 561, RG 94, National Archives.

Chapter 8

1. "Talks with Transients," August 16, 1891, St. Paul. Clipping, Dr. H.R. Porter's Scrapbook.
2. Ronald H. Nichols, *Men with Custer*, 87–8.
3. Ibid., 382.
4. "In Reno's Defense," *Bismarck Daily Tribune*, January 17, 1888.
5. Nichols, *Men with Custer*, 87–8.
6. W. A. Graham, *The Custer Myth*, 125–49.
7. *Bismarck Tri-weekly Tribune*, January 31, 1878
8. "Whitaker's Custer," *Bismarck Weekly Tribune*, February 7, 1877.
9. Ernest Haycox, *Bugles in the Afternoon* (New York: Bantam, [1944] 1946), 338–57; also, Dee Brown, *Showdown at Little Big Horn* (Lincoln: University of Nebraska Press, [1964] 2004).
10. Nichols, ed., *Men with Custer*, 246–47.
11. "A Complicated Case," *Bismarck Tribune*, November 4, 1878.
12. "The Mystery of Mrs. Noonan," *Bismarck Tribune*, November 11, 1878.
13. "Straight Through the Heart," *Bismarck Tribune*, December 2, 1878.
14. "From out of the Depths of Hell," *Bismarck Tribune*, December 30, 1878.

Chapter 9

1. James Grassick, *North Dakota Medicine Sketches and Abstracts* (Grand Forks: North Dakota Medical Association, 1926), 235.
2. Elwyn B. Robinson, *History of North Dakota* (Lincoln: University of Nebraska Press, 1966), 132.
3. *Bismarck Weekly Tribune*, January 24, 1877.
4. *Bismarck Weekly Tribune*, March 14, 1877.
5. "The Fire," *Bismarck Weekly Tribune*, March 21, 1877.
6. W.A. Falconer, "History of Bismarck Closely Associated with Building of the Railroad," *Bismarck Tribune*, July 25, 1931.
7. Kenneth M. Hammer, *The Westerners Brand Book* 7, no. 3 (1960): 55–8.
8. *Bismarck Semiweekly Tribune*, April 18, 1877.
9. Linda W. Slaughter, "Fortress to Farm, or, Twenty-three Years on the Frontier," *Bismarck Daily Tribune*, March 31, 1894.
10. *Bismarck Tri-Weekly Tribune*, June 20, 1877.
11. "Colonel Sheridan's Report," in W.A. Graham, ed., *The Custer Myth*, 373–5.
12. Paul A. Hutton, *Phil Sheridan and His Army* (Lincoln: University of Nebraska Press, [1985] 1986), 328–9. See "The River," *Bismarck Tri-Weekly Tribune*, July 13, 1877.
13. "River News," *Bismarck Tri-Weekly Tribune*, July 27, 1877.
14. "Another Indian Massacre," *Bismarck Tri-Weekly Tribune*, June 20, 1877.
15. Alvin M. Josephy, Jr., *The Nez Perce Indians and the Opening of the Northwest* (Boston: Houghton Mifflin, [1965] 1997), 517.
16. Custer's remains, if properly identified, were in a pine coffin aboard the *J.G. Fletcher* that returned to Bismarck from Bighorn along with those of ten other officers for a total of eleven, not thirteen as stated in the *Tribune* (unless two were not officers), for shipment first to Fort Abraham Lincoln and then east for burial (*Bismarck Tri-Weekly Tribune*, July 27, 1877). Generals Phil Sheridan and George A. Forsyth were passengers on the *Silver City*, which arrived in Bismarck July 27. The two generals reported that they had visited the Custer Battlefield on July 21, 1877, with seventy soldiers and with Sioux guides who had been in the battle, had examined thoroughly any bodies and bones, and had carefully buried them. See W.A. Graham, *The Custer Myth*, 370–1. Elizabeth Custer was assured by Major Joseph G. Tilford of the 7th Cavalry that the remains shipped east were those of her husband. The Custer remains were stored in a vault in Poughkeepsie, NY, until a funeral and reburial at the United States Military Academy occurred on October 10, 1877. See Thom Hatch, *The Custer Companion*, 232–5, for information on burials. The remains of Captain G.W. Gates, Captain T.W. Custer, Lieutenant J. Calhoun,

Lieutenant D. McIntosh, and Lieutenant A.E. Smith were forwarded to Fort Leavenworth, KS, where they were buried with full military honors on August 4, 1877. See *Bismarck Tri-Weekly Tribune*, August 8, 1877.

17. *Bismarck Tri-Weekly Tribune*, July 27, 1877.

18. "Bismarck's Big Hotel," *Bismarck Tri-Weekly Tribune*, July 2, 1877.

19. Cathy A. Langemo, *Images of America: Bismarck, North Dakota* (Chicago: Arcadia, 2002), 69.

20. *Oberlin (OH) Weekly News*, September 6, 1877.

21. Patricia Ann Hoagland McEwen, *Robert McEwen: Scottish Exile in America 1685 and His Descendants in the Line of His Grandson Gershom McEwen, Junior of Winchester, Connecticut* (Palo Alto, CA: Privately Printed, 1991), 74–86.

22. *Alumni Register: Graduates and Former Students, Teaching and Administration Staff 1833–1960* (Oberlin, OH: Oberlin College, November 1, 1960), 225.

23. Wedding details are furnished by two letters; both are written on the same pages by Samantha Viets and Sarah Viets to Helen V. Fairchild in Bismarck, dated August (sic, September) 6, 1877, and September 7, 1877, Wyman Family Papers, Lucy Wyman, Lancaster, NH.

24. *Bismarck Tri-Weekly Tribune*, September 21, 1877.

25. *Bismarck Tri-Weekly Tribune*, October 15, 1877.

26. *Bismarck Tri-Weekly Tribune*, November 14, 1877.

27. "Out West," *Bismarck Tri-Weekly Tribune*, August 1, 1877.

28. Ibid.

Chapter 10

1. Bob Blaisdell, ed., *Great Speeches by Native Americans* (Mineola, NY: Dover, 2000), 148.

2. Alvin M. Josephy, Jr., *The Nez Perce Indians and the Opening of the Northwest* (Boston: Houghton Mifflin, [1965] 1997), 631.

3. Fred G. Bond, "Flatboating on the Yellowstone, 1877," *North Dakota History* 12, no. 4 (1945): 172–3.

4. "Joseph's Arrival," *Bismarck Tri-Weekly Tribune*, November 21, 1877.

5. Bond, "Flatboating on the Yellowstone, 1877," 201.

6. Ibid.

7. "Gen. Miles," *Bismarck Tri-Weekly Tribune*, November 21, 1877.

8. Luther S. "Yellowstone" Kelly (1849–1928) learned the Sioux language while trapping and hunting along the Yellowstone River and served as chief of scouts for Miles. A native of New York State, he was well educated before going west. He served as agent of the San Carlos Indian Reservation after his scouting days on the Yellowstone. He was buried on Kelly Mountain, Billings, MT. The author was privileged to know his great-nephew, the late Dr. Luther S. Kelly, Charlotte, NC. Dr. Kelly's widow, Susan, and his daughter, Mary Luther Leatherman, still have "Yellowstone's" sword. See http://www.fpcc.net/~sgrimm/yellowstone_kelly.htm. Accessed October 29, 2003.

9. "Joseph's Arrival," *Bismarck Tri-Weekly Tribune*.

10. Ibid.

11. David Lavender, *Let Me Be Free: The Nez Perce Tragedy* (New York: HarperCollins, 1992), 330.

12. "Joseph's Arrival," *Bismarck Tri-Weekly Tribune*.

13. George W. Sweet arrived in what would be Bismarck on May 13 and found that land previously selected for the town site "was [already] held and occupied by other parties." He thus located another site for Bismarck on May 14, 1872, and drew the first plat as attorney for the Puget Sound Land Company. See "Early Days of Bismarck," *Bismarck Tribune*, June 18, 1883. Sweet Avenue in Bismarck is named for him. He died in Fort Benton, MT, in 1898. See "George Sweet Dead," *Bismarck Daily Tribune*, March 19, 1898. Also, "History of Bismarck Closely Associated with Building of Railroad," *Bismarck Tribune*, July 25, 1931.

14. Josephy, *The Nez Perce Indians and the Opening of the Northwest*, 521.

15. "Joseph's Banquet," *Bismarck Tri-Weekly Tribune*, November 23, 1877.

16. Ibid.

17. Ibid.

18. "Banqueting Joseph," *Bismarck Tri-Weekly Tribune*, November 23, 1877.

19. Ibid.

20. "Chief Joseph," *Bismarck Tri-Weekly Tribune*, November 21, 1877.

21. Two accounts make no mention of the banquet in Bismarck for Chief Joseph. See Mark H. Brown, *The Flight of the Nez Perce* (New York: G.P. Putnam's Sons, 1967), and Harvey Chalmers, *The Last Stand of the Nez Perce: Destruction of a People* (New York: Twayne, 1962), 239. The latter notes: "The people of Bismarck received the Wallamwatkins (Non-Christian Nez Perce) with cordiality and kindness. The Indians responded. For a few days everyone was happy. Then came an order from the Secretary of War directing that Joseph

and his people be sent by train to Fort Leavenworth, Kansas."

Chapter 11

1. "Articles of Association," *Bismarck Tri-Weekly Tribune*, November 28, 1877.
2. "The Narrow Gauge Road to the Hills," *Bismarck Tri-Weekly Tribune*, March 5, 1878.
3. "Dissolution of Corporation," *Bismarck Tribune*, April 2, 1880.
4. "Fairchild's House Burned," *Bismarck Tri-Weekly Tribune*, December 18, 1877.
5. H.R. Porter to Surgeon General U.S. Army, January 8, 1878. Entry 561, RG 94, National Archives, Washington, DC.
6. *Bismarck Tri-Weekly Tribune*, February 16, 1878.
7. Ibid.
8. *Bismarck Weekly Tribune*, March 26, 1878.
9. *Bismarck Tri-Weekly Tribune*, January 10, 1878.
10. *Bismarck Tri-Weekly Tribune*, January 25, 1878.
11. *Bismarck Tri-Weekly Tribune*, March 16, 1878.
12. This land is NW 1/4, Section 8, Township 139, range 80, Tax List, Burleigh County, 1881, page 93.
13. "This is Business," *Bismarck Tribune*, November 25, 1878.
14. *Bismarck Tri-Weekly Tribune*, April 6, 1878.
15. "Bismarck to Lake Kampeska," *Bismarck Tri-Weekly Tribune*, March 30, 1878.
16. *Bismarck Weekly Tribune*, August 21, 1878.
17. *Bismarck Tribune*, October 16, 1878.
18. Undated clipping, Dr. H.R. Porter's Scrapbook.
19. Photograph 0264-27, State Archives and Historical Research Library, State Historical Society of North Dakota, Bismarck.
20. Theodore Roosevelt, *Hunting Trips of a Ranchman: Sketches of Sport on the Northern Cattle Plains* (New York: Modern Library [1885] 1998), 15, 112.
21. Ibid.
22. "In the Local Political Pot," *Bismarck Tribune*, October 16, 1878; "Burleigh County Election Returns—Official," *Bismarck Tribune*, November 11, 1878.
23. "The County Ticket," *Bismarck Tribune*, October 15, 1880; "Dakota: Burleigh County," *Bismarck Tribune*, November 5, 1880.
24. "The Business of Bismarck," *Bismarck Tribune*, November 25, 1878.
25. Ibid.

Chapter 12

1. Ronald H. Nichols, *In Custer's Shadow*, 217–9.
2. Ibid., 245–55, 266–87.
3. "Summoned to Chicago," *Bismarck Tribune*, December 30, 1878.
4. Undated clipping, Dr. H.R. Porter's Scrapbook.
5. *Bismarck Tribune*, January 6, 1879.
6. Undated clipping, Dr. H.R. Porter's Scrapbook.
7. Nichols, *In Custer's Shadow*, 274.
8. Ibid.
9. A person facing downstream with the right bank on one's right side determines the bank of a stream.
10. "Reno at the Custer Massacre," *New York Times*, January 24, 1879.
11. "Reno's Run," *Chicago Times*, January 25, 1879.
12. Transcript of *Chicago Times*, January 13–24, 1879, Box 5, File 43-5-40, Frank L. Anders Papers, Elwyn B. Robinson Department of Special Collections, Chester Fritz Library, University of North Dakota, Grand Forks, ND.
13. "News Cobbled from All Over the World," *Bismarck Tribune*, January 27, 1879.
14. W.A. Graham, *The Reno Court of Inquiry: Abstract of the Official Record of Proceedings* (Mechanicsburg, PA: Stackpole Books, [1954] 1995), 266.
15. Brian Pohanka, Introduction to W.A. Graham, *The Reno Court of Inquiry: Abstract of the Official Record of the Proceedings*, xxxiii–xxxiv.
16. "Talks with Transients," Clipping, August 16, 1891, Dr. H.R. Porter's Scrapbook.
17. Frank Anders to R. A. Burnside, October 21, 1951, Box 5, File 43-5-4, Frank Anders Papers.

Chapter 13

1. *Bismarck Tribune*, May 17, 1879.
2. *Bismarck Tribune*, July 19, 1879.
3. *Elyria (OH) Republican*, April 3, 1879. Henry Viets gave Lottie J. Porter parts of lot 35, known as subs 180, 181, Oberlin Village valued at $4,000.
4. George H. Fairchild to Mary Fairchild, March 30, 1879, George H. Fairchild Papers, SHSND 227/1/1.
5. Original Tax List, Personal 1882, Burleigh County, ND. Based on this assessment with the assumed valuation of $60 per share, Asa Fisher held 77 shares; Henry Viets, Lottie's father, 67; Lottie Porter, 43; Helen Viets Fairchild, 40; Dr. Henry R. Porter, 37; Dr. Henry

Norton Porter, 10; Mrs. Henry Norton Porter, 3; George H. Fairchild, 2; Dr. James H. Fairchild, 2; and in addition other members of the Fairchild family held a few shares.

6. "The First National," *Bismarck Tribune*, August 9, 1879.

7. Fannie Dunn Quain, "Shall Bismarck Become of Age?" 1946, Fannie Dunn Quain Papers, SHSND A23/1/2, Bismarck.

8. *Bismarck Daily Tribune*, August 23, 1879.

9. "Early Days in Bismarck," *Bismarck Daily Tribune*, July 26, 1908.

10. "Extension Excursionist," *Bismarck Tribune*, September 5, 1879.

11. *Bismarck Tribune*, September 19, 1879.

12. Sergeant Michael Madden, who underwent amputation of his right leg below the knee by Dr. Porter on June 26, 1876, at Little Big Horn, received a pension of $18 per month beginning August 29, 1876. It was increased to $24 per month in 1883 and to $30 per month in 1886. See Ronald H. Nichols, ed., *Men with Custer*, 202.

13. "Report of the Condition of the First National Bank of Bismarck," *Bismarck Tribune*, January 9, 1880.

14. George H. Fairchild to James H. Fairchild, December 30, 1879. George H. Fairchild Papers, SHSND Box A227/1/1; Two of Porter's cards are in the Fannie Dunn Quain Papers, SHSND A23/1/2, Bismarck. One is inscribed, "H.R. Porter, George H. Fairchild, New Years [sic] Day 1877" in Porter's handwriting; the other engraved, "Dr. H.R. Porter," January 1, 1889, written on the lower left corner.

15. "New Year's Calls," *Bismarck Daily Tribune*, January 6, 1875.

16. "Early Days in Bismarck," *Bismarck Daily Tribune*, July 26, 1908.

17. M.H. Jewell, *Jewell's First Annual Directory of the City of Bismarck* (Bismarck, DT: M.H. Jewell, 1879).

18. George H. Fairchild to James H. Fairchild, April 16, 1880, George H. Fairchild Papers, SHSND A227/1/2.

19. Ibid., January 5, 1881.

20. George H. Fairchild to James H. Fairchild, May 9, 1881, George H. Fairchild Papers, SHSND A227/1/2.

21. "Regular Local Lay," *Bismarck Tribune*, April 2, 1880.

22. Ibid.

23. "Montana and Dakota: Two Territories United by the North Pacific R.R," *Bismarck Tribune*, November 12, 1880.

24. *Bismarck Tribune*, May 27, 1881.

25. George H. Fairchild to Mary Fairchild, May 23, 1881, George H. Fairchild Papers, SHSND A227/1/2.

26. "The Programme," *Bismarck Tribune*, June 24, 1881.

27. "Sitting Bull," *Bismarck Tribune*, August 5, 1881. See Markus H. Lindner, "Family, Politics, and Show Business: The Photographs of Sitting Bull," *North Dakota History* 72, nos. 3 and 4 (2005): 4 for photograph of Sitting Bull by O.S. Goff on July 31, 1881 wearing goggles. Also, in the same article, on page 2, is a photograph of Sitting Bull on the back of a Nicholson and (H.R.) Porter Drugstore business card.

28. "A Pleasant Trip," *Bismarck Tribune*, August 5, 1881.

29. George H. Fairchild to James H. Fairchild, July 20, 1881, George H. Fairchild Papers, SHSND A227/1/2.

30. *Bismarck Daily Tribune*, August 26, 1881.

Chapter 14

1. George H. Fairchild to Mary Fairchild, January 22, 1882, George H. Fairchild Papers, SHSND A227/1/3.

2. "The River," B*ismarck Tribune*, June 2, 1882.

3. "Who Threw Bricks," *Bismarck Tribune*, Undated clipping, Dr. H.R. Porter's Scrapbook. One of the earliest settlers, Henry Suttle, as early as 1869 supplied steamboats with wood from his yard five miles south of Bismarck near Sibley Island. See W.A. Falconer, "History of Bismarck Closely Associated with Building of Railroad," *Bismarck Tribune*, July 25, 1931.

4. "Curious Accident," *Bismarck Tribune*, July 14, 1882.

5. *Bismarck Tribune*, October 27, 1882.

6. H.R. Porter, "Fracture of Clavicle Treated Without Apparatus," *Medical Record* 21, April 8, 1882: 391.

7. Colonel William Thompson, a native of Pennsylvania, served in the 30th and 31st U.S. Congress representing southern Iowa, acted as chief clerk of the House of Representatives in 1861, volunteered in the 18th Iowa Cavalry where he was elected to a captaincy, made colonel of the regiment in the spring of 1864, and joined Custer in the spring of 1865 as a brevet brigadier general of U.S. volunteers. After the Civil War, he was appointed captain in the 7th Cavalry under Custer but resigned from the army in December 1875 to pursue agricultural interests in the Dakota Territory. See "Col. Wm. Thompson," *Bismarck Tri-weekly Tribune*, July 25, 1877. Orlando Scott Goff (1843–1916) served in the Civil War in the 10th Connecticut Infantry, learned photography in Lyons, NY, first worked at Portage, WI, and Yankton before arriving in Bismarck in 1873.

He moved later that year to become post photographer at Fort Abraham Lincoln. He toured the Plains' forts in 1878 and left his studio in Bismarck to be run by David F. Barry. Goff was the first to photograph both Sitting Bull and Chief Joseph after their surrenders. He ran for mayor of Bismarck in the early 1880s and when defeated reportedly said, "God, deliver me from my friends." See Fannie Dunn Quain Papers, SHSND A23/1/2. He later operated studios in Fort Custer, Havre, and Fort Assiniboine, all in Montana, before retiring in 1900. He died in Boise, ID, October 17, 1916, and was buried in Morris Hill Cemetery in that city. Of interest, he was a distant cousin of the poet Hart Crane (1899–1932), whose mother was a Goff. See Gwen Goff Hobbes, "Goffe-Goff-Gough Family From Wethersfield, Connecticut to Manifest Destiny and Beyond-Eighth Generation." *http://freepages.genealogy.roots web.com/~guineve60/goff/pafg19.htm#24735*. Accessed June 2, 2004.

8. "The Dakota Block," *Bismarck Tribune*, November 17, 1882.

9. "The Business Thermometer," *Bismarck Tribune*, June 9, 1882.

10. *Bismarck Tribune*, October 13, 1882.

11. "The Banner City," *Bismarck Tribune*, October 20, 1882.

12. "Real Estate Boomlets," *Bismarck Tribune*, November 17, 1882.

13. "Bismarck's Bridge," *Bismarck Tribune*, January 6, 1882.

14. "First Train over the Missouri," *Bismarck Tribune*, October 20, 1882.

15. George H. Fairchild to Mrs. James H. Fairchild, November 5, 1882, George H. Fairchild Papers, SHSND A227/1/3.

16. George H. Fairchild to James T. Fairchild, December 26, 1882, George H. Fairchild Papers, SHSND A227/1/3.

17. "The First National Bank," *Bismarck Tribune*, December 8, 1882.

18. "Bismarck," *Bismarck Tribune*, January 5, 1883.

19. "Snow Above," *Bismarck Tri-Weekly Tribune*, March 16, 1878.

20. *Bismarck Tri-Weekly Tribune*, March 16, 1878.

21. *Bismarck Tribune*, January 5, 1883.

22. "General Information," *Bismarck Weekly Tribune*, March 2, 1883.

23. "Crop Reports of 1882," *Bismarck Tribune*, March 2, 1883.

24. *Bismarck: The Commercial Centre of Western North Dakota and State Capital* (Bismarck, ND: Cushing, 1906). Institute of Regional Studies, North Dakota State University, Fargo.

25. George H. Fairchild to Helen V. Fairchild, February 11, 1883, Wyman Family Papers, Lucy Wyman, Lancaster, NH.

26. George H. Fairchild to Helen V. Fairchild, February 15, 1883, SHSND A227/1/3.

27. George H. Fairchild to Helen V. Fairchild, March 4, 1883, Ibid.

28. George H. Fairchild to Helen V. Fairchild, undated filed with 1882–83 correspondence, Ibid.

29. George H. Fairchild to Helen V. Fairhild, April 4, 1883, Wyman Family Papers, Lucy Wyman, Lancaster, NH.

30. George H. Fairchild to Helen V. Fairchild, April 29, 1883, SHSND A227/1/3.

31. George H. Fairchild to Helen V. Fairchild, May 2, 1883, Ibid.

32. George H. Fairchild to Helen V. Fairchild, May 11, 1883, Wyman Papers, Lucy Wyman, Lancaster, NH.

33. "Fisher's Addition," *Bismarck Tribune*, May 11, 1883.

34. "A Magnificent Building," *Bismarck Daily Tribune*, September 5, 1883.

35. *Bismarck Daily Tribune*, September 5, 1883.

36. "Sitting Bull's Party," *Bismarck Daily Tribune*, September 5, 1883.

37. Robert M. Utley, *The Lance and the Shield: The Life and Times of Sitting Bull* (New York: Henry Holt, 1993), 261. Sitting Bull, Spotted-Horn-Bull, Gray Eagle, Flying By, Long Dog, and Crow Eagle with some wives performed on the stage in New York City in 1884 as part of the "Sitting Bull Combination." Spotted-Horn-Bull was killed in the melee with Indian police when Sitting Bull died in 1890. See Robert M. Utley, *The Lance and the Shield*, 263, 301.

38. "Bismarck," *Bismarck Daily Tribune*, September 5, 1883.

Chapter 15

1. James Grassick, *North Dakota Medicine: Sketches and Abstracts* (Grand Forks: North Dakota Medical Association, 1926), 234–5.

2. Dr. William A. Bentley served as mayor of Bismarck, adjutant-general on the staff of Governor Andrew H. Burke (1891–93), and was elected to the North Dakota legislature as a Republican. See "Biographical Sketches," *Bismarck Daily Tribune*, January 5, 1893.

3. George H. Fairchild to Mary Fairchild, June 13, 1884, George H. Fairchild Papers, SHSND A227/1/4.

4. George H. Fairchild to James H. Fairchild, April 10, 1884, Ibid.

5. George H. Fairchild to James T. Fairchild, August 18, 1884, Ibid.

6. George H. Fairchild to James H. Fairchild, December 15, 1884, Ibid.
7. George H. Fairchild to James H. Fairchild, July 18, 1885, Ibid.
8. George H. Fairchild to Dr. H.R. Porter, March 2, 1885, Ibid.
9. "The Fairchild Agency," *Bismarck Daily Tribune*, July 4, 1885.
10. *Bismarck Daily Tribune*, August 7, 1885.
11. *Seventy Fifth Anniversary St. Alexius Hospital, Bismarck, N.D., 1885–1960*, Institute of Regional Studies, North Dakota State University, Fargo; Kevin A. Hessinger, "The Development of Health Care Systems in Bismarck, 1872–1937," *North Dakota History* 53, no. 1 (1986): 3–11.
12. "Board of Health," *Bismarck Daily Tribune*, August 23, 1885.
13. "Bound for the Battlefield," *Bismarck Daily Tribune*, June 23, 1886.
14. David Frances Barry (1854–1934) came to Bismarck in 1878 to work as an apprentice to O.S. Goff, photographer, 18 Main Street, later at the Dakota Block on Main Street. He traveled over the Dakota Territory photographing famous Indian chiefs including Sitting Bull, Rain in the Face, Gall, Red Cloud, and Shooting Star, military officers, and important forts and battlefields including Little Bighorn. He later took over the business from Goff and advertised as a photographer and gallery owner with the "finest collection" of Indian photographs in the world. See "D.F. Barry, Photographer," *Bismarck Daily Tribune*, December 5, 1885. He left Bismarck in 1890 for Superior, WI. See "Photographer Barry Will Leave," *Bismarck Daily Tribune*, April 12, 1890. After his death the Denver Public Library purchased the original glass negatives and prints from his collection. See "David F. Barry," http://photoswest.org/exib/barry/barry.htm. Accessed June 2, 2004.
15. Clipping in Dr. H.R. Porter's Scrapbook, dated June 25 (1886), noted in the clipping, "Special to the (St. Paul) *Globe*."
16. W.A. Graham, ed., *The Custer Myth* (Harrisburg, PA: Stackpole Books, 1953), 87–9.
17. Ibid.
18. "Custer's Last Fight," clipping dated June 25 (1896), twentieth anniversary of the battle, Dr. H.R. Porter's Scrapbook.
19. Graham, *The Custer Myth*, 91–2.
20. "Returned from the Battlefield," *Bismarck Daily Tribune*, June 29, 1886.
21. Ibid.
22. "Struck by Lighting," *Bismarck Daily Tribune*, July 9, 1886.
23. "Brilliant Wedding," *Mitchell* (SD) *Daily Republican*, October 31, 1886.
24. "A Catechism," *Dakota Settler*, January 10, 1888, Dr. H.R. Porter's Scrapbook.

25. Kenneth J. Carey, "Alexander McKenzie, Boss of North Dakota" (master's thesis, University of North Dakota, 1949), 2–33.
26. "Moffet vs. Griffin," *Bismarck Daily Tribune*, May 28, 1890.
27. *Bismarck Daily Tribune*, May 31, 1890.
28. William Porter Moffet, "Story of Henry R. Porter," typescript, undated, Dr. H.R. Porter Papers.
29. "Gone Dry," *Bismarck Daily Tribune*, October 4, 1889.
30. *Bismarck Daily Tribune*, October 4, 1889.
31. "Twenty Years Ago," *Bismarck Daily Tribune*, April 17, 1910.
32. George H. Fairchild to James H. Fairchild, December 31, 1887, George H. Fairchild Papers, SHSND A227/1/5.
33. The dried leaf of the purple foxglove used at that time as a "powerful sedative — diminishing the velocity of the pulse, diuretic and sorbefacient." See Robley Dunglison, *Dictionary of Medical Science* (Philadelphia: Lea, 1874), 317.
34. George H. Fairchild to James H. Fairchild, December 31, 1887, SHSND A227/1/5.
35. George H. Fairchild to Mrs. James H. Fairchild, October 28, 1888, George H. Fairchild Papers, Ibid.
36. *Bismarck Daily Tribune*, January 6, 1888.
37. "Social News," *Bismarck Daily Tribune*, August 7, 1888.
38. Lucy Wyman, telephone conversation March 27, 2006.
39. George H. Fairchild to Mary Fairchild, January 2, 1889, George H. Fairchild Papers, SHSND A227/1/5.
40. George H. Fairchild to Mary Fairchild, January 22, 1889, Ibid.
41. George H. Fairchild to James H. Fairchild, March 23, 1889, Ibid.
42. George H. Fairchild to Lucy Fairchild Kenaston, June 22, 1889, SHSND A227/1/5.
43. Edgar Erskine Hume, ed., *The Golden Jubilee of the Association of Military Surgeons of the United States: A history of its first half-century 1891–1941* (Washington, DC: Association of Military Surgeons, 1941), 268–72.
44. George H. Fairchild to Mrs. James H. Fairchild, September 8, 1889, Ibid.

Chapter 16

1. George H. Fairchild to Mary Fairchild, January 7, 1890, George H. Fairchild Papers, SHSND A227/1/5.
2. George H. Fairchild to James H. Fairchild, August 13, 1890, George H. Fairchild Papers, Ibid.

3. "A Good Joke on Dr. Porter," *Bismarck Daily Tribune*, April 20, 1890.
4. *Bismarck Daily Tribune*, June 13, 1890.
5. Clipping, dated June 20 [1890], Dr. H.R. Porter's Scrapbook.
6. Clipping, dated July 19, 1890, Ibid.
7. Clipping, Ibid.
8. Clipping, Ibid.
9. George H. Fairchild to Mary Fairchild, February 14, 1891, George H. Fairchild Papers, SHSND A227/1/5.
10. George H. Fairchild to Mary Fairchild, June 4, 1891, Ibid.
11. "Of Local Interest," *Bismarck Daily Tribune*, October 13, 1891.
12. Pioneer settler in the territory in 1869 who farmed and ran an omnibus route between Fort Abraham Lincoln and Bismarck. See "Returns to Bismarck," *Bismarck Daily Tribune*, April 8, 1910.
13. Ibid.
14. George H. Fairchild to Mary Fairchild, October 20, 1891, George H. Fairchild Papers, SHSND A227/1/5.
15. *Bismarck Daily Tribune*, December 1, 1891.
16. *Bismarck Daily Tribune*, March 1, 1892.
17. Clipping, undated. Dr. H.R. Porter's Scrapbook. The author has determined the date of this clipping to be May 29, 1889, based on an identical report that appeared in the Portland [OR] *Morning Oregonian* on May 30, 1889. The government bought the property for the zoo for $119,914.16 at "a low cost per acre" with funds appropriated by the 51st Congress. See "The National Zoo," *Freeborn County Standard* (Albert Lea, MN), July 29, 1891.
18. George H. Fairchild to Grace Fairchild, May 20, 1892, George H. Fairchild Papers, SHSND A227/1/5.
19. Katherine M. Fairchild Diary, Lucy Wyman, Lancaster, NH.
20. George H. Fairchild to Mary Fairchild, November 9, 1892, Ibid.
21. Dr. H.R. Porter to Helen Davis, July 13, 1892, Porter Family Papers.
22. Clipping, dated October 11, 1892. Dr. H.R. Porter's Scrapbook.
23. Katherine M. Fairchild Diary, Lucy Wyman, Lancaster, NH.

Chapter 17

1. George H. Fairchild to Mary Fairchild, March 13, 1893, George H. Fairchild Papers, SHSND A227/1/5.
2. George H. Fairchild to Mary Fairchild, April 6, 1893, Ibid.
3. George H. Fairchild to Mary Fairchild, April 11, 1893, Ibid.

4. *Bismarck Daily Tribune*, April 14, 1893.
5. David Blackstead et al., eds., *Bismarck 100: Official Publication of Bismarck Centennial Association* (Fargo, ND: Institute of Regional Studies, North Dakota State University, 1972), 27.
6. Katherine M. Fairchild Diary, Lucy Wyman, Lancaster, NH.
7. *Bismarck Daily Tribune*, July 6, 1893.
8. "The Ladies Concert," *Bismarck Daily Tribune*, May 10, 1993.
9. "Lounsberry Lost," *Bismarck Daily Tribune*, June 2, 1893.
10. U.S. Department of State Certificate, dated June 17, 1893. Dr. H.R. Porter's Scrapbook.
11. *Bismarck Daily Tribune*, August 6, 1893.
12. Clipping, undated, "Dr. Porter Abroad," Dr. H.R. Porter's Scrapbook.
13. Clipping, "Delightful Vienna," dated October 9, [1893]. Dr. H.R. Porter's Scrapbook.
14. William M. Pye, early real estate man in Bismarck and official of the Bismarck City Bank. "Bismarck, Dakota Territory," *Bismarck Daily Tribune*, December 22, 1875.
15. Hannafin came from Ireland when he was ten years old, lost his father by death on the crossing, and settled in Buffalo, New York, where he supported his family. After participating in Sherman's march to the sea, he worked with the Union Pacific Railroad, but primarily made a living by gambling. He was a squatter on 80 prime acres of land that would become Bismarck, then opened a saloon. He made a fortune by staking a claim on a vein of coal in 1873. See "Dennis Hannafin, Irishman," *Dakota Datebook*, March 16, 2004, North Dakota Public Radio. http://www.prairiepublic.org/programs/datebook/bydate/04/0304/031604.jsp. Accessed April 17, 2004. Also, see "Thoroughbred Sports," *Bismarck Tribune*, March 11, 1881. This article describes his legendary gambling and concludes, "He 'plays the limit' to win, and scarcely ever fails."
16. At Monte Carlo," *Bismarck Daily Tribune*, November 11, 1893.

Chapter 18

1. "Reorganization of Northern Pacific Railroad Co.," *New York Times*, September 2, 1896.
2. "District Court News," *Bismarck Daily Tribune*, December 12, 1893.
3. "Verdict for Fisher," *Bismarck Daily Tribune*, December 13, 1893.
4. Katherine M. Fairchild Diary, Lucy Wyman, Lancaster, NH.
5. "Wanted to see Venice Again," *Bismarck Daily Tribune*, November 27, 1893.

6. Dr. Porter is in Rome," *Bismarck Daily Tribune*, December 19, 1893.
7. "He Sees the Pope," *Bismarck Daily Tribune*, January 4, 1894.
8. Mr. H.R. Porter to [Nell] Helen Workman Davis and Sarah Porter Davis, January 1, 1894, Porter Family Papers.
9. Don Gifford with Robert J. Seidman, *Ulysses Annotated: Notes for James Joyce's Ulysses*, 2nd ed. (Berkeley: University of California Press, 1988), 599.
10. James Joyce, *Ulysses* (New York: Vintage, 1986), 598.
11. "Live and See Naples," *Bismarck Daily Tribune*, February 11, 1894.

Chapter 19

1. "Among the Pyramids," *Bismarck Daily Tribune*, February 15, 1894.
2. "Mr. Fairchild Dead," *Bismarck Tribune*, February 9, 1894. Fairchild was buried in Westwood Cemetery in Oberlin, Ohio, in the Fairchild family plot just across the road from Lottie Porter. His wife, Helen Viets Fairchild, was buried in the Fairchild plot in 1923 as were their daughters, Gertrude Viets Fairchild (1869–70) and Katherine Fairchild Leslie (1881–1959).
3. H.R. Porter to Helen Workman Davis and Sarah Porter Davis, February 12, 1894, Porter Family Papers.
4. *Bismarck Daily Tribune*, March 24, 1894.
5. "On the Upper Nile," *Bismarck Daily Tribune*, March 19, 1894.

Chapter 20

1. Jaffa, an ancient seaport on the Mediterranean shore, merged with Tel Aviv in 1950.
2. Baldwin Locomotive Works of Philadelphia was founded in 1831 and built locomotives for the Pennsylvania Railroad, Northern Pacific, the Baltimore and Ohio, the Atchison, Topeka, & Santa Fe, and other railroads in North America and overseas. See John K. Brown, *The Baldwin Locomotive Works, 1831–1915* (Baltimore: Johns Hopkins University Press, 1995), and Fred Westing, *The Locomotives that Baldwin Built* (New York: Bonanza, 1966).
3. "In the Holy Land," *Bismarck Daily Tribune*, April 18, 1894.
4. Clipping, "Letter from Turkey," undated, Dr. H.R. Porter's Scrapbook.
5. The French Messageries Maritimes (M.M.) liner *Senegal* was an iron screw, bark-rigged steamship that was 390 feet long and had a beam of forty feet. It was built at Marseilles in 1872 and served the Mediterranean trade until it was damaged severely by a harbor mine in Smyrna May 22, 1913. See "French Liner Struck Submerged Harbor Mine," *Fort Wayne* (IN) *News*, May 22, 1913.
6. "No Earthquake Yet," *Bismarck Daily Tribune*, May 9, 1894.
7. "Greek Earthquakes," *Middletown* [NY] *Daily Argus*, April 23, 1894.
8. *Bismarck Daily Tribune*, May 13, 1894.
9. Clipping, "Among the Grandees," undated, Dr. H.R. Porter's Scrapbook.

Chapter 21

1. "A Washington Letter," *Bismarck Daily Tribune*, June 2, 1894.
2. Ibid.
3. Katherine M. Fairchild Diary, Lucy Wyman, Lancaster, New Hampshire.
4. "C.B. Little House — New Home for SBAND," *The Gavel*, January 2005, 12–15
5. Clipping, dated in Porter's hand "Sept. 17, '95." Dr. H.R. Porter's Scrapbook.
6. "Sioux and Arab," *Washburn* (ND) *Leader*, Dr. H.R. Porter's Scrapbook. Joseph Henry Taylor, author of *Sketches of Frontier and Indian Life on the Upper Missouri and Great Plains* (1889), was editor of the paper as well as being a hunter and trapper of renown.
7. Bigelow Neal, "Tomcat Burial Was Big Boyhood Event Half Century Ago," *Bismarck Tribune*, Golden Jubilee Edition, August 15, 1939.
8. *Bismarck Daily Tribune*, January 29, 1896.
9. *Bismarck Daily Tribune*, March 5, 1896.
10. Robley Dunglison, *Dictionary of Medical Science*, 2nd ed. (Philadelphia: Lea, 1868), 208.
11. "The Very Worst," *Bismarck Daily Tribune*, November 28, 1896.
12. Dr. H.R. Porter to Helen W. Davis, December 16, 1896, Porter Family Papers.
13. Clipping, untitled, dated October 31, 1897, Dr. H.R. Porter's Scrapbook.
14. *Compendium of History and Biography of North Dakota* (Chicago: Ogle, 1900), 164.
15. Clipping, undated, "Should Ministers Pay Doctors?" *Medical Record*, Dr. H.R. Porter's Scrapbook.
16. Martin N. Johnson to Dr. H.R. Porter, March 15, 1898, Dr. H.R. Porter's Scrapbook. Also see John Adelson Porter (secretary to the president) to Martin N. Johnson, March 17, 1898, Dr. H.R. Porter's Scrapbook.
17. Clipping, "He Comes of Fighting Stock," March 19 [1898], Dr. H.R. Porter's Scrapbook.

18. *Bismarck Daily Tribune*, March 21, 1898.
19. Robert M. Utley, *The Lance and the Shield: The Life and Times of Sitting Bull* (New York: Henry Holt, 1993), 162.
20. "Portrait of Sitting Bull," *Bismarck Daily Tribune*, January 20, 1898.
21. Katherine M. Fairchild Diary.
22. "Some of the Losses," *Bismarck Daily Tribune*, August 10, 1898.
23. "The Big Fire at Bismarck," *New York Times*, August 10, 1898.
24. Frank Vyzralek, "Capital crimes and criminals executed in Northern Dakota Territory and North Dakota, 1885–1905," *North Dakota Supreme Court News* http//www.court.state.nd/court/news/executed.htm. Accessed October 3, 2003.
25. *Bismarck Daily Tribune*, March 24, 1899.
26. Clipping, undated, Dr. H.R. Porter's Scrapbook.
27. *Bismarck Daily Tribune*, September 26, 1899.
28. *Bismarck Daily Tribune*, October 14, 1899.
29. *Compendium of History and Biography of North Dakota* (Chicago: Ogle, 1900), 164.
30. See Appendix A.
31. Dr. H.R. Porter's Scrapbook.
32. Ibid.
33. Paul W. Freise, *The Story of Quain and Ramstad Clinic* (Bismarck: Tribune, 1972), 9–10.
34. Clipping, dated December 1900, Dr. H.R. Porter's Scrapbook.

Chapter 22

1. Clipping, February 2, 1901, Dr. H.R. Porter's Scrapbook.
2. "The City," *Bismarck Daily Tribune*, March 14, 1901.
3. Clipping, Dr. H.R. Porter's Scrapbook.
4. *Bismarck Daily Tribune*, April 13, 1901.
5. Katherine M. Fairchild Diary, Lucy Wyman, Lancaster, New Hampshire.
6. Lucy Wyman, Personal Interview, May 10, 2006, Lancaster, New Hampshire.
7. *Bismarck Daily Tribune*, September 9, 1901; also, "The History of St. John's Northwestern Military Academy — St. John's Military Academy." http://studentweb.uwstout.edu/kollerm/Templates/SJMA_history.html. Accessed August 8, 2005.
8. Katherine M. Fairchild Diary, Lucy Wyman, Lancaster, New Hampshire.
9. *Bismarck Daily Tribune*, August 7, 1902.
10. "Building Proposals Asked," *Bismarck Daily Tribune*, February 28, 1902.
11. *Bismarck Daily Tribune*, May 2, 1902.

12. William Porter Moffet, "Story of Henry R. Porter, M.D.," Typescript, undated. Library, State Historical Society of North Dakota.
13. John J. Jackman, who was with the original survey party of the Northern Pacific Railroad, learned of the point where the railroad would cross the Missouri River, resigned his job, and with Major William Woods, Colonel J.H. Richards, E.N. Corey, and George Sanborn left Fargo during the night of March 24–25, 1872, to pre-empt the land ahead of the company's agents and arrived a few hours ahead of Colonel Sweet's party. This forced the railroad to take land back from the riverfront. See "Early Days of Bismarck," *Bismarck Tribune*, June 8, 1883; also see H.E. Stevens, "Jamestown to Bismarck in 1872," *Bismarck Daily Tribune*, July 28, 1910. In 1875 Jackman was one of two U.S. court commissioners in Bismarck. "Bismarck, Dakota Territory," *Bismarck Daily Tribune*, December 22, 1875.
14. William Thomas Fee to Judge John Bowen, January 21, 1904, Wyman Family Papers.
15. *Bismarck Daily Tribune*, March 9, 1903.
16. "Letter from Calcutta," *Bismarck Daily Tribune*, March 18, 1903.
17. "What Time is It?" *Bismarck Daily Tribune*, April 1, 1903, also, "Dr. Porter's Death Recalled," *Bismarck Daily Tribune*, August 20, 1903.
18. John M. Carroll, "Surgeon Henry R. Porter," *Newsletter, Little Big Horn Associates* 23:4 (August) 1989.
19. "Death of Dr. H.R. Porter," *Bismarck Daily Tribune*, March 5, 1903.
20. "Remains are Interred," *Bismarck Daily Tribune*, March 9, 1903.
21. William Thomas Fee to John Bowen, January 21, 1904, Wyman Family Papers.
22. Editorial, "Death of Dr. Porter," *Bismarck Daily Tribune*, March 5, 1903.
23. Copy of H.R. Porter Will of July 15, 1902, Porter Family Papers.
24. Copy of Appeal, F.H. Register and H.F. Douglas[s] vs. H.V. Porter, Dated January 27, 1906, Porter Family Papers.
25. "Hal Porter in Paris," *Bismarck Daily Tribune*, January 29, 1908.
26. Porter, H.V., to Helen W. Davis, February 12, 1908, Porter Family Papers.
27. "A Good Sale," *Bismarck Daily Tribune*, October 4, 1910.
28. "Pioneer Doctor's Son Visits Capital City," *Bismarck Daily Tribune*, June 8, 1916.
29. His tombstone is inscribed: Henry Viets Porter, Born May 23, 1881, Bismarck, North Dakota [sic, Dakota Territory], Died June 30, 1968, Mansfield, Conn., Son of Henry Renaldo [sic] Porter and Charlotte Viets Porter.

Chapter 23

1. Ted Quanrud, "Forgotten Hero of Little Big Horn," *Bismarck Tribune*, April 6, 1986.
2. "Leaves From the Early History of Burleigh County," *Bismarck Daily Tribune*, February 3, 1912.
3. Ronald H. Nichols, ed., *Men with Custer*, 396.
4. Henry R. Porter to Dr. and Mrs. Henry Norton Porter, November 25, 1870, Porter Family Papers.
5. "Death of Dr. Porter," *Bismarck Daily Tribune*, March 5, 1903.
6. Henry R. Porter to Henry Norton Porter, November 16, 1870, Porter Family Papers.
7. David Lavender, *Let Me Be Free: The Nez Perce Tragedy* (New York: HarperCollins, 1992), 330.
8. "Joseph's Arrival," *Bismarck Tri-weekly Tribune*, November 21, 1877.

Epilogue

1. Winston Churchill, *Savrola: A Tale of the Revolution in Laurania* (London and Bombay: Longmans, Green, 1900), 43.

Bibliography

Alumni Register: Graduates and Former Students, Teaching and Administrative Staff 1833–1960. Oberlin, OH: Oberlin College, 1960.

Anders, Frank L. Papers. Elwyn B. Robinson Department of Special Collections, Chester Fritz Library, University of North Dakota, Grand Forks, ND.

Atlas of Oneida County, New York. Philadelphia: Beers, 1874. Reprint. Churchville, NY: Wehle, 1974.

Babcock, William A. "Historical Resource Survey, Glendive, Montana." Prepared for the Glendive Chamber of Commerce and Agriculture, Glendive, MT, 1987.

Bangor (Maine) *Daily Whig and Courier.*

Barnard, Sandy. *I Go with Custer: The Life and Death of Reporter Mark Kellogg.* Bismarck, ND: Bismarck Tribune, 1996.

Bismarck Commercial Club. *Bismarck: The Commercial Centre of Western North Dakota and State Capital.* Bismarck, ND: Cushing, 1906.

Bismarck Directory, 1908. Fargo, ND: Northwestern Directory, 1908.

Bismarck Tribune.

Blackstead, David, Richard Palmer, Pat de Forest, Robert L.H. Stukenbruck, Tom Baker, and Harold Derrick. *Bismarck 100: Official Publication of Bismarck Centennial Association.* Bismarck, ND: Bismarck Centennial Association, 1972.

Blaisdell, Bob, ed. *Great Speeches by Native Americans.* Mineola, NY: Dover, 2000.

Boatner, Mark M. III. *The Civil War Dictionary.* New York: McKay, 1959.

Bond, Fred G. "Flatboating on the Yellowstone, 1877." *North Dakota History* 12, No. 4 (1945).

Bordin, Ruth. *The University of Michigan: A Pictorial History.* Ann Arbor: University of Michigan Press, 1967.

Bourke, John G. *On the Border with Crook.* Reprint, New York: Time-Life, (1891) 1980.

Brandt, Nat. *The Town that Started the Civil War.* Syracuse, NY: Syracuse University Press, 1990.

"Brave Doctor." *Big Horn-Yellowstone Journal* 2, No. 4 (1993).

Brininstool, E.A. *Troopers with Custer: Historic Incidents at the Battle of Little Big Horn.* Mechanicsburg, PA: Stackpole Books, (1952) 1994.

Brown, Dee. *Showdown at Little Big Horn.* Lincoln: University of Nebraska Press, (1964) 2004.

Brown, John K. *The Baldwin Locomotive Works, 1831–1915: A Study of American Industrial Practice.* Baltimore: Johns Hopkins University Press, 1995.

Brown, Mark H. *The Flight of the Nez Perce.* New York: Putnam, 1967.

"The Buffalo Soldiers." *http://ushist.com/buffalo-soldiers.htm.*

Bulfinch, Thomas. *Bulfinch's Mythology.* New York: Modern Library, (1855) 1998.

Burleigh County, Original Tax List, Personal Taxes, 1882.

Burlington (IA) Hawk-Eye.

Camp, Walter M. *Custer in '76: Walter Camp's Notes on the Custer Fight.* Edited by Kenneth Hammer. Norman: University of Oklahoma Press, (1976) 1990.

Carey, Kenneth J. "Alexander McKenzie."

Master's thesis, University of North Dakota, 1949.

Carley, Kenneth. *The Dakota War of 1862: Minnesota's Other Civil War*. 2nd ed. St. Paul: Minnesota Historical Society Press (1976), 2000.

Carroll, John M. "Surgeon Henry R. Porter." *Newsletter, Little Big Horn Associates* 23, No. 4 (August 1989).

Cella, Mathew, and Jon Ward. "Columbia Hospital to Close." *Washington Times*, May 8, 2002. http://www.washtimes.com/metro/20020508.html (accessed November 20, 2002).

Chalmers, Harvey. *The Last Stand of the Nez Perce: Destruction of a People*. New York: Twayne, 1962.

Chicago Times.

Child, Hamilton. *Gazetteer and Business Directory of Oneida County for 1869*. Syracuse, NY: Printed at the Journal Office, 1869.

Chorne, Laudie J. *Following the Custer Trail of 1876*. Rev. ed. Bismarck: Trails West, 2001.

Churchill, Winston. *Savrola: A Tale of the Revolution in Laurania*. London, Bombay: Longmans, Green, 1900.

Cochran, Thomas C. *Railroad Leaders, 1845–1890: The Business Mind in Action*. New York: Russell and Russell, 1953.

Cody, William F. *The Life of Hon. William F. Cody Known as Buffalo Bill: An Autobiography*. Lincoln: University of Nebraska Press, (1879) 1978.

Compendium of History and Biography of North Dakota: Containing a History of North Dakota. Chicago: Ogle, 1900.

Cookinham, Harry J. *History of Oneida County, New York: from 1700 to the Present Time*. Vol. 1. Chicago: Clarke, 1912.

Crook, George. *General Crook, His Autobiography*. Edited and annotated by Martin F. Schmitt. Norman: University of Oklahoma Press, 1946.

Dakota Settler.

"Dennis Hannafin, Irishman." Dakota Datebook. March 16, 2004, North Dakota Public Radio. http://www.prairiepublic.org/programs/datebook/bydate/04/0304/031604.jsp.

"Descendents of Simon DeWolf." http://guweb2gonzaga.edu/~dewolf/perry/chapter2.htm and "The DeWolf Family of Bristol, Rhode Island — Part I, http://rhodeisland-philatelic.com/rhodeisland/stampless66.htm.

DeWolf, James W. "The Diary and Letters of Dr. James W. DeWolf." Edward S. Luce, ed. *North Dakota History* 25, Nos. 2 and 3 (1958).

Dictionary of American Medical Biography. Edited by Martin Kaufman, Stuart Galishoff, Todd L. Savitt, and Joseph Carvalho III, editorial associate. 2 vols. Westport, CT: Greenwood Press, 1984.

Dorland, W.A.N. *The American Illustrated Medical Dictionary*, 22nd ed. Philadelphia: Saunders, 1951.

"Doctor H.R. Porter, Thrilling Incidents in the Life of a Bismarck Physician, A Remarkable Steamboat Ride." *Plains Talk* 3, no. 4, new series, 1972.

Dunglison, Robley. *Medical Lexicon: A Dictionary of Medical Science*. 2nd ed. Philadelphia: Lea, 1868.

_____. *Medical Lexicon: A Dictionary of Medical Science*. Rev. ed. Philadelphia: Lea, 1874.

Durant, Samuel W. *History of Oneida County, New York: Illustrations and Biographical Sketches of Some of its Prominent Men*. Philadelphia: Everts and Fariss, 1878.

Eliot, Johnson, Herbert Boardman, and R.D. DeL. French. *Addresses Delivered to the Twenty-third Annual Commencement of the Medical Department of Georgetown College*. Washington, DC: Tomlinson, 1872.

Elyria (OH) *Republican*.

Fairchild, George H. Papers. State Historical Society of North Dakota, Bismarck, ND.

Fairchild. Katherine M. [Frost] [Leslie] Diary. Lucy Wyman, Lancaster, NH.

Fargo (ND) *Record*.

First Presbyterian Church, Bismarck, ND. MSS Collection 1873–1900, 1957. MSS 20490. State Historical Society of North Dakota.

Fletcher, Robert S. *A History of Oberlin College from Its Foundation Through the*

Civil War. 2 vols. Oberlin, NY: Oberlin College, 1943.

"Fort Buford State Historic Site, North Dakota." http://www.ourheritage.net/index_page_stuff/Following_Trails/Chief_Joseph/11_Nov77/1.

Fort Wayne (IN) *News.*

Forsyth, James W., and Frederick D. Grant. *Report of an Expedition Up the Yellowstone River, Made in 1875.* Washington, DC: Government Printing Office, 1875.

Fox, Richard A. Jr. *Archaeology, History, and Custer's Last Battle: The Little Big Horn Reexamined.* Norman: University of Oklahoma Press, 1993.

Freeborn County (Albert Lea, MN) *Standard.*

Freise, Paul W. *The Story of the Quain and Ramstad Clinic, Bismarck, North Dakota, 1900–1972.* Bismarck, ND: Bismarck Tribune, 1972.

The Gavel. (Bismarck, ND) January 2005, 14–5.

Georgetown College. *Catalogue of the Officers and Students of Georgetown College, District of Columbia for the Academic Year, 1871–72.* Baltimore: Murphy, 1872.

Gifford, Don, with Robert J. Seidman. *Ulysses Annotated: Notes for James Joyce's Ulysses.* 2nd ed., rev. and expanded. Berkeley: University of California Press, 1988.

Gillett, Mary C. *The Army Medical Department, 1865–1917.* Washington, DC: Government Printing Office, 1995.

Godfrey, Edward S. "Custer's Last Battle." In *The Custer Reader,* Paul Andrew Hutton ed., Lincoln: University of Nebraska Press, 1992.

Graham, W.A. *The Custer Myth: A Source Book of Custeriana.* Harrisburg, PA: Stackpole Books, 1953.

_____. *The Reno Court of Inquiry: Abstract of the Official Record of Proceedings.* Mechanicsburg, PA: Stackpole Books, (1954) 1995.

Grassick, James. *North Dakota Medicine Sketches and Abstracts.* Grand Forks: North Dakota Medical Association, 1926.

Gray, John S. "Medical Service on the Little Big Horn Campaign." *Westerners Brand Book* 24, no. 11 (Los Angeles Westerners: Los Angeles, 1968).

Gray, John S. *Centennial Campaign: The Sioux War of 1876.* Norman: University of Oklahoma Press, (1976) 1988.

Greene, Jerome A., ed. *Battles and Skirmishes of the Great Sioux War, 1876–1877: The Military View.* Norman: University of Oklahoma Press, 1993.

Hammer, Kenneth. "Frontier Doctor." *The Westerner's Brand Book* 7, No. 3, *New York Posse* (The Westerners, New York: 1960).

Hanson, Joseph Mills. *The Conquest of the Missouri: The Story of the Life and Exploits of Captain Grant Marsh.* Mechanicsburg, PA: Stackpole Books, (1909) 2003.

Hardorff, Richard G. *Hokahey! A Good Day to Die: The Indian Casualties of the Custer Fight.* Lincoln: University of Nebraska Press, (1993) 1999.

Haycox, Ernest. *Bugles in the Afternoon.* New York: Bantam, (1944) 1946.

Hedren, Paul L., ed. *The Great Sioux War 1876–77: The Best from Montana, the Magazine of Western History.* Helena: Montana Historical Society Press, 1991.

Helena (MT) *Independent.*

Hessinger, Kevin A. "The Development of Health Care Systems in Bismarck, 1872–1937." *North Dakota History* 53, no. 1 (1986).

Hillsdale (MI) *Standard.*

Hobbs, Gwen Goff. "Goffe-Goff-Gough Family From Wethersfield, Connecticut to Manifest Destiny and Beyond-Eighth Generation." http://freepages.genealogy.rootsworld.com/~guineve60/goff/pafg19.htm#24735.

Hume, Edgar E., ed. *The Golden Jubilee of the Association of Military Surgeons of the United States: A History of its First Half Century 1891–1941.* Washington, DC: Association of Military Surgeons, 1941.

Hutton, Paul A. *Phil Sheridan and His Army.* Lincoln: University of Nebraska Press, (1985) 1986.

_____, ed. *The Custer Reader.* Lincoln: University of Nebraska Press, 1992.

Hyde, C.W.G., and William Stoddard, eds. *History of the Great Northwest and its Men of Progress*. Minneapolis: Minneapolis Journal, 1901.

"Immigrants to Canada, The Voyage over on a Ship of the Allan Line." *http://ist.uwaterloo.ca/~marj/genealogy/allan.html*.

Indiana (PA) Democrat.

Innis, Ben. "Bottoms Up! The Smith and Leighton Store Ledger of 1876." *North Dakota History* 51, no. 3 (1984).

"James P. Corry and Company." *http://fp.redduster.f9.co.uk/corry.htm*.

Jewell, Marshall H. *Jewell's First Annual Directory of the City of Bismarck, Dakota*. Bismarck, D.T.: Jewell, 1879.

Johnson, Roy P. "Jacob Horner of the 7th Cavalry." *North Dakota History* 16, no. 2 (1949).

Jones, Pomroy. *Annals and Recollections of Oneida County*. Rome, NY: Self-published, 1851.

Josephy, Alvin M. *The Nez Perce Indians and the Opening of the Northwest*. Boston: Houghton Mifflin, (1965) 1997.

Joyce, James. *Ulysses*. New York: Vintage, 1986.

Keen, William W., and J. William White, eds. *An American Text-book of Surgery*. Philadelphia: W.B. Saunders, 1900.

King, Charles R. "James L. Neame at Fort Berthold, Dakota Territory, 1875–1885." *North Dakota History* 58, no. 4 (1991).

Knox, John Jay, Bradford Rhodes and Elmer Youngman. *A History of Banking in the United States*. New York: Rhodes, 1900.

Langemo, Cathy A. *Images of America: Bismarck, North Dakota*. Chicago: Arcadia, 2002.

Lavender, David S. *Let Me Be Free: The Nez Perce Tragedy*. New York: HarperCollins, 1992.

Lord, George E. Papers, Surgeon General of the Army, RG94, National Archives.

Lindner, Markus H. "Family, Politics, and Show Business: The Photographs of Sitting Bull." North Dakota History 72, nos. 3 and 4, (2005).

Map of Lee Center, NY, 1858. Oneida County Historical Society, Utica, NY.

Marion (OH) *Daily Star*.

Mathews, Mitford M., ed. *Dictionary of Americanisms on Historical Principles*. 2 vols. Chicago: University of Chicago Press, 1951.

McEwen, Patricia Ann Hoagland. *Robert McEwen: Scottish Exile in America 1685 and his Descendants in the Line of Grandson Gershom McEwen, Junior of Winchester, Connecticut*. Palo Alto, CA: Privately Printed, 1991.

McGreevy, Patrick S. "Surgeons of Little Big Horn." *Surgery, Gynecology, and Obstetrics* 140, No. 5 (1975).

Medical Fortnightly, August 1896.

Michno, Gregory F. *Lakota Noon: The Indian Narrative of Custer's Defeat*. Missoula, MT: Mountain Press Publishing Company, 1997.

Middletown (NY) *Daily Argus*.

Mitchell (SD) *Daily Republican*.

Moffet, William Porter. "Story of Henry R. Porter." Typescript, undated, 7 pages, State Historical Society of North Dakota, Bismarck, ND.

Monaghan, Jay. *Custer: The Life of General George Armstrong Custer*. Lincoln: University of Nebraska Press, (1959) 1971.

Morris, Edmund. *The Rise of Theodore Roosevelt*. New York: Coward, McCann & Geoghagen, 1979.

"Moses Gunn, Corydon Ford and the Clandestine Cargoes." *Michigan Today*. *Http://www.umich.edu/~newsinfo/MT/99/Fa199/mtlf99c.html*.

Murphy, Edward C. "The Northern Pacific Railway Bridge at Bismarck." *North Dakota History* 62, no. 2 (1995): 2–19.

New York Herald.

New York Times.

Nichols, Ronald H. *In Custer's Shadow: Major Marcus Reno*. Norman: University of Oklahoma Press, (1999) 2000.

____, ed. *Men with Custer*. Hardin, MT: Custer Battlefield Historical and Museum Association, 2000.

North Dakota History: Journal of the Northern Plains.

Norway-Heritage: Hands Across the Sea, "The Anchor Line and Allan Line Agents, 1870 newspaper campaign."

(100 years of Emigrant Ships from Norway), http://www.norwayheritage.com/ships/allan-anker.htm.

Nugent, William David. "From Memory's Store." Typescript, May 13–14, 1933. Frank Anders Papers. Grand Forks, ND.

Oberlin (OH) *Weekly News*.

Olch, Peter D. "Medicine in the Indian-Fighting Army, 1866–1890." *Journal of the West* 21, no. 3 (1982).

Panther Primitives. "Catalogue of Panther Primitives." http://www.pantherprimatives.com/pdf/67.pdf.

Peckham, Howard H. *The Making of the University of Michigan*. Ann Arbor: University of Michigan Press, 1967.

Petersen, Edward S. "Surgeons of the Little Big Horn." *The Westerners Brand Book* 31, no. 6 (Los Angeles Westerners: Los Angeles, 1974).

Porter Family Papers.

Porter, Henry R. "Fracture of Clavicle Treated Without Apparatus," *Medical Record* 21, (1882).

———. "A Soldier with Crook, the Letters of Henry R. Porter." Gene Gressley ed. *Montana, the Magazine of Western History* 8, No. 3 (1958): 33–47.

Porter, Dr. Henry R. Papers. State Historical Society of North Dakota, Bismarck.

Porter, Henry R. Papers, Surgeon General of the Army, Entry 561, RG94, National Archives.

Porter, Dr. Henry R. Scrapbook. State Historical Society of North Dakota, Bismarck.

Porter, Joseph W. *A Genealogy of the Descendants of Richard Porter who settled at Weymouth, Massachusetts 1635*. Bangor: Barr & Robinson, 1898.

Portland [OR] *Morning Oregonian*.

Prohaska, Brian. "Introduction" to W.A. Graham, *The Reno Court of Inquiry: Abstract of the Official Record of the Proceedings*. Mechanicsburg, PA: Stackpole Books, (1954) 1995.

Quain, Fannie Dunn. Papers. State Historical Society of North Dakota, Bismarck, ND.

Rankin, Charles E., ed. *Legacy: New Perspectives on the Battle of Little Bighorn*. Helena: Montana Historical Society Press, 1996.

Reno, Ottie W. *Reno and Apsaalooka Survive Custer*. New York: Cornwall, 1997.

Robinson, Charles M. III. *General Crook and the Western Frontier*. Norman: University Of Oklahoma Press, 2001.

Robinson, Elwyn B., *History of North Dakota*. Lincoln: University of Nebraska Press, 1966.

Roosevelt, Theodore. *Hunting Trips of a Ranchman: Sketches of Sport on the Northern Cattle Plains*. New York: Modern Library, (1885) 1998.

St. Joseph (MI) *Herald*.

Sanford, Wilmot P. "The Fort Buford Diary of Private Sanford, 1876–1877." Michael Hill and Ben Innis, eds. *North Dakota History* 52, no. 3 (1985).

San Francisco Chronicle.

Scott, Douglas D., R.A. Fox, Jr., M.A. Conner, and Dick Harmon. *Archaeological Perspectives on the Battle of Little Big Horn*. Norman: University of Oklahoma Press, 1989.

Scott, Douglas D., P. Willey, and M.A. Conner. *They Died with Custer: Soldier's Bones from the Battle of Little Big Horn*. Norman: University of Oklahoma Press, 1998.

"Seminary Had Its Origin in Old Oneida Institute." Typescript, June 23, 1931. Oneida County Historical Society, Utica, NY.

"Seventy-fifth Anniversary St. Alexius Hospital, Bismarck, North Dakota, 1885–1960," May 6, 1960.

Sides, Hampton. *Blood and Thunder: An Epic of the American West*. New York: Doubleday, 2006.

Sklenar, Larry. *To Hell with Honor: Custer and the Little Big Horn*. Norman: University of Oklahoma Press, 2000.

Slaughter, Linda W. *Linda W. Slaughter's "Fortress to Farm or Twenty-three Years on the Frontier."* Hazel Eastman, ed. New York: Exposition Press, 1972.

S/S Australia. 100 Years of Emigrant Ships from Norway. http://www.norwayheritage.com/p_ship.asp?sh+austl.

Stewart, Edgar I. *Custer's Luck*. Norman: University of Oklahoma, 1955.

Swenson, Fern E., and Walter L. Bailey. "Camp Hancock: Archeological and Historical Perspectives." *North Dakota History* 58, no. 1 (1991).

Taylor, Joseph H. *Sketches of Frontier and Indian Life on the Upper Missouri and Great Plains.* Pottstown, PA: Self-published, 1889.

Taylor, William O. *With Custer on the Little Bighorn: A Newly Discovered First-Person Account.* New York: Viking, 1996.

"Tax Assessments for Town of Lee, 1852 thru 1858, P thru Z." *http://freepages. history.rootsweb.com/~townoflee/misc/a ssessment52–58p.html.*

Tocqueville, Alexis de. *Democracy in America.* Edited and translated by Harvey C. Mansfield and Delba Winthrop. Chicago: University of Chicago Press, 2002.

Traverse City (MI) *Grand Traverse Herald.*

Urbinato, David. "London's Historic 'Pea-Soupers,'" U.S. Environmental Protection Agency, History. *http:// www.epa.gov/history/topics/perspect/ london.htm.*

U.S. Census 1880. *http://www.rootsweb. com/~usgenweb/nd/burleigh/census/ 1880/082–07.gif.*

U.S. War Department. *Camp Hancock and Camp Sykes Post Returns, 1872–1877.*

U.S. War Department. *Fort Abraham Lincoln Medical History, 1872–1891.*

Utica (NY) *Daily Observer.*

Utley, Robert M. *Custer and the Great Controversy.* Pasadena: Westernlore, 1980.

_____. *Cavalier in Buckskin: George Armstrong Custer and the Western Military Frontier.* Norman: University of Oklahoma Press, 1988.

_____. *The Lance and the Shield: The Life and Times of Sitting Bull.* New York: Henry Holt, 1993.

Vaughn, J.W. *With Crook at the Rosebud.* Mechanicsburg, PA: Stackpole Books, (1956) 1994.

"Village of Lee Center." *http://freepages. history.rootsweb.com/~townoflee/Lee Centerer/leecenter.html.*

"Visit Saltcoats." The History of Saltcoats. *http://www.visitsaltcoats.com/ history.html.*

Vyzralek, Frank. "Capital crimes and criminals executed in Northern Dakota Territory and North Dakota, 1885–1905." *North Dakota Supreme Court News.* *http://www.court.state.nd.us/ court/news/executened.htm.*

Walker, L.G. Jr. "Military Medicine at Little Bighorn." *Journal of the American College of Surgeons* 202, no. 1 (2006).

Wengert, James W. "The Contract Surgeon." *Journal of the West* 36, No. 1 (1997).

Westing, Fred. *The Locomotives that Baldwin Built.* New York: Bonanza, 1966.

Weymouth Historical Society. *History of Weymouth Massachusetts.* Boston: Wright and Potter, 1923.

Whitestown Seminary. *Catalogue of the Officers and Students of the Whitestown Seminary at Whitestown, Oneida County, New York for the Year Ending March 1869.* Utica, NY: Roberts, 1869.

"Whitestown Seminary Reunion 1881–1931" Typescript, 1931, Various Records Collected for the Dunham Public Library by a Member of the Class of 1881, Oneida County Historical Society, Utica, NY.

Winks, Robin W. *Frederick Billings: A Life.* New York: Oxford University Press, 1991.

Wyman Family Papers, Lucy Wyman, Lancaster, NH.

"Yellowstone Kelly." *http://www.fpcc.net/ ~sgrimm/yellowstonekelly.htm.*

Young, Clyde L. *85 Years: The First Presbyterian Church, Bismarck 1873–1958.* Bismarck, ND: Bismarck Tribune, 1958.

Index

Abington, MA 4
Adams, Mary 63–64
Agra 175–77, 183
Alabama claims 18, 192n25
Alexandria, Egypt 153
Allan, Alexander, Jr. 10, 12, 14–15
Allan, Alexander, Sr. 10
Allan, Mrs. Alexander, Jr. 14–15
Allan, Robert 14
Allan Line 10, 12
American Fur Company 46
American Heritage Center 193n29
Anchor Line 10–11, 14
Anders, Frank 104
Ann Arbor 8–9
Antwerp 136
Apache Indians 20, 22–23, 25–28
Arizona Territory 1, 20, 24–26, 29, 32, 181
Army Medical Corps 98
Army Medical Museum 19, 63
army pay 194n58
art work: European 137, 160; Vatican 142
Ashland, WI 128, 134–35, 162
Ashton, Isaiah 47, 63, 197n7
Asiatic cholera 110
Association of Acting Assistant Surgeons, U.S. Army 127
Aswan 149, 150
Athens 157–59
Auburn Theological Seminary 6
Austen, Jane 80
S.S. *Australia* 10
Ayr 12
Ayrshire 3, 12, 14

Baker, I.P. 92
Baker, Stephen 35
Baldwin Locomotive Works 31, 153–54, 205n2
Bank of Bismarck 32
Barry, David F. 55, 121–22, 203n14
Beale Springs, Arizona Territory 25
Bear Paw, MT 83
Beirut 156

Belfast 15, 17
Belknap, William Worth 44
Bell, Emily 96
Bennett, James C. 63
Benteen, Frederick 2, 47, 54–57, 59, 68–69, 71, 96, 99, 104, 121, 182
Bentley, William A. 76, 86–87, 91, 95, 119, 183, 202n2
Berlin 137
Bethlehem 154
Bigelow, Arizona Territory 95
Bill Williams Mountain 23, 27
Bismarck: beginnings 1, 2, 30–41; churches 114; early days 76–77, 81, 89–90, 94–95, 107, 109, 113–14; fires 76–77, 167; frontier town 29, 39, 115; hotels 81; state capital 127; territorial capital 117–18, 164; weather 107, 115, 165
Bismarck, Prince Otto 30
Bismarck and Lake Kampeska Railroad 93
Bismarck, Fort Lincoln and Black Hills Railroad 91
Bismarck National Bank 92
Bismarck Tribune 32, 38, 40, 42, 49, 66, 72, 74, 76, 79, 81, 88–89, 91, 92, 94, 107–10, 113, 115, 117–18, 121–22, 125, 128–30, 132, 137, 139, 142, 147, 149, 152, 159, 166–68, 173–74, 177, 180
Black Hills 91–92
Bloody Knife 68–70
Bly, E.H. 79
Boardman, Herbert 20
Bogue, H.P. 168
Bond, Fred 85
Boots and Saddles 67
Bouguereau, Adolphe W. 165
Bourke, John G. 24, 49
Bowen, John B. 34, 93, 128–29, 173, 177
Boyd, Eliza (Mrs. Robert Workman) 13
Boyer, Mitch 50
Bozeman Trail 45
Bragg, Justus 108
Braun, Frank 63
British Cantonment Cemetery 176

215

Index

Brockmeyer, Wesley 65
Brown, Dee 73
Brown, Helen Workman (Mrs. John Brown) 11, 14
Brown, John 11, 14
Brown, W.S. 34–35
Bugles in the Afternoon (Haycox) 73
Burleigh County 30, 92, 105, 107, 121, 123, 125, 133, 159, 178
Burns, Robert 12, 14

Cairo 147–52, 178
Calcutta 173–75
Calhoun, James 35, 62, 64, 78
Calhoun, Margaret 35, 63–64
S.S. *Cambria* 192n20
Camp Apache 25
Camp Crittenden 27
Camp Date Creek 25
Camp Grant 25, 27–28
Camp Greeley 32
Camp Hancock 29–30, 32, 38–40, 65, 163, 181
Camp Huston 108
Camp Hualpai 22–23, 25–26
Camp McDowell 24–26
Camp Mt. Graham 27
Camp Verde 24–25
Camp Whipple 25
Capital National Bank of Bismarck 163
Carnahan, John M. 34, 58
Centralia, WA 125
Chamberlain, Joshua 51
Chapman, Arthur 87
Cheyenne Indians 51, 122
Chicago 42, 91, 96–97, 135, 175
Chicago and Northwestern Railroad 93, 114
Chicago Medical School 52
Chicago, Milwaukee, and St. Paul Railroad 114
Chicago Times 96, 99, 101–3
Chicago Tribune 44
Chrysostrom, Father 74
Churchill, Benjamin F. 104
Churchill, Winston 184
Clair, Elihu F. 57
Clark, E.J. 39, 47
Clark, William 43
Clarke, Mr. and Mrs. James W. 128, 135
Clinton Seminary 6
Clymer Committee 44
coccidiodes immitis 193n30
Cochise 27
Cody, Buffalo Bill 135
Coe, H.W. 119
Cole, James W. 168
Collier Publishing Company 165
S.S. *Columbia* 146
Columbia Hospital for Women 20
Columbian Exhibition 135
A Complete Life of Custer (Whittaker) 73
Constantinople 156–58, 178

Cooke, Jay 31
Cooke, William W. 35, 55, 62, 64, 68, 78, 99
Cooney, David 63
Cornish, J. 5
Corry, Sir William 10, 15–56
Crane, Charles H. 29
Crazy Horse 55, 76
Crazy Mountains 45
Crittenden, John J. 64
Crook, George 20, 22–25, 28, 46–47, 49, 51, 55, 163
Crow Eagle 118
Crow Indians 43, 78, 122
Cummington, MA 4
Curley 121–22
Cushman, C.M. 91
Custer, Boston 35, 62, 64
Custer, Elizabeth (Mrs. George A. Custer) 34–35, 63, 67, 73, 127
Custer, George Armstrong: Belknap hearings 44–45; Black Hills Expedition 33–34; Civil War 2, 45; death and burial 78, 198n16; Fort Abraham Lincoln 32, 35, 40, 76–77; Little Bighorn 1, 2, 39, 54–58, 61–62, 64, 67–73, 96–99, 104, 110, 122, 182; Terry-Custer column 45, 47, 49, 51, 74
Custer, Thomas W. 34, 35, 57, 62, 64, 78
The Custer Myth (Graham) 122

Dakota Block 105, 111–12, 169, 182
Dakota Territory 1, 2, 81, 92, 108, 121, 181
Damascus 153, 155
"Dandy" 68
Dandy, George Brown 36
Darjeeling 175
Dartmouth College 163
Davis, David Melling 13, 19, 178
Davis, H. Porter 178
Davis, Helen Workman 9–10, 165, 178
Davis, Sarah 19
Deadwood 2, 38, 76, 91, 94
Deadwood Champion 38
Delafield, WI 173
Delamater, Josiah 34–35
Detroit Lake, MN 127
Devils Lake, N.D. 66
DeWolf, James W. 40, 46, 48–52, 57, 61, 64, 71, 78, 195n30
Dietrich, Joe 130, 204n12
Dock, George 136
Donoughue, John F. 66–73
Dorman, Isaiah 70
Douglass, Henry F. 34–35, 63, 109, 113, 116–17, 131, 134, 162, 177, 178
Dresden 137–38
Dunn, Fannie (Mrs. Eric P. Quain) 36, 60, 105
Dunn, John P. 37–38, 91, 95, 105, 159

Early, John 20

Eckford, Mrs. P.M. 107
Edgerly, Winfield S. 35, 70, 121
Edinburgh 12, 14
Edwinton 30
Egypt 147–52
Ehrenburg, Arizona Territory 21
Eisenburg, Dan 105, 117, 141
El Paso 130
Elliot, Johnson 20

Fairchild, George H.: banking 76, 81, 92, 105, 107–8, 111, 116, 120, 141; Bismarck 32–33, 36–37, 41, 64, 91, 108–10, 113, 115–16, 119, 126, 128, 131, 164, 193n16; death 149, 205n2; financial problems 120–21, 125–27, 132, 142; illnesses 80, 113, 120, 125, 129, 133, 142
Fairchild, Gertrude 109
Fairchild, James H. 32, 80, 121, 193n16
Fairchild, James T. 113, 120
Fairchild, Katherine M. 109–10, 126–27, 129–30, 132–33, 142, 149, 162–64, 167, 170, 172–73, 179
Fairchild, Lucy (Kenaston) 127
Fairchild, Mary F. 105, 108, 125–26, 129
Fancher, Frederick B. 169
Far West (steamboat) 49–50, 57–59, 61–64
Fee, William T. 177
5th Cavalry 22, 97
5th Infantry 65
First Annual Directory of Bismarck (Jewell) 107
1st Infantry 84
First National Bank of Bismarck 105, 107–8, 110–11, 117, 132, 141, 163, 167–68, 182, 200n5
First Presbyterian Church, Bismarck 35
Fisher, Asa 105, 117, 120–21, 123, 131, 141–42, 182
Flannery, George P. 34, 64, 92, 108, 117, 198n16
Florence 137, 140
Flying-By 118
Ford, Corydon L. 8
Ford, Esther 4
Forsyth, James W. 42–43, 78
Fort Abercrombie 96
Fort Abraham Lincoln 1, 30, 32–33, 35–36, 39–40, 44, 46–47, 58–63, 64, 67, 72–73, 76, 81, 83, 104, 107
Fort Benton 113–14
Fort Berthold 58
Fort Buford 49, 58, 61, 83, 85, 92, 109
Fort Ellis 44–45
Fort Fetterman 44, 46
Fort Keogh 94, 114
Fort Laramie 46–47
Fort Leavenworth 83, 89, 183
Fort Lincoln and Black Hills Railroad 91
Fort McKeen 32
Fort Randall 52

Fort Sarpy 45
Fort Snelling 52
Fort Stevenson 58
Fort Whipple 22
Fort Yates 109, 113, 117, 121
Fort Yuma 21
Fouch, J.B.C. 89
4th Infantry 46
Francis, Jud 123
Freemasonry 168
French, R.D. Del. 20
Frett, John 104
S.S. *Friesland* 136
Frost, John 5

Gage, J.R. 141
Gale, George W. 5
Gall, Chief 121–23, 167
Garyowen 46
Gebhart, Jacob H. 59
General Meade (steamboat) 110
General Sherman (steamboat) 109
Geneva Medical College 4, 8
Genoa 137, 140, 159
George, William M. 61
Georgetown College 19
Gibbon, John 2, 45, 49–50, 59, 67
Gilbert, Lyman D. 97, 100–3
Girard, Frederic F. 104
The Girl I Left Behind Me 46
Glasgow 10, 13–14, 16, 136
Glendive, MT 132, 173, 176, 182
Glover, Ralph 179
Godfrey, Edward S. 54, 60, 70, 73, 121, 182
Goff, Orlando S. 1, 35, 111, 201n7
Golden, Patrick M. 71
Gordon, Henry 57
Graham, Sylvester 4
Grant, Frederick D. 42–43
Grant, Orvil 44
Grant, Ulysses S. 20, 42, 44
Grass (Sioux Indian) 167
Gray Eagle 118
Great Dakota Boom 76, 92, 108, 117–18, 163–64
Greely, Horace 32
Greenock 17
Griffin, L.N. 124–25
Groves, D.P. 9
Gunn, Moses 8
Gurley, C. 63

Hackett, Edmund 91
Hammer, Kenneth M. 177
Hanauer, Joe 129
Hannafin, Dennis 140, 204n15
Hardisty, Huntington 176
Hare, Luther R. 68
Harrington, Henry M. 51, 64
Harrisburg, PA 97

Hartsuff, Albert 46
Harvard Law School 163
Harvard Medical School 52
Havana 171
Haycox, Ernest 73
Helena Independent 46
Herendeen, George B. 73, 104
Hodgson, Benjamin H. 51, 64, 70, 78
Hoffman House 165
Hogg, Andrew 95
Hong Kong Telegraph 173
Horner, Jacob 61
Hot Springs, AR 130
Howard, Oliver O. 27
Hualpai Indians 22
Hughes, Robert H. 71
Hull, John 4
Hunting Trips of a Ranchman (Roosevelt) 94

Jackman, John J. 173, 206n13
Jaffa 153, 205n1
Jamestown Alert 128
Jamestown, ND 128–29
Jerusalem 153–55, 178
Jewell, Marshall H. 107–8, 129–30, 149, 162, 173, 180
John G. Fletcher (steamboat) 78
Johnson, Edwin F. 30
Johnson, Martin N. 166–67
Johnston, R.E. 84
Jones, James K. 166
Joseph, Chief 79, 83–91, 183, 199n21
Josephine (steamboat) 42–43, 49, 63

Kanipe, Daniel Alexander 57
Kelley, Douglas 176
Kellogg, Marcus H. 49, 64
Kelly, John P. 64
Kelly, Luther S. 85, 199n8
Kelly, Patrick 64
Kendrick, F.D. 133
Keogh, Myles W. 35, 49, 62, 64, 78
Kilwinning, Scotland 11–12
King, John H. 97
Knox College 5
Kom Ombo 149

Lake Chautauqua, NY 164
Lake Geneva, WI 129
Lamborn Hotel 121
Lavender, David 86
Lee, Jessie M. 97, 99, 102
Lee Center, NY 3–4, 191n2
Lee, MA 5
Leo XIII, Pope 144–45
Lewis and Clark Expedition 42
Lincoln, Abraham 30
Little, Clarence B. 163
Little Big Horn Associates 176–77, 183

Little Bighorn 1–2, 5, 21, 41, 46–47, 51, 60, 66–73, 96–104, 108, 167, 176, 180
Livingston, MT 128
Loch Katrine 14
Loch Lomand 12
London 16
Londonderry 14
Long Dog 118
Long Soldier 118
Lord, George E. 35, 49, 51–52, 54–56, 61–62, 64, 79, 182, 195n28
Lounsberry, Clement A. 32, 40, 58, 91, 93, 108, 135

Madden, Michael P. 58, 61, 63, 201n12
Madrid 159–61
Maguire, Edward 101
Mandan, ND 81, 106, 108, 111, 113, 129, 131, 132, 168, 182
Manila 173–74
Mann, J.S. 35
Mann, Walter 105
Marryat, Fredrick 73
Marsh, Grant 42–43, 50, 58–59, 197n9
Mason, Julius 22–23
Massachusetts General Hospital 8
Matthews, H.M 28, 193n32
McCaskey, W.S. 63
McDougall, Thomas M. 55, 57, 69, 121
McIntosh, Donald 55, 64, 70, 78
McKenzie, Alexander 107, 116–17, 123–24, 164
McKenzie, M.J. 178
McKenzie, S. 79
McLaughlin, James 117
McLean, John A. 91
Meador, Thomas E. 59
Medal of Honor 180, 197n4
Medical Record 166
Men with Custer (Nichols) 177
Merchants Bank of Bismarck 92
Merchants Bank of Glendive 117, 178
Merritt, Wesley 97
Mexico City 131
Meyer, William D. 57
Middleton, J.V.D. 30, 63
Miles, Nelson A. 83, 85–86, 88–90
Miles City 114
Minneapolis, MN 92, 134, 178
Minneapolis Tribune 110
Missouri Medical Society 119
Missouri River 2, 29–31, 34, 81, 106–7, 113–14, 142
Mitchell, Thomas J. 91, 93
Moffet, William P. 123, 125
Mont Blanc 136
Montana: The Magazine of Western History 25
Montana Territory 1, 108
Monte Carlo 137, 139–40
Moore, Orlando H. 50, 65
Morgan, George 65

Mount Everest 175
Moylan, Myles 49, 64
Muchos Canyon 22
Mullins Station, A.T. 21–22

Naples 145, 159
National Bank of Commerce 92
National Museum of Health and Medicine 63
New Orleans 114
New York Herald 73
New York Mills, NY 3–4, 19, 25, 28–29, 63, 80, 96, 162, 168, 191n2
New York, NY 10, 13–14, 131, 135–36, 138, 175
New York Stock Exchange 134
New York Times 47, 99
S.S. *Newbern* 21
Nez Perce Indians 78–79, 83, 85, 87, 90, 183
Nicholson, O. 38
Nickel Plate Road 168
9th Infantry 46, 97
Noonan, John 73–75
North Dakota 167, 170, 173, 178, 183
North Dakota Bar Association 163
North Dakota Historical Society 168–69, 178–79
Northern Pacific Railroad 2, 29–31, 42, 76, 79, 81, 85, 91, 94, 108, 111, 113–15, 117, 133, 141, 164
Northwestern Stage Company 77
Nowlin, Henry J. 78
Nugent, William D. 59

Oberlin College 32, 76, 80, 163–64
Oberlin, OH 32, 36–37, 64, 76, 79, 116, 119, 125–26, 128, 142, 162–63, 167, 176–77, 179
Omaha 114
Oneida County Medical Society 4
Oneida Institute 5

Palmer House 97
Panic of 1873 31
Panic of 1893 131, 134, 141, 152
Paris 136–38, 178
Patzki, Julius H. 46
Paulding, Holmes O. 35, 45
Pennell, Joe 81
Pennsylvania Bar Association 97
Pennsylvania Railroad 106
Penwell, George B. 121
Pierce, Gilbert 123
Pittsburgh, PA 175
Pohanka, Brian C. 103
Polk, James K. 3
Polson, Janet Stewart 13
Polson, John 4, 13
Pompeii 145
Pope Leo XIII 144–45
Poplar River Indian Agency 108
Port-au-Prince 170
Porter Avenue 180–81

Porter, Frances Emogene (sister of H.R. Porter) 4, 12, 17, 162, 178
Porter, Helen Polson (mother of H.R. Porter) 3–4, 17, 162, 168
Porter, Henry Norton (father of H.R. Porter) 3–4, 13, 16–17, 162, 168
Porter, Henry Rinaldo: birth and early education 3–7, 191n2; business and farming activities 76–95, 105, 110, 113, 115–17, 120–21, 131–32, 141, 181–82; contract surgeon in Arizona Territory 20, 29, 39, 163; death 175–76, 183; death of wife 182; early life in Bismarck 30–41, 116, 124, 133; estate 177–78; at Georgetown College 19–20; internship 20; life in Washington, DC 162–63, 183; Little Bighorn 46–60, 66, 78, 91, 93, 108–9, 121–22, 167, 177, 179, 181, 183; marriage 76, 79–81; medical practice 76, 92–93, 105, 110–11, 119, 121, 124–25, 127, 129, 164, 169, 181–82; return to Bismarck 163; sited for gallantry 28; travels from Bismarck 120, 129–31, 133, 135–40, 142–61, 170–75, 183; travels to Scotland, England, and Ireland 10–18; at University of Michigan 8–9
Porter, Henry Viets (son of H.R. and Charlotte Porter) 108–9, 119–20, 123–24, 126–27, 128–31, 133–35, 142, 162–64, 170, 171–73, 176–79, 182, 206n29
Porter, Jacob 4
Porter, James E. 62, 64, 79
Porter, John 4
Porter, Noah 4
Porter, Norton 4
Porter, Richard 4
Porter, Samuel 4
Porter, Sarah (Mrs. David Melling Davis; sister of H.R. Porter) 4, 13–15, 126, 162, 178
Powell, Junius 46
Power, T.C. 92
Pride and Prejudice (Austen) 80
Princess Victoria Louise 170–71
Pye, William M. 139, 204n14

Quain, Eric P. 169
Queens College 17

Rain-in-the-Face 57, 135, 167
Raymond, J.W. 32, 34, 36, 64, 81, 91–92, 109–10
Raymond, Rachael 64
Rea, John 91
Reed, Harry Armstrong 54, 64
Reed, Maria 63
Register, Francis H. 178
Reily, William V.W. 62, 64, 78
Reno, Marcus A. 36, 47, 50–51, 54–57, 59–60, 64, 67–73, 96–105
Reno Inquiry 96–104
Reynolds, Charles A. 37, 50, 55, 64, 70, 194n40

Index

Rinaldo 4–5
Rock Creek Cemetery 168
Rome 137, 142–45, 159, 178
Roosevelt, Theodore 93–94, 133, 166
Rosebud, battle 51, 55
Royall, W.B. 97
Running Antelope 167
Rush Medical School 8, 119
Rutter, A.T. 175–76

St. Alexius Hospital 169
St. John's Military Academy 173
St. Louis, MO 114
St. Paul Globe 67, 96
St. Paul, MN 29, 89, 104–5, 116–17, 119, 169
St. Paul Pioneer Press 88
Saltcoats 3, 11, 13
San Francisco 20–21, 28, 175
Sanborn, John B. 64
Sanford, Wilmot P. 61
Schuyler, Walter 28
Scott, Sir Walter 14, 15
2nd Cavalry 45–46
S.S. *Senegal* 158, 205n5
The Settler (Bismarck) 123, 167
7th Cavalry 40, 44, 46, 49, 51, 54, 59, 61, 63, 66, 75, 84–85
7th Infantry 45
Shaved Head 86–87, 183
Shaw, W.B. 35
Shaw, Mrs. W.B. 107
Sheridan, Michael V. 78
Sheridan, Philip H. 42, 44, 78, 83
Sheridan House 79–80, 85–86, 91–92, 107, 116, 164, 167, 183
Sherman (steamboat) 109
Sherman, William T. 44, 83, 127
Showdown at Little Big Horn (Brown) 73
Sibley stove 49, 195n14
Silver City (steamboat) 78
Sioux Indians 43–44, 51, 57, 86, 121, 163
Sipe, Robert T. 44
Sitting Bull 46–48, 76, 89, 102, 107, 109, 117–18, 135, 166–67, 201n27
6th Infantry 49–50
Sketches of Frontier and Indian Life on the Upper Missouri and Great Plains (Taylor) 163
Slaughter, Benjamin F. 30, 32, 76, 95, 111, 181
Slaughter, Linda 30, 77–78
Sloan, I.O. 35–36, 194n29
Smith, Algernon E. 35, 62, 64
Smith, Edward W. 58, 64
Smith, George 15
Smith, Nellie 35
Smith, Robert 10, 14
Smith, Mrs. Robert 12, 14
Smith, Whiting 4
Smith, William M. 63
Smithsonian Institution 131

smog 192n24
Smyth, Francis R. 164
S.S. *Somali* 174
Spain 159–61
Spanish American War 166, 168
Spotted-Horn-Bull 118
Spurgeon, Charles H. 17–18, 180
Square Butte 93
stagecoaches 76, 92, 94, 115
Standing Rock Agency 109, 117
Statehood, North Dakota 127
steamboats 107, 114
Stevens, Richard H. 46
Stirling 15
Storrs, CT 179
Stoyell, John A. 91, 105, 121
Sturgis, James G. 62, 64, 79
Superstition Mountains 26, 28
Suttle, Henry 110, 201n3
Sweet, George W. 86–87, 91, 93, 183, 199n13
Swett, L.H. 35

Tall-as-the-Clouds 118
Taylor, Joseph H. 163, 197n6
Territorial Capital, Dakota 116–18
Terry, Alfred 44–46, 49–51, 57, 63–64, 67–68, 72
3rd Cavalry 46–47, 97
Thompson, Frank 106
Thompson, Richard 35
Thompson, William 91, 93, 108, 111, 201n7
Thorpe, Hans 168
Tilford, Joseph G. 74
Tipperary, Ireland 66
Tocqueville, Alexis de 3
Tomahawk 118
Treaty of Guadalupe Hidalgo 3
22nd Infantry 65
Two Bears 118

Umatilla Indian 87
U.S. Army 1, 179, 196n35
University of Michigan 8–9
Ute Indians 25
Utley, Robert M. 167
Utica Herald 25
Utica, NY 19

varioloid 110
Varnum, Charles A. 70, 98–99
Venice 137, 139, 142
Vermont Medical College 4
Vienna 137–38
Viets, Charlotte (Mrs. Henry R. Porter) 33, 35, 37, 77, 79–80, 96, 105, 108–9, 113, 115–17, 119–20, 123–24, 126–27
Viets, Edward 79
Viets, Helen Josephine (Mrs. George M. Fairchild) 33–36, 64, 76, 80, 107, 113, 115–16, 131, 149, 162–63, 170, 172

Viets, Henry (father of Charlotte Viets Porter) 79, 126, 200n3
Viets, Henry Shelton 79
Viets, Samantha (mother of Charlotte Viets Porter) 40, 79–80, 119, 126
Viets, Sarah Elizabeth 79–80
Voight, Henry C. 59
Vyzralek, Frank 31, 167

Wadsworth, Emma 35
Wadsworth, Nellie 35
Wallace, J.F. 105–6, 108
Warn, John 106
Warnton, ND 106
Washburn Leader 163
Washington, DC 19, 28–29, 131–33, 135, 159, 162–63, 170, 178
Watertown Arsenal 52
Watson, Emily 35
Wealth of Nations (Smith) 116
weapons at battle 54
Weir, Thomas B. 35, 99
Wells, N.S. 34
Wessagusset, MA 4
Westmoreland, NY 4
Westwood Cemetery 126, 176, 179
Weymouth, England 4

Weymouth, MA 4
Whetstone Agency 52
White Bird, Chief 78
Whitestown Seminary 5–7, 191n13
Whittaker, Frederick 73
Williams, J.W. 47
Wilson, Robert 38
Wilton, ND 173
Winchester, Walter 133, 141, 168
Winney, Dewitt 71
Wirth, Carl 111
Wollemborn, Les 176
Workman, Helen (Mrs. John Polson) 4, 13
Workman, Robert 13, 16
Workman, Mrs. Robert 17

Yankton 114, 116
Yanktonais Indians 118
Yates, George W.M. 62, 64, 78
Yellow Bull 86, 183
Yellow Wolf 86–87, 183
Yellowstone Park 106, 117, 120
Yellowstone Supply Depot 74
Young Fireheart 118
Yuma 21
Yuma Indians 25

www.ingramcontent.com/pod-product-compliance
Ingram Content Group UK Ltd.
Pitfield, Milton Keynes, MK11 3LW, UK
UKHW041951140426
5217IPUK00014B/740